Obstetric anaesthesia

Published and forthcoming Oxford Specialist Handbooks

General Oxford Specialist Handbooks
A Resuscitation Room Guide (Banerjee and Hargreaves)

Oxford Specialist Handbooks in End of Life Care
Cardiology: From advanced disease to bereavement (Beattie, Connelly, and Watson eds.)
Nephrology: From advanced disease to bereavement (Brown, Chambers, and Eggeling)

Oxford Specialist Handbooks in Anaesthesia
Cardiac Anaesthesia (Barnard and Martin eds.)
Neuroanaesthesia (Nathanson and Moppett eds.)
Obstetric Anaesthesia (Clyburn, Collis, Harries, and Davies eds.)
Paediatric Anaesthesia (Doyle ed.)

Oxford Specialist Handbooks in Cardiology
Cardiac Catheterization and Coronary Angiography (Mitchell, West, Leeson, and Banning)
Pacemakers and ICDs (Timperley, Leeson, Mitchell, and Betts eds.)
Echocardiography (Leeson, Mitchell, and Becher eds.)
Heart Failure (Gardner, McDonagh and Walker)
Nuclear Cardiology (Sabharwal, Loong, and Kelion)

Oxford Specialist Handbooks in Neurology
Epilepsy (Alarcon, Nashaf, Cross, and Nightingale)
Parkinson's Disease and Other Movement Disorders (Edwards, Bhatia, and Quinn)

Oxford Specialist Handbooks in Paediatrics
Paediatric Gastroenterology, Hepatology, and Nutrition (Beattie, Dhawan, and Puntis eds.)
Paediatric Nephrology (Rees, Webb, and Brogan)
Paediatric Neurology (Forsyth and Newton eds.)
Paediatric Oncology and Haematology (Bailey and Skinner eds.)
Paediatric Radiology (Johnson, Williams, and Foster)

Oxford Specialist Handbooks in Surgery
Cardiothoracic Surgery (Chikwe, Beddow, and Glenville)
Hand Surgery (Warwick)
Neurosurgery (Samandouras)
Operative Surgery (McLatchie and Leaper eds.)
Otolaryngology and Head and Neck Surgery (Warner and Corbridge)
Plastic and Reconstructive Surgery (Giele and Cassell eds.)
Renal Transplantation (Talbot)
Urological Surgery (Reynard, Sullivan, Turner, Feneley, Armenakas, and Mark eds.)
Vascular Surgery (Hands, Murphy, Sharp, and Ray-Chaudhuri eds.)

Obstetric anaesthesia

Edited by

Paul Clyburn
Consultant Anaesthetist,
University Hospital of Wales,
Cardiff, UK

Rachel Collis
Consultant Anaesthetist,
University Hospital of Wales,
Cardiff, UK

Sarah Harries
Consultant Anaesthetist,
University Hospital of Wales,
Cardiff, UK

Stuart Davies
Consultant Anaesthetist,
Swansea NHS Trust, UK

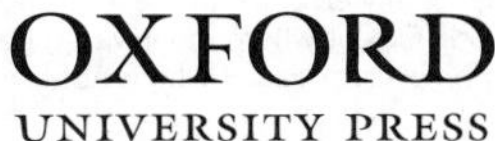

OXFORD
UNIVERSITY PRESS

Great Clarendon Street, Oxford OX2 6DP

Oxford University Press is a department of the University of Oxford. It furthers the University's objective of excellence in research, scholarship, and education by publishing worldwide in

Oxford New York

Auckland Cape Town Dar es Salaam Hong Kong Karachi Kuala Lumpur Madrid Melbourne Mexico City Nairobi New Delhi Shanghai Taipei Toronto

With offices in

Argentina Austria Brazil Chile Czech Republic France Greece Guatemala Hungary Italy Japan Poland Portugal Singapore South Korea Switzerland Thailand Turkey Ukraine Vietnam

Oxford is a registered trade mark of Oxford University Press in the UK and in certain other countries

Published in the United States by Oxford University Press Inc., New York

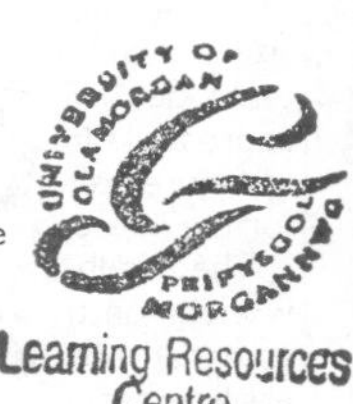

First published 2008

British Library Cataloguing in Publication Data
Data available

Library of Congress Cataloging in Publication Data
Data available

Typeset by Newgen Imaging Systems (P) Ltd., Chennai, India
Printed in China through
Asia Pacific Offset

ISBN 978–0–19–920832–6 (flexicover: alk.paper)

10 9 8 7 6 5 4 3 2 1

Oxford University Press makes no representation, express or implied, that the drug dosages in this book are correct. Readers must therefore always check the product information and clinical procedures with the most up-to-date published product information and data sheets provided by the manufacturers and the most recent codes of conduct and safety regulations. The authors and the publishers do not accept responsibility or legal liability for any errors in the text or for the misuse or misapplication of material in this work. Except where otherwise stated, drug dosages and recommendations are for the non-pregnant adult who is not breast-feeding.

Preface

There are many fine obstetric anaesthesia textbooks available of varying size and complexity. Our intention was not just to replicate the available texts but, wherever possible, to take a fresh and less conventional approach. Although not directly referenced, most sections end with a list of key references for further reading which should act as a starting point for the interested reader.

The handbook is aimed at the anaesthetic trainee to help them when working on the labour ward and doing their obstetric module. It is also essential reading for preparation for the FRCA examination. However, its easily accessible style makes it useful to other members of the labour ward team including midwives, obstetric trainees and consultant anaesthetists who have responsibility without regular sessions on the labour ward. The style and layout are meant to make navigation easy for quick reference, with emphasis on the practical and how to manage problems. With this in mind, we have allowed a certain degree of duplication of detail in different sections rather than expect readers to follow extensive cross-referencing when seeking guidance on the more common and urgent clinical scenarios. We hope it is also easily read as a study guide in more relaxed situations.

In addition to conventional chapters covering maternal physiology, pathophysiology and obstetric regional and anaesthetic techniques, there is practical and useful advice on how to survive on the labour ward and anticipate potential problems. An important and often neglected area is the antenatal identification and preparation of mothers with potential for anaesthetic problems during childbirth, and there is a chapter dedicated to this important topic. Postnatal review of the mothers who have received attention from the anaesthetist during delivery is another area comprehensively covered.

One of the biggest challenges for the anaesthetist is recognizing and managing the sick mother. There is much practical advice on caring for the sick mother suffering major haemorrhage, hypertensive and embolic diseases, and a chapter is devoted to managing the collapsed and compromised parturient.

The final section is a comprehensive and easily navigated A–Z of the less common conditions encountered in mothers on the labour ward, including a couple of key references on each topic for further reading.

This book is the result of collaboration with a number of contributors, and we are indebted to the many authors for all their hard work in getting their contribution to us on time.

Paul Clyburn, Rachel Collis, Sarah Harries and Stuart Davies
May 2008

Dedication

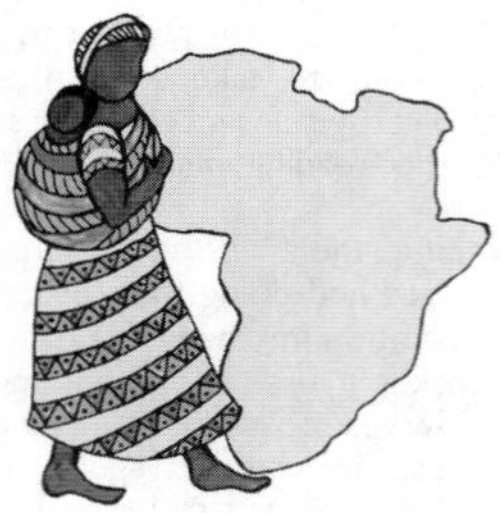

This handbook is dedicated to all mothers in Africa who aspire to receive first world healthcare.

The Department of Anaesthetics in Cardiff is supporting education and training of healthcare professionals in the poorest countries of Africa through its registered charity:

Mothers of Africa
Registered No 1114509

Contents

Contributors

Korede Adekanye
Consultant Anaesthetist
University Hospital of Wales
Cardiff, UK

Rafal Baraz
SpR, Anaesthetics
Welsh School of
Anaesthesia

Fiona Benjamin
Consultant Anaesthetist
Princess of Wales Hospital
Bridgend, UK

Val Billing
SpR, Anaesthetics
Welsh School of Anaesthesia

Sue Catling
Consultant Anaesthetist
Singleton Hospital
Swansea, UK

Monica Chawathe
Consultant Anaesthetist
Princess of Wales Hospital
Bridgend, UK

Karthikeyan Chelliah
Consultant Anaesthetist
Princess of Wales Hospital
Bridgend, UK

Doddamanegowda Chethan
SpR, Anaesthetics
Welsh School of Anaesthesia

Paul Clyburn
Consultant Anaesthetist
University Hospital of Wales
Cardiff, UK

Rachel Collis
Consultant Anaesthetist
University Hospital of Wales,
Cardiff, UK

Christine Conner
Consultant in Obstetrics and
Fetal Medicine
University Hospital of Wales
Cardiff, UK

Stuart Davies
Consultant Anaesthetist
Swansea NHS Trust,
UK

Libby Duff
SpR, Anaesthetics
Welsh School of Anaesthesia

Kath Eggers
Consultant Anaesthetist
Princess of Wales Hospital
Bridgend, UK

Caroline Evans
SpR, Anaesthetics
Welsh School of Anaesthesia

Moira Evans
Consultant Anaesthetist
Singleton Hospital
Swansea, UK

Claire Farley
SpR, Anaesthetics
Welsh School of Anaesthesia

Martin Garry
Consultant Anaesthetist
Singleton Hospital
Swansea, UK

Shubhranshu Gupta
SpR, Anaesthetics
West of Scotland School of
Anaesthesia

Sarah Harries
Consultant Anaesthetist
University Hospital of Wales,
Cardiff, UK

David Hill
Consultant in Anaesthesia and Pain Management
The Ulster Hospital,
Belfast, UK

Felicity Howard
SpR, Anaesthetics
Welsh School of Anaesthesia

Jon Hughes
Consultant Anaesthetist
Princess of Wales Hospital
Bridgend, UK

Saira Hussain
SpR, Anaesthetics
Welsh School of Anaesthesia

Aravindh Jayakumar
SpR, Anaesthetics
Welsh School of Anaesthesia

Eleanor Lewis
SpR, Anaesthetics
Welsh School of Anaesthesia

Anthony Murphy
Consultant Anaesthetist
Singleton Hospital
Swansea, UK

Vinay Ratnalikar
Consultant Anaesthetist
Singleton Hospital
Swansea, UK

Shilpa Rawat
SpR, Anaesthetics
Welsh School of Anaesthesia

Dan Redfern
SpR, Anaesthetics
Welsh School of Anaesthesia

Alun Rees
Consultant Anaesthetist
Withybush General Hospital
Haverfordwest, UK

Leanne Rees
Consultant Anaesthetist
University Hospital of Wales
Cardiff, UK

Hywel Roberts
SpR, Anaesthetics
Welsh School of Anaesthesia

Anette Scholz
Consultant Anaesthetist
University Hospital of Wales
Cardiff, UK

Raman Sivasankar
SpR, Anaesthetics
Welsh School of Anaesthesia

Stephen Stamatakis
StR, Anaesthetics
Welsh School of Anaesthesia

Gavin Sullivan
SpR, Anaesthetics
Welsh School of Anaesthesia

Daryl Thorp-Jones
SpR, Anaesthetics
Peninsula School of Anaesthesia

Matthew Turner
SpR, zAnaesthetics
Welsh School of Anaesthesia

Ramesh Vasoya
StR, Anaesthetics
Welsh School of Anaesthesia

Viju Varadarajan
SpR, Anaesthetics
Welsh School of Anaesthesia

Dave Watkins
SpR, Anaesthetics
Welsh School of Anaesthesia

Shreekar Yadthore
StR, Anaesthetics
Welsh School of Anaesthesia

Detailed contents

Symbols and abbreviations

↑	increased
↓	decreased
≈	approximately
AAGBI	Association of Anaesthetists of Great Britain and Ireland
ABG	arterial blood gas
AC	abdominal circumference
ACE	angiotensin-converting enzyme
ACTH	adrenocorticotrophic hormone
ADP	accidental dural puncture
A&E	Accident and Emergency
AF	atrial fibrillation
AFE	amniotic fluid embolus
AFI	amniotic fluid index
AFV	amniotic fluid volume
AITP	autoimmune thrombocytopenic purpura
ALS	advanced life support
ALT	alanine aminotransferase
AoDP	aortic diastolic pressure
APTT	activated partial thromboplastin time
ARDS	adult respiratory distress syndrome
ARF	acute renal failure
ARM	artificial rupture of membranes
AS	aortic stenosis
ASD	atrial septal defect
AST	aspartate aminotransferase
AVA	aortic valve area
AVM	arteriovenous malformation
BD	twice a day
BMI	body mass index
BMR	basal metabolic rate
BP	blood pressure
bpm	beats per minute
CDP	computerized dynamic posturography
CEMACH	Confidential Enquiry into Maternal and Child Health
CEMD	Confidential Enquiry into Maternal Deaths
CHD	congenital heart defect

cLMA	classic laryngeal mask airway
CNS	central nervous system
CO	cardiac output
COP	colloid oncotic pressure
CP	cerebral palsy
CPAP	continuous positive airway pressure
CPP	coronary perfusion pressure
CPR	cardiopulmonary resuscitation
CS	caesarean section
CSE	combined spinal–epidural
CSF	cerebrospinal fluid
CSM	Committee on the Safety of Medicines
CT	computed tomography
CTG	cardiotochograph
CTPA	CT pulmonary angiography
CVP	central venous pressure
DDAVP	1-desamino-8D-arginine vasopressin
DIC	disseminated intravascular coagulation
DVT	deep vein thrombosis
EBP	epidural blood patch
ECG	electrocardiograph
ECV	external cephalic version
EDF	end-diastolic flow
EEG	electroencephalograph
EF	ejection fraction
EFL	epidural for labour
EFM	electronic fetal monitoring
ENT	Ear, Nose and Throat
EXIT	*ex utero* intrapartum treatment
FBC	full blood count
FBS	fetal blood sample
FFP	fresh frozen plasma
FHR	fetal heart rate
FRC	functional residual capacity
FSE	fetal scalp electrode
FSH	follicle-stimulating hormone
GA	general anaesthesia
GCS	Glasgow Coma Score
GFR	glomerular filtration rate
GIT	gastrointestinal tract
GTN	glyceryl trinitrate
GTP	gestational thrombocytopenia of pregnancy

Hb	haemoglobin
HbF	fetal haemoglobin
HC	head circumference
hCG	human chorionic gonadotrophin
HDU	High Dependency Unit
HELLP	haemolytic anaemia, elevated liver enzymes and low platelets
HIT	heparin-induced thrombocytopenia
HIV	human immunodeficiency virus
HPV	human papillomavirus
HR	heart rate
5-HT	5-hydroxytryptamine
ICP	intracranial pressure
ICU	Intensive Care Unit
Ig	immunoglobulin
IGP	intragastric pressure
IM	intramuscular
INR	international normalized ratio
IPPV	intermittent positive pressure ventilation
ITP	idiopathic thrombocytopenic purpura
ITU	Intensive Therapy Unit
IUGR	intrauterine growth restricition/retardation
IV	intravenous
IVC	inferior vena cava
IVF	*in vitro* fertilization
JVP	jugular venous pressure
LA	local anaesthesia
LAP	left atrial pressure
LBP	low back pain
LEHPZ	lower oesophageal high pressure zone
LFT	liver function test
LH	luteinizing hormone
LMA	laryngeal mask airway
LMWH	low molecular weight heparin
LSCS	lower segment caesarean section
LV	left ventricle
LVEDP	left ventricular end-diastolic pressure
LVF	left ventricular failure
MAC	minimum alveolar concentration
MAP	mean arterial pressure
MAS	meconium aspiration syndrome
MCQ	multiple choice questions
MPAP	mean pulmonary arterial pressure

MR	mitral regurgitation
MRI	magnetic resonance imaging
MSL	meconium-stained liquor
MVP	mitral vein prolapse
NeP	neuropathic pain
NICE	National Institute for Health and Clinical Excellence
NIPP	non-invasive positive pressure ventilation
NMDA	*N*-methyl-D-aspartate
NNT	number needed to treat
NOAD	National Obstetric Anaesthetic Database
NSAID	non-steroidal anti-inflammatory drug
NYHA	New York Heart Association
OAA	Obstetric Anaesthetists' Association
ODP	operating department practitioner
PCA	patient-controlled analgesia
PCEA	patient-controlled epidural analgesia
PCWP	pulmonary capillary wedge pressure
PDA	patent ductus arteriosus
PDPH	postdural puncture headache
PE	pulmonary embolism
PEA	pulseless electrical activity
PET	pre-eclampsia toxaemia
PFO	patent foramen ovale
PG	prostaglandin
PIH	pregnancy-induced hypertension
PO	per os (orally)
PPH	postpartum haemorrhage
PR	per rectum
PT	prothrombin time
PTH	parathyroid hormone
PVR	pulmonary vascular resistance
QDS	four times a day
RBBB	right bundle branch block
RBC	red blood cell
RRT	renal replacement therapy
RV	right ventricle
RVF	right ventricular failure
SC	subcutaneous
SEP	somatosensory evoked potential
SFG	small for gestational age
SFH	symphyseal fundal height
SIRS	systemic inflammatory response syndrome

SLE	systemic lupus erythematosus
SNP	sodium nitroprusside
STAN	ST analysis of the fetal ECG
SV	stroke volume
SVD	spontaneous vaginal delivery
SVR	systemic vascular resistance
T_3	tri-iodothyronine
T_4	thyroxine
TB	tuberculosis
TBG	thyroxine-binding globulin
TEG	thromboelastography
TENS	transcutaneous electrical nerve stimulation
TIBC	total iron binding capacity
TID	three times a day
TORCH	toxoplasmosis, rubella, cytomegalovirus and herpes simplex
TSH	thyroid-stimulating hormone
TTP	thrombotic thrombocytopenic purpura
TV	tidal volume
UA	umbilical artery
U&E	urea and electrolytes
UFH	unfractionated heparin
URTI	upper respiratory tract infection
UTI	urinary tract infection
VBAC	vaginal delivery after caesarean section
V/Q	ventilation/perfusion
VR	venous return
VSD	ventricular septal defect
vWF	von Willebrand factor
WCC	white cell count

Chapter 1

Thinking about obstetric anaesthesia

Rachel Collis, Shreekar Yadthore
and Caroline Evans

Ramesh Vasoya, Rachel Collis

Surviving the labour ward

The labour ward can be a stressful and demanding experience for all anaesthetists, junior and senior alike. Start off by seeing yourself as part of a team comprising anaesthetists, midwives and obstetricians. Your level of seniority will often determine how you are viewed within that team, but the principles of team-working are always the same.

Obstetricians and midwives may need an anaesthetist to aid in the safe delivery of mother and baby, as well the multidisciplinary management of a whole host of complications associated with childbirth. The anaesthetist, however, cannot work effectively, dealing with the multitude of problems on the delivery suite, without the skills of both midwives and obstetricians. No one is better or more important than anyone else; only experience should change how you function within the team.

When the anaesthetist starts working on the delivery suite for the first time, it can feel like one of the most frightening and out of control places in the hospital. The anaesthetist can feel they are working to their maximum capability, at flat out pace with heightened emotion in nearly every setting. By the end of a shift it can be natural to feel exhausted and perhaps grateful that no major mistakes have been made, and both mothers and babies are safe.

Before you start, think how you can function optimally. The best way to start is to think ahead. This means not only familiarizing yourself with local protocols and the layout of the maternity unit before your first shift but also constantly thinking ahead as each situation arises. You need to minimize the tendency to react to a situation and start to learn to anticipate potential problems. You will feel more in control, and that control will enable you to work in a calmer and more effective manner.

The A–Z layout sets out ways that can help you cope without emphasizing one point above others. No single suggestion is more important than another and no single action will help without taking into account many of the others.

A–Z of survival

A

- ***Advice***: ask for advice if you are not sure. Never be afraid to ask. It may be a very simple question but, if you don't know the answer, it can lead to problems later on.
- ***Anaesthetic alert***: has the patient been to an anaesthetic antenatal clinic? If so, what are the likely anaesthetic problems and what is the plan? Familiarize yourself with the local mechanism of alert; there may be clinic letters, special anaesthetic alert pages in the maternity notes or a separate folder kept on the labour ward.
- ***Anticipate***: almost all problems on the labour ward can be anticipated. The '*crash section*' is rarely so, it's that you only just found out about it and now everything has to be done immediately in a hurry.
- ***Assessment***: before you perform any general or regional anaesthetic, always preoperatively assess the patient. It is routine practice in all other fields of anaesthesia but can be overlooked on the labour ward. Learn to do it the same on every occasion so nothing is missed, even if time is of the essence.

B

- ***Bleeps***: give your bleep number to the midwife who is co-ordinating the labour ward. Make sure that the bleep numbers of consultants, ODPs and senior cover are known to you and clearly displayed on the contact information board. Most units have one. If you have duties away from the labour ward, inform the senior midwife how best to get hold of you.
- ***Blood***: blood loss can be rapid. Find out local blood policy: how to get hold of it in a hurry, who to ask and what forms need to be filled out. Most hospitals will provide O negative blood, group-specific blood and full cross-match depending on the urgency. Give a clear account to the blood bank of how urgent the situation is and find out how long the blood will take to reach the labour ward. If the situation changes and becomes more or less urgent, inform the blood bank.
- ***Board***: all labour wards have a board with details of patients, current obstetric progress and management. Abbreviations are nearly always used and there could be over 30 different ones. Some are universal such as P for parity or a number for centimetres of cervical dilatation. Some others can be unique to an individual unit. Make sure you know what every one means, otherwise you could be missing an essential piece of information. If you don't know, ask. The information on the board can change rapidly. Review it regularly.
- ***Breaks***: it is important to sit down and have a drink and something to eat as often as you can, even if it is only for a few minutes. When the delivery suite is busy it can be difficult to get to the hospital canteen, so bring some snacks to work. Don't spend long periods of time away from a busy unit during a break as you can be caught unawares regarding pending problems.
- ***Busy***: if the labour ward is very busy, let another anaesthetist in the hospital know if possible, so help can be quickly summoned if required.

C

- ***Calm***: if you stay outwardly calm, even if inwardly you feel the opposite, the people around you will trust you and stay calmer themselves, thus making a difficult situation easier to handle.
- ***Caesarean section (CS)***: find out the urgency for surgery. This can be categorized into:
  1. Threat to life of mother or baby that requires immediate delivery.
  2. Compromise to mother or baby that requires early delivery.
  3. Early delivery where neither the baby nor mother is compromised.
  4. Elective CS.

  This classification does not dictate the type of anaesthetic you should give, but provides an approximate time frame for you to give a safe anaesthetic in the situation.
- ***Communicate***: clear and concise communication with the ODP, midwife and other members of the labour ward team is crucial. Take adequate time to communicate with the mother and her birthing partner. Taking a little time early on can save time later. Inadequate communication is the basis for many legal claims.
- ***Confrontation***: this can quickly arise, especially in a stressful situation. It never helps, so take a deep breath and don't get involved. If there is a point you feel strongly about, be polite or get someone more senior to deal with it. Sort out ongoing confrontation later and away from the clinical setting when there is plenty of time for a long discussion.
- ***CTG***: the cardiotochograph is a printed record of the fetal heart rate (FHR) with a pressure gauge reading of the mother's contractions. Knowing the basic patterns associated with fetal well-being and impending fetal compromise will allow you to think ahead as you provide epidural analgesia or anaesthesia for CS.
- ***Consent***: this should be obtained before all anaesthetic procedures, either written or verbal informed consent. There is much debate regarding the capacity of a labouring woman to give informed consent, therefore it is good practice to ensure that consent is witnessed by the attending midwife and her birthing partner, if present.

D

- ***Debrief***: things do go wrong. Sometimes you may feel responsible and sometimes you are an onlooker. In all situations, talk to someone senior about it.
- ***Drugs***: draw up all drugs that may be required in an emergency. Label each syringe with content, concentration and the time and date that the drug was drawn up; remember that a different anaesthetist may have to use them. Store them in a drug fridge.
  - Find out where non-anaesthetic emergency drugs are kept, particularly those used for eclampsia.
  - Familiarize yourself with the entire content of the drug cupboard. Know what is routinely kept on delivery suite and how they are stored, e.g. alphabetically or groups of drugs by function.

E

- ***Emotions***: happiness, sadness, fear, aggression and helplessness are all normal and commonly encountered emotions on the labour ward. You will feel them in yourself and see them in others. Work out how you can cope with them before they happen, and stay focused. If you become distracted, you can miss something important.
- ***Epidural***: almost every labour ward will have an epidural policy. Follow it, even if you have used something different elsewhere. All the other staff will be used to it and it is dangerous to do your own thing. If you want to make changes, talk to the policy makers.
- ***Equipment***: always check all anaesthetic equipment at the beginning of the shift. This must include the anaesthetic machine, monitoring and airway equipment. You may need to use them in a hurry later on.
- ***Experience***: appreciate the limitations of your expertise. When you reach your limit, ask for help.

F

- ***Fear***: this is a normal reaction to a situation that you don't understand, is happening too quickly or is outside your control or competence. Recognize the signs early and ask for help before it gets the better of you.
- ***Flag issues***: if you are concerned about a particular problem, flag it up early with a senior midwife, obstetrician or a senior anaesthetist.
- ***Fluids***: know where they are kept, what to give and when. Fluid requirements can be difficult to estimate in a labouring mother.
- ***Forceps delivery***: find out the local policy on where they should be carried out—delivery room or operating theatre. Always get involved, even if the mother does not want or already has an epidural. You can at least make an assessment of the situation so you are not completely caught out when forceps delivery turns into a 'crash section'.

G

- ***Guidelines***: most delivery suites have them. Find out where they are kept, read them before you start and refer back to them regularly.

H

- ***Handovers***: usually happen at the beginning of the morning shift, at ~5:00 pm and at the start of the night shift. They should involve midwives, obstetricians and anaesthetists, and will provide useful information about women who have not required anaesthetic intervention at that time. You may also find out about potential problems that are on the ante- or postnatal wards, medical wards or A&E.
    - Within your shift pattern there should be adequate time for anaesthetic handover. Make full use of it.
- ***Help***: where is it? Who is it? How long will it take to get to you?
- ***Helpful***: if what you have been asked to do is within your competence, be helpful when you have time, even if you think it is not your direct responsibility. If you genuinely don't have time to help, be polite.

I

- ***Information***: labour is a dynamic process. Situations progress and change rapidly. Stay well informed about all mothers in labour, not just the ones with an epidural.
- ***Intravenous access***: make sure you use a 14G or 16G drip in all mothers who have an epidural or need an obstetric anaesthetic.

J

- ***Jehovah's Witness***: there are Association of Anaesthetists of Great Britain and Ireland (AAGBI) and local guidelines for the management of a Jehovah's Witness. You should be informed when a Jehovah's Witness is admitted, and have a management plan.

K

- ***Knowledge***: keep up to date and discuss controversial issues surrounding patient management.

L

- ***Labels***: label all syringes and infusions with the drug name and concentration.
- ***Labour***: understand the normal and abnormal patterns of labour. Abnormally prolonged labour very frequently requires anaesthetic intervention at some time.

M

- ***Meetings***: attend the multidisciplinary labour ward meeting or organize it if you don't have one. It is a forum to raise concerns and issues.
- ***Multidisciplinary team***: you are a member of a team. Don't work in isolation. Understand what you are expected to do during a major obstetric emergency.

N

- ***Notes***: legible notes are very important. Discuss and document plans, procedures and advice received. '*If you have not written it down, you have not done it*'. Every entry should be timed and dated with a legible signature. If notes are written in retrospect, make that clear.
  - Read the patients notes, especially if there is additional medical information and a high-risk obstetric plan.

O

- ***Obstetric emergencies***: there are a number of obstetric emergencies including antenatal and postpartum haemorrhage, shoulder dystocia and eclampsia which you may see and will be expected to be involved with. Find out what you need to do in each and ask about teaching or 'obstetric fire drills' when it is quiet.
- ***Organize***: Organize your workload for the shift by prioritizing and delegating to others if appropriate. If a mother is thinking about an epidural, it is usually possible to tell her and her midwife whether you anticipate other more pressing anaesthetic procedures. Remember you can only be in one place at a time.

- ***Oxytocics and prostaglandins***: give these drugs slowly. Find out how the different drugs should be given and diluted. Be aware as you step up the therapeutic ladder from oxytocin bolus to oxytocin infusion to prostaglandin that blood loss can be considerable and difficult to estimate. An obstetric patient will appear to be cardiovascularly stable until she has lost 25–30% of her blood volume, and blood loss can be insidious.

P

- ***Passwords***: in many hospitals, blood results and X-rays can only be accessed electronically. Familiarize yourself with the computerized system and have an up-to-date access code and password.
- ***Position***: make sure the mother is in the ideal position for your regional technique. Taking your time and being patient, especially if she is in a lot of pain, will save time later.

  When sitting or lying a mother down, take great care to avoid aorto-caval compression. Explain to the mother why this is important.
- ***Problem epidural***: work out what you are going to do if an epidural for labour is not working well. Replace it early if you have got time, or recognize that you may need to do a spinal anaesthetic should the mother need a CS.

Q

- ***Questions***: there must be time for patients to raise concerns. Always ask mothers if they have any questions.

R

- ***Rapport***: build a rapport with the midwives. They can help you a lot.
- ***Resuscitaire***: this is where a baby that requires resuscitation is placed. They can be complex to use, but find out how to operate the basic functions. Babies are frequently born unexpectedly, requiring help, and with good airway skills the anaesthetist is ideally placed to give initial resuscitation until a paediatrician can attend. Find out about the basic principles of neonatal resuscitation and how they differ from other life support algorithms.
- ***Risk management***: this is a part of clinical governance and is important for patient safety. Raise any concerns and report them to the appropriate person, who is frequently one of the senior midwives.

S

- ***Smile***: it may seem a small thing but to appear relaxed and friendly will go a long way on a labour ward.
- ***Stress***: the labour ward can be a very stressful place to work and fear can be a normal response. Accept it and have a way of coping with it.

T

- ***Teach***: teaching and training—get involved and show initiative. Valuable informal teaching should take place with midwives looking after a mother with an epidural and with midwifery and medical students. A midwife who understands more about an epidural will call you to troubleshoot less often.

- ***Time***: there is a tendency for the obstetrician to demand a general anaesthetic when time is short. The question in reply should be 'how quickly does the baby need to be delivered?'

U

- ***Use***: use quiet time to practise difficult scenarios or learn about equipment you are less familiar with.
- ***Utilize***: utilize all your resources. The haematologist, general physicians and surgeons can all be invaluable in an emergency or when there are complex management issues with a sick mother.

V

- ***Value***: value the opinion of midwives and others in the team. Many will be more experienced than you and can offer an opinion that, although different from yours, can be equally valid and helpful in the long run.
- ***Vulnerable***: the patient can feel vulnerable, which can come across as rude and aggressive behaviour. Put yourself in her place.

W

- ***Ward rounds***: all mothers who have had an obstetric anaesthetic should be followed-up. Feedback is important and you will learn a lot from listening to her.

X

- ***(E)Xpectations***: it is easy to underestimate the mother's expectations in a stressful environment like the labour ward. She may not be able to differentiate one doctor from the other. Introduce yourself, be courteous and be clear. For the doctors, one situation can merge into the next. For the mother, she will remember her personal experiences for many years.

Y

- ***Y***: why are you doing what you are doing? Watch and learn from others to improve your own practice.

Z

- ***Plan Z***: always have one before things go wrong.

Asking the right questions OR where do you look for the answers?

There are different questions that should be directed to the patient, obstetrician and midwife. The questions you ask will depend upon the time you have, but most of the information below will need to be obtained, even if time is very short. Directing your questions to the right person can save time.

The midwife

Has the pregnancy and labour been normal? The midwife will have carefully reviewed the mother's notes and will be aware of problems that may alter your anaesthetic management:
- History of blood pressure (BP) problems or pre-eclampsia, which could cause clotting or platelet abnormalities.
- History of low platelets (ITP).
- History of thrombosis. Is the mother on heparin?

The midwife will also be able to tell you if the pattern of labour up to that point has been normal or abnormal and if the CTG has been reassuring or suggestive of fetal compromise.

- ***Is this a first or subsequent labour***? A mother who has laboured before is more likely to deliver quickly, and this may alter your anaesthetic management.
- ***Is this a spontaneous or induced labour***? An induced labour is more likely to be slow and complicated.
- ***How many centimetres of cervical dilatation has the labour progressed to?*** An early request for an epidural may already indicate a slow labour with excessive pain from an occipito-posterior presentation of the fetal head. An epidural will need to be effective for many hours. You may consider late requests for an epidural to be inappropriate as delivery is possibly imminent. However, it may reflect major obstetric difficulties in the latter stages of labour, when epidural analgesia can be difficult to achieve and operative delivery is likely.
- ***Has the mother had a previous CS?*** If so, she is more likely to have another one.
- ***Is this labour slow and is augmentation with oxytocin likely?*** If so, an epidural may to be required for many hours and needs to be effective.
- ***Is the CTG normal or abnormal?*** If it is abnormal, is fetal scalp blood sampling or early operative delivery anticipated?

The obstetrician

There will be overlap between the questions you can direct towards the midwife and obstetrician, especially about the obstetric history, but a clearer overview of the labour and likelihood of operative delivery can usually be obtained from the obstetrician.

- ***How long do I have to do this anaesthetic?*** Is the anaesthetic urgent for fetal blood sampling or operative delivery, or can I take more time?
- ***When do you anticipate obstetric intervention?*** This may be in the next few minutes or in several hours if there has been inadequate progress in labour.
- ***Is it likely the baby will be born by forceps or caesarean delivery?*** If an operative vaginal delivery is likely, is there a high risk of proceeding to CS? In which case the anaesthetic needs to be effective for both procedures before the obstetrician starts.

The mother

The mother will be able to tell you if she has any past medical complications. There is usually a tick box questionnaire in her notes that will have been filled out in early pregnancy, but there may be a need for clarification. The mother should also tell you what she understands about the procedure you have been asked to carry out.

- ***What do you know about epidurals?*** There are issues about consent in labour, but it is important that the mother understands the major issues. If she tells you that she has read the information from a well-recognized source and discussed it with a midwife or anaesthetist in the antenatal period, the information you need to give her is brief. If she says she knows nothing, you must spend some time in giving her a good explanation.
- ***What are your expectations?*** The mother may have very high or unrealistic expectations. Listen carefully and give good information back. If she has low expectations, be reassuring.

A systematic review of questions

Many obstetric units have a dedicated obstetric anaesthetic chart because the information that needs to be documented is different from other theatre work. It is helpful if the chart is subdivided into systems and has some tick boxes so a history and examination can be carried out quickly without overlooking important factors.

Past medical history

- ***Medical problems***: systems review.
- ***Previous surgery***: what?
- ***Anaesthesia***: any previous problems with regional or general anaesthetic?

Drug

- ***Current medication:*** diabetic, hypertensive or epileptic?
- ***Heparin or gastric acid prophylaxsis*** given recently?
- ***Allergies*** especially latex and antibiotics.

Obstetric history

- ***Gravidity (G)***: the number of pregnancies.
- ***Parity (P)***: the number of births.
  - P0 long labour, high expectation compared with P3 short labour, higher risk of uterine atony/postpartum haemorrhage (PPH).

- ***Mode of delivery***: spontaneous vaginal delivery (SVD), elective caesarean section (LSCS), emergency LSCS and why?
- ***Mode of anaesthesia***: nil, epidural for labour (EFL) ± top-up/spinal/combined spinal–epidural (CSE).

Any complications from any of the above.

Current pregnancy

Problems—mother, placenta or fetus.

- ***Mother***: raised BP, proteinuria, diabetes.
- ***Placenta:*** insufficiency, praevia; minor or major, anterior or posterior
- ***Fetus***: congenital anomaly requiring early delivery or transfer to another unit, multiple pregnancy, poly/oligohydramnios, large/small baby, prematurity.

Planned delivery

SVD, LSCS and why?

Examination

Examination of the patient can provide a lot of answers. Particular attention should be given to:

Airway: higher incidence of failed intubation 1:250.

Assessment includes Mallampati score and mouth opening, dentition, thyromental distance, occlusion of the teeth and neck movement. In pregnancy, a high body mass index, oedema and large breasts can also present greater difficulties.

Body mass index (BMI): is becoming an increasing problem in obstetrics and may predict a difficult regional and general anaesthetic.

Systems examination

CNS, HR, BP, heart sounds: be aware of the cardiovascular changes in normal pregnancy and how maternal disease will influence your findings (see Chapter 3).

Respiratory: breath sounds. Physiological changes that underline the importance of pre-oxygenation

GIT: reflux. Note the delayed gastric emptying in labour. Look at your labour ward starvation policy. Prescribe ranitidine and don't forget to give sodium citrate prior to emergency anaesthesia.

Spine: increased lumbar lordosis and higher BMI, deformed anatomy, previous spinal surgery. Look and feel for lumbar spaces.

Investigations

The majority of mothers requesting a routine epidural for labour do not need current investigations. Women have a large number of investigations in pregnancy, which screen for complications such as a low haemoglobin or platelet count. The likelihood of picking up further pathology during labour if the pregnancy has proceeded without other complications is minimal and will only delay analgesia and anaesthesia when required.

- The midwife should know the results from the mother's most recent tests, which could be 8 weeks old.
- If the mother has signs or symptoms of pre-eclampsia, a platelet count within the last 4h should be known before an epidural or spinal is inserted. U&Es, LFTs and a clotting screen can also be useful.
- If a mother has a history of a low platelet count, other than from pre-eclampsia, then a platelet count within the last 12h should be known before an epidural or spinal is inserted.
- An emergency anaesthetic may need to be given before recent investigations are known. Unless major abnormalities are suspected, then the lack of blood results should not delay you.
- In cases of emergency anaesthesia, make sure that a full blood count and at least a blood 'group and save' is on its way to the laboratories.

Dealing with difficult behaviour

The labour ward is a stressful environment. Problems can progress rapidly and this can lead to patients, partners and colleagues behaving in a difficult and inappropriate manner. It helps to try and understand why they may be behaving in this way. Think, however, how your behavior may appear to others, to prevent yourself becoming the problem.

The midwife

- Senior midwives and those in charge of the labour ward often have the most direct and assertive personalities. Don't take things too personally; they do a difficult job.
- Midwives can be thought of by some as difficult people. The reality is that they are highly qualified professionals, working in the best interests of the mother and baby and therefore may have a forceful but valid opinion.
- High workload is a big factor affecting behaviour; midwives may be looking after more than one patient and juggling other tasks.
- It is highly stressful to look after a difficult or demanding patient for many hours.
- The difficult behaviour of a patient may be taken out on you. Take a deep breath.
- Lack of breaks. Many labour wards suffer from midwifery shortages. This can lead to inadequate or absent breaks, not even time for a drink. Try to be sympathetic.
- Lack of skill and inexperience can also make people behave aggressively.

How you can help

- Try and help out; be calm and polite. Do not behave aggressively in return.
- If a particular midwife is always a problem, speak to your seniors and ask if they can help.

The obstetrician

- High work intensity can lead to behavioural changes.
- You may recognize that the obstetrician is inexperienced, out of their depth or has lost time perspective.

How you can help

- You can help by being non-confrontational and offering support. Remember there may be occasions where you need their help.
- They may see calling for help as a failure on their part; constructively suggest senior or additional assistance if inexperience is leading to difficult behaviour as the situation will only become worse.

The mother

- A mother may spend the majority of her pregnancy worrying about how she will cope with labour and the responsibility of a new baby. This can spill out into apparently difficult behaviour.
- Most difficult behaviour during labour is caused by pain.
- Fear for her unborn baby can also be a major concern.
- A mother may have had very little preparation for her experience. This is most common during a first labour, but can also happen unexpectedly when a labour is very different from one already experienced.
- Individual preconceived ideas, media, social and cultural background can contribute to the mother's attitude.
- There can be a real sense of disappointment that labour and analgesia choices have not gone to plan.

How you can help

- The pain of labour is made worse by anxiety. If a mother observes competency and efficiency in the staff dealing with her, confidence can be more easily gained.
- Give full but concise information.
- Never shout back.
- Sometimes the simple act of sitting down, coming properly into the mother's view and taking time to allay anxiety will transform the situation.
- Stay calm.
- If the mother is finding it very difficult to listen, then only one person must talk to her. It may be better to leave the room and let a confident midwife regain control.
- A lot of communication by an anaesthetist is from behind a face mask and from behind the mother. If she is finding it difficult to understand and co-operate, walk round in front of her, remove your mask and talk face to face.

The partner

A birthing partner is a person who has been designated by the mother to accompany them in labour. It is well recognized that a calm and supportive birthing partner can reduce anxiety, which in turn can lead to a better outcome in labour. Unfortunately, many birthing partners are ill prepared for the experience, and their anxiety can easily become difficult behaviour.

- The hospital environment can be frightening and alien.
- Sometimes medical and nursing staff as patients can be the most difficult. It is somehow expected that they should know about labour and hospitals, but they may not have been on a labour ward for many years. The environment may seem as alien to them as to someone who has never been to hospital before.
- Confusion may arise from the large number of individuals involved in the mother's care.

- The partner may feel fearful for the unborn child and the labouring mother.
- They want to be protective but can't.
- A partner may have a job where they control a work situation or a workforce. They can find themselves unable to control the pain their loved one is experiencing, or control the midwifery and medical staff who are in attendance.
- The birthing experience of a mother accompanying her daughter may be helpful, but can also result in overprotective behaviour.
- There can also be real disappointment that the labour and anticipated analgesia have not gone to plan.

How you can help

- It is important that difficult and overanxious behaviour is rapidly diffused to prevent the labouring woman also becoming anxious and difficult herself.
- Introduce yourself clearly by name and explain the role you have in attending the mother.
- Bring the partner into the conversation.
- Bring the partner into the decision making.
- Explain clearly what you are doing and why.
- Never shout back.
- Occasionally, it is better to have a conversation with the partner away from the labouring woman, especially if there are raised voices.
- Very occasionally, the partner may be aggressive or confrontational whatever you do. Tell them calmly that you feel their behaviour is unacceptable and that measures will be taken to remove them from the ward. Don't get into personal arguments over this; senior midwifery staff will help. They frequently have a great deal of experience in dealing with these problems.

Dealing with malformation and death

Fetal malformations are common and always cause great anxiety to the mother and birthing partner. The degree of malformation may not reflect the degree of anxiety, and minor or trivial abnormalities can cause significant emotional problems. Most severe congenital anomalies will be picked up on antenatal ultrasound scanning, but many minor problems will not. Some mothers will choose not to have antenatal scans and, occasionally, babies will be born with unexpected significant major problems.

Some large maternity centres will look after many mothers who are known to carry babies with major abnormalities because of regional fetal medicine and neonatal surgical services. The anaesthetist working on such units will meet these mothers on an almost daily basis and needs to understand rapidly the specific needs of the baby's parents.

Maternity units that deal with these problems will frequently have staff who are specifically trained to counsel the parents. The anaesthetist should be guided by the experts and listen carefully to any advice offered.

Expected malformation

The mother and partner have been told about the malformation, but they may or may not have come to terms with it.

Mid-trimester termination of pregnancy

In the UK, a mother has a right to choose to end her pregnancy up to the 24th week gestation for social reasons. A mother can undergo a termination of her pregnancy for significant fetal anomalies at any gestation, although it is uncommon after ~24 weeks gestation as most problems are picked up on a 20-week anomaly scan. If the pregnancy is beyond 21 weeks plus 6 days when a decision is made to terminate the pregnancy, a specially trained obstetrician undertakes a feticide, where potassium is injected through the mother's abdominal wall into the fetal heart so that the baby is delivered dead. The mother will then be given prostaglandins to induce labour.

- Formal anaesthesia or major sedation is not usually required for feticide procedures so the anaesthetist will not have to be directly involved. See Chapter 13 for further details on feticide management.
- It is recognized that some anaesthetists, because of strongly held moral or religious views, do not give anaesthesia or sedation for these procedures. If as a professional you feel unable to be involved, your views must be made known to the service providers so alternative arrangements can be made.
- You have a moral obligation as a professional to ensure the mother receives the best care there is, which could require you personally to find an alternative anaesthetist.
- Some anaesthetists will not directly involve themselves in the termination or feticide but will provide necessary analgesia or anaesthesia for complications such as a retained placenta. Make sure your colleagues and the midwife in charge knows what you are prepared to do.

- It is never right to impose your views on the situation, as the mother and partner will already have had time to reflect, be counselled and have made their choice.
- Many mothers will have significant pain during the labour of a mid-trimester termination. They have a right, like any labouring mother, to have a choice of analgesia.
- Many women find regular opioid-based analgesia enough, whilst others may request an epidural.
- An epidural can safely be given, but the usual safety aspects of providing it must be rigorously upheld.

When providing analgesia in these situations, there is frequently a very difficult atmosphere in the delivery room. There is often a real sense of guilt and grief. The usual rules about the number of birthing partners are frequently flouted, and you can find yourself addressing a large number of people.

- Be sensitive to the situation.
- Never voice personal views.
- Don't be judgemental.
- Talk primarily to the patient but make sure everyone else understands what you are doing.
- It can be useful to find out who are friends and family members. The midwife looking after the patient usually knows.
- If you find the situation difficult or upsetting, talk to someone about your feelings.

Term deliveries of a baby with known congenital malformation

The anaesthetist may be involved in providing regional analgesia during labour but is also frequently involved when anaesthesia for CS is required. During a CS, it is usual for the anaesthetist to take on the role of primary carer of the mother from the midwife. This is considerably more demanding when the baby has congenital abnormalities. The anaesthetist will then meet the mother again during a postnatal ward round. The mother is frequently distressed, but it is important to ascertain that there has been good recovery from the anaesthetic and that analgesia is effective. The mother must have the opportunity to talk over problems or concerns she may have about her anaesthetic, just as every mother should.

- Before you get involved, find out from the obstetrician and midwife the nature and degree of abnormality.
- Is the baby expected to live or die?
- Is the baby expected to need neonatal resuscitation and transfer to a special care neonatal unit?
- Talk to the mother very carefully about what type of anaesthetic (general or regional) she wants for her CS.
- It is normal for any patient to be anxious about being awake for a CS.
- This normal anxiety is heightened when the baby is known to have an anomaly.
- Most mothers, however, do want to be awake when their baby is born; it may be very important so that the mother and partner can more quickly come to terms with the problem.
- This is especially so if the baby is likely to die or need immediate transfer to the neonatal unit.
- A general anaesthetic may seem the easier option, but it is only moving the emotional problems out of the operating theatre and from the anaesthetist's view.
- Some parents want to see the defect immediately and others want the baby carefully wrapped, therefore hiding the problem. Listen very carefully to their wishes.
- Partners need to be made welcome and feel included.
- Acknowledge the malformation if appropriate.
- Some mothers become very remote after the baby is born, while others want to talk. Facilitate the emotion she wants to show at that time.
- Dealing emotionally with this situation can be very difficult for a doctor who has not had to deal with this situation before. Talk to someone about it afterwards.

Unexpected malformation

Babies are quite frequently born with obvious abnormalities that have not been picked up on routine antenatal ultrasound screening. The abnormalities that are picked up at birth are usually highly visible and therefore distressing, but may also become apparent over the first few minutes of life when a baby that is expected to be healthy fails to breath or to become pink because of an underlying respiratory or cardiac problem.

- Always acknowledge to the mother and partner that there is a problem. They will have already noticed that the baby is causing concern to the staff and will immediately know if they are lied to.
- The parents are likely to be extremely shocked and may behave in a difficult or overtly emotional way.
- The midwife will always be involved but it is possible that she will have only just met the parents. Work together.
- A paediatrician will usually be involved but they may also be inexperienced in dealing with the situation.
- Be informative about the abnormality if it is within your knowledge, but don't be reassuring if you are not certain.
- If the partner wants to see the baby and the baby is stable, invite him/her to the resuscitaire.
- It may be difficult for the mother to see the abnormality even if she wants to. A simple explanation is appropriate at this stage.
- Sometimes the partner wants to stay with the mother and support her; sometimes he may become emotionally detached and even leaves the operating theatre or delivery room. In the latter situation, the mother will need additional support from the medical and midwifery staff. Never be critical of the partner.
- Dealing emotionally with this situation can be very difficult for a doctor who has not had to deal with this situation before. Talk to someone about it afterwards.

The death of a baby

The admission of a mother whose baby is found to have died *in utero* is sadly common. The death of a baby at any gestation can be devastating for the mother and partner. A common euphemism for death is 'loss' or 'lost'. Be very careful when using these words because they may also imply a degree of carelessness. The mother may already have a huge feeling of guilt associated with her baby's death, and the use of these words may aggravate this.

The anaesthetist frequently becomes involved with these mothers because labour has to be induced and may be prolonged and painful. She is also less likely to cope with labour pain.

The anaesthetist may encounter the death of a baby whilst administering an anaesthetic for fetal distress when the paediatricians cannot resuscitate the baby.

General anaesthesia

- If the mother needs a general anaesthetic, don't become distracted. Stay focused on the anaesthetic and keep the mother safe.
- She will have gone to sleep knowing that there was a problem; she is likely to ask about it as soon as she awakes. Be truthful.

Regional anaesthesia

- The mother may have had a regional technique and her partner may be with her. They will be immediately aware that there is a significant problem.
- The mother and partner must not be allowed to interfere with the resuscitation, but it is acceptable that they are allowed to look on from a distance. If the parents can see that the medical staff are working effectively and calmly to save their baby's life, it can help them to come to terms with the baby's death later.
- The anaesthetist and midwife must form a link between the resuscitation and the couple.

Aftermath

- It is natural to feel extremely sad. Expressing how you feel in a controlled fashion can help the couple, as they will appreciate your empathy.
- You must carry on communicating with them as they are in an alien hospital environment and will need emotional support.
- Some parents want to see the baby straight away and some may not wish to see the baby until they are quietly together after the delivery is over. Help facilitate whatever the parents want.
- It is common to want to criticize your anaesthetic technique and feel a personal sense of guilt. Did you do everything possible to save the baby's life? Don't express these feelings to the parents at this time.
- Never start blaming other medical personnel in front of the parents, even if you feel that their actions may have contributed to the baby's death. These types of concerns need to be discussed at length with senior medical and midwifery staff later.
- As soon as possible afterwards, write down the sequence of events with times from the start of your involvement in the death. There will almost certainly be an internal enquiry and occasionally there may be a formal complaint or court case.
- Dealing emotionally with this situation can be very difficult for a doctor who has not had to deal with this situation before. Talk to someone about it afterwards.
- Remember that your anaesthetic assistant may not have faced death before; they may need to talk afterwards too.

The death of a mother

Thankfully, the unexpected death of a mother in the peripartum period is uncommon in the UK (1:10 000). Her death, however, is nearly always catastrophic and unexpected. The death of a baby is relatively common and many midwives will have plenty of experience dealing with bereaved parents and will help you. However, it is very unlikely that there is anybody immediately available who has much experience of dealing with a maternal death.

- Stay focused and professional.
- Stay calm.
- Ask for help from a senior colleague.
- You will feel deeply upset, and it is usual to experience guilt if you have been either a passive onlooker or deeply involved in the mothers care.
- Recriminations and blame are common. Don't get emotionally involved; there will be plenty of time afterwards for proper reflection.

The relatives

- Senior staff must present a unifying front to the relatives and provide accurate information.
- It is important that the relatives do not feel that there is a cover-up from the hospital staff.

The aftermath

- A proper debriefing is essential for all staff involved. This is best carried out the following day. If you feel very distressed, talk to someone sooner.
- As soon as possible afterwards, write down the sequence of events with times from the start of your involvement in the death. There will be an internal enquiry and coroner's inquest.
- It is a personal decision as to whether you feel able to carry on to the end of your shift. However, if you have been closely involved, arrangements should be made for you to hand over duties and go home.

The mother who does not speak English

The mother who does not speak English on a labour ward can be either a visitor, or a legal or an illegal resident. She is likely to come from an ethnic group with a different social and cultural background, with varying views on childbirth and pain relief. These views can sometimes lead to many problems, as well as not having the same language in common.

She may find all aspects of her care difficult to understand, and the problems of pain and anxiety seen in many labouring mothers will make communication more difficult.

Translators

- It is common for the mother's birthing partner to speak more English than she does.
- The birthing partner can be a husband or female relative. A female partner may be from the husband's family and can sometimes forcefully express the husband's viewpoint.
- Sometimes the partner's views can be strongly felt and divergent from those of the medical staff.
- In this situation, it is important that an independent translator is used if at all possible. The mother must be told in accurate terms what she is to expect, otherwise her care could be compromised.
- Most hospitals provide some type of independent translation service, although this can be language dependent.
- It is common and acceptable to use hospital staff in these situations. Some hospitals organize training and a register of staff that are willing to help. This is particularly helpful in the emergency situation.
- Registered translators are routinely used in many antenatal clinics, but it is unusual to have these translators available on a 24h basis.
- Some hospitals subscribe to a 24h telephone translation service. It can be difficult to talk via a third unseen party on the telephone but can be useful and should be used if available.
- The Obstetric Anaesthetist Association (OAA) has a number of translated patient information leaflets relating to obstetric analgesia and anaesthesia on their web site www.oaa-anaes.ac.uk. There are detailed information booklets as well as simple sheets with common words and useful diagrams. The latter are more useful in an emergency. All are free to download.
- In a real emergency, translation services can be difficult to use and an English-speaking member of the family may have to be used.

General advice

- Remember that the mother's expectations of childbirth may be as high as those of many English-speaking mothers. It is your duty as a professional to facilitate the care that she needs.
- Assess the level of English she can speak and understand. Women may understand much more English than they are willing to speak. Sometimes plenty of signs and the use of simple words are all that is required.
- Use non-verbal communication to establish a rapport; a simple handshake or smile can help.
- It is especially difficult to inform in the usual detail about regional techniques for labour analgesia and CS. This should not mean that the mother should not have an epidural or that she must have a general anaesthetic for an operative delivery. There are risks associated with deviating from your usual practice simply because it cannot be explained easily to the patient. Use a translation service if at all possible.
- Inability to understand the language, pain and fear can make behaviour appear difficult. The tone of your voice and a sympathetic manner in which you approach the mother can help her cope in this situation.
- Keep the relatives informed, but always address the mother even if the relatives seem to be doing all the talking.
- Do provide time for any questions from the mother or the relatives. All mothers experience the same feelings and emotions through labour, wherever they are from. It is easy to underestimate this.

Audit in obstetric anaesthesia

Audit is an integral part of medical practice, acting as a means of improving service delivery, as an aid to research, as a means of accountability and quality control, and to facilitate efficient management.

Definition and principles of use

'Audit is a quality improvement process that seeks to improve patient care and outcomes through systematic review of care against explicit criteria and the implementation of change' (NICE/CHI 2002).

Audit vs research

There is a clear distinction between the processes of audit and research. Audit is a process of quality control; in medicine it is taken as the systematic peer review of clinical practice with the object of maintaining and improving the quality of that practice. Research, in contrast, is the process of improving medical care by expanding knowledge in the known areas of medicine.

Audit it generally easier to set up, more quickly performed and may lead to rapid conclusions.

Research	Clinical audit
Asks what we should be doing	Asks whether we are doing what we should
Creates new knowledge (evidence)	Assesses whether best practice (often informed by research evidence) is being used
Often experimental	Never experimental
Hypothesis generated	Measures against predetermined standards
May involve new or untried treatment	Treatment always previously evaluated
Often involves randomization of patients to treatment and use of placebos	No randomization (patient choice). No placebo
Uses statistical tests and power analysis	Descriptive statistical analysis only

The audit cycle

The audit cycle is a description of how audit ought to work in clinical practice, with continual assessment and feedback:

- Set a standard.
- Measure performance against that standard.
- Diagnose reasons why the standard is not met, which will broadly fall into four subheadings:
  - knowledge
  - skills
  - attitude
  - organization.
- Implement corrective change.
- Return to the measurement of performance to confirm that the changes have brought about improvement.

The audit cycle is frequently broken. The measure of performance against a standard is easily determined, but analysing the reasons behind a poor performance is complex and caused by many factors. Implementing change can be challenging, and a return to the remeasuring of performance may demonstrate how difficult it is to implement change in clinical practice.

Data collection

- **Quantitative data**: provide information on activity within a service and are important to establish adequate staffing levels and denominator numbers for qualitative audit.
- **Qualitative data**: provide information on the quality of a service and the incidence of side effects.

Even at a hospital level, accurate information can be difficult to collect. Complicated forms and numerical coding systems can lead to erroneous results and loss of data. Many local audits are still conducted using manual data collection, as many NHS database systems are not set up to extract useful information on quality issues.

Topics for audit

It is useful to think about your chosen audit topic based on one of the classifications below. This type of classification allows a clearer understanding of the process and diagnosis of the problem if the standard is not met.

- **Structure**: the healthcare facilities available.
- **Process**: the management given to the patient.
- **Outcomes**: the result for the patient.
- **Patient satisfaction**.

Audit in obstetric anaesthetic practice

A high standard of care within obstetric anaesthesia is essential to achieve acceptable levels of maternal satisfaction and a low incidence of complications, and to maintain a high degree of safety within the service.

Audit in obstetric anaesthetic practice should be carried out at a departmental level to assess local practice against a nationally agreed standard and the incidence of common side effects. Audit at a regional level assesses uniformity of practice and standards, and at a national level monitors rare complications and makes broad recommendations on standards in general.

Departmental audits

The Royal College of Anaesthetists has drawn up a list of audits that should be regularly carried out and re-audited. The focus is generally on quality issues and compliance with national guidelines.

- Adequacy of staffing.
- Timely anaesthetic involvement in the care of high risk mothers.
- Information about obstetric anaesthesia and analgesia.
- Pain management in labour.
- Consent given by women during labour.
- Response times for the provision of intrapartum analgesia and anaesthesia.
- Monitoring levels for regional analgesia.
- Technique of anaesthesia for CS.
- Pain relief after CS.
- Monitoring of obstetric patients in recovery and the High Dependency Unit (HDU).
- Airway and intubation problems during general anaesthesia for CS.
- Anaesthetic complications and side effects such as postdural puncture headache (PDPH) rate and regional to general anaesthesia conversion rates.
- The use of antacid prophylaxis in labour and for CS.

Regional audits

- Regional audits allow analysis of a much larger data set.
- Larger numbers can increase inaccuracies within the data collected—especially quantitative numbers—but are very good at looking at relatively rare problems and complications within obstetric anaesthesia.
- They are probably a more satisfactory way of looking at trends.
- The setting up of a regional database will also improve communications between neighbouring maternity units and will facilitate service development as it can more easily justify a need when a problem is relatively rare.

National audits

National audits usually have a broad framework and have looked in general terms at setting up good maternity services and analysing the risks associated with very rare complications.

National postal questionnaires

- A useful network of key personnel that provide obstetric anaesthetic services in the UK has been set up through the OAA.
- Are helpful adjuncts to local audit.
- Provide a snapshot of current practice across a large number of units and allow current local practice to be evaluated against national trends.
- Most published surveys have a response rate >70%, which is thought to give an acceptable spread of views.

National Obstetric Anaesthetic Database (NOAD)

- NOAD was set up in 1998 with the aim of establishing a framework for collecting national obstetric anaesthetic data considered useful and relevant by obstetric anaesthetists.
- This initial project provided useful information that was fed into the National Maternity Record project and has led to work on the design and content of obstetric anaesthetic records.
- It has produced reports on PDPH, requirement for high dependency care, baseline obstetric anaesthetic data, and rare complications of difficult intubation and high regional blocks.

CEMACH (Confidential Enquiry into Maternal and Child Health)

- Is the longest running audit project in the world.
- Previously known as CEMD (Confidential Enquiry into Maternal Death), this audit was started in 1952.
- Reports every 3yrs, and highlights main factors responsible for maternal mortality.
- CEMACH has probably had one of the greatest influences in reducing mortality relating to general anaesthesia in obstetrics.
- Recommendations on the broader involvement of anaesthetic services within maternity services have reduced maternal mortality relating to a number of obstetric emergencies including the management of PPH.
- This UK-based audit has had far-reaching influence across the world relating to maternity care, and many countries have used it to set their own standards.

Tips to the trainee doing audit

- Participation in audit is a contractual requirement for all anaesthetists.
- Select a topic and set a time limit.
- Ask for consultant input.
- Ask other healthcare professionals to help in data collection: nurses, midwives and colleagues.
- Use computers in data collection and analysis if appropriate.
- Present at an appropriate multidisciplinary meeting where a discussion to implement change can take place.
- Make someone responsible and accountable for seeing through the necessary change. Frequently, the best person to do this is a manager.
- Make arrangements for the audit to be repeated after an appropriate time interval to assess progress and close the audit loop.

Further reading

Principles for Best Practice in Clinical Audit. National Institute for Clinical Excellence. www.nice.org.uk

The Royal College of Anaesthetists. *Raising the Standard: A Compedium of Audit Recipes*, 2nd edn. Section 8. The Royal College of Anaesthetists, London, 2006.

Urqurhart J. Audit in obstetric anaesthesia. In: Collis R, Platt F, Urquhart J, ed. *Textbook of Obstetric Anaesthesia*. Greenwich Medical Media Ltd, London, 2002, 39–46.

National Obstetric Anaesthesia Database, Obstetric Anaesthetists' Association. www.oaa-anaes.ac.uk.

Confidential Enquiry into Maternal and Child Health. www.cemach.org.uk.

Chapter 2

Confidential Enquiry into Maternal and Child Health

Sarah Harries, Raman Sivasankar
and Paul Clyburn

Introduction

- In 1952, the system of local reporting of maternal deaths by Medical Officers of Health directly to the Ministry was replaced by an enhanced national system of regional and national assessment by clinicians. The first triennial report of these maternal deaths, covering the years 1952–1954, was published in 1957.
- Since then, a report of maternal deaths in the UK has been produced every 3yrs, with specific recommendations to guide future improvements in clinical practice on a worldwide scale.
- The Confidential Enquiry into Maternal Deaths (CEMD) is the longest running audit of practice in the UK.
- Fifty years later, the overarching organization and responsibility for producing the triennial report for 2000–2002 was handed over to the Confidential Enquiry into Maternal and Child Health (CEMACH).
- CEMACH is now commissioned by the National Institute for Health and Clinical Excellence (NICE), with regional CEMACH report managers responsible for data collection, and regional CEMACH assessors responsible for assessing the standard of care delivered in each individual case.

Maternal deaths

Maternal death is defined as 'the death of a woman while pregnant or within 42 days of termination of pregnancy, from any cause related to or aggravated by the pregnancy or its management, but not from accidental or incidental causes'.

They can be further subdivided into:

- Direct deaths.
- Indirect deaths.
- Late deaths.
- Coincidental deaths.

Direct deaths

Direct maternal deaths are those resulting from conditions, complications or their subsequent management that are unique to pregnancy, occurring during the antenatal, intrapartum or postpartum period, e.g. thromboembolism, haemorrhage or pre-eclampsia.

Indirect deaths

Indirect maternal deaths are those resulting from previously existing disease or disease that develops during pregnancy, which is not due to a direct obstetric cause, but was aggravated by the physiological effects of pregnancy, e.g. cardiac disease.

Late deaths

These are deaths occurring between 42 days and 1 year after abortion, miscarriage or delivery that are due to direct or indirect causes. Identifying late deaths enables lessons to be learned from deaths in which a woman had problems that began during the pregnancy, even if she survived for greater than 42 days after its end. The number of late deaths collected in recent reports has been enhanced by linking with data from the Office of National Statistics.

Coincidental deaths

These are deaths from unrelated causes, which happen to occur in pregnancy or the puerperium, e.g. domestic violence, road traffic accidents.

Enquiry objectives

The objectives of the enquiry are:

- To assess the main causes of and trends in maternal deaths.
- To identify any avoidable or substandard factors contributing to the death.
- To promulgate these findings to all relevant healthcare professionals.
- To improve the care that pregnant and recently delivered women receive and to reduce maternal mortality and morbidity rates still further, as well as the proportion of deaths due to substandard care.
- To make recommendations concerning the improvement of clinical care and service provision, including local audit, to purchasers of obstetric services and professionals involved in caring for pregnant women.
- To suggest directions for future areas for research and audit at a local and national level.

Maternal mortality trends

Maternal mortality rapidly declined from the 1930s to the 1980s—from 989 per million maternities in 1951 to 86 deaths per million maternities in 1984. However, the mortality rate has plateaued since the 1985–1987 triennium. The beginning of the 21st century has seen a small rise in reported deaths, which is not simply a consequence of improvements in data collection.

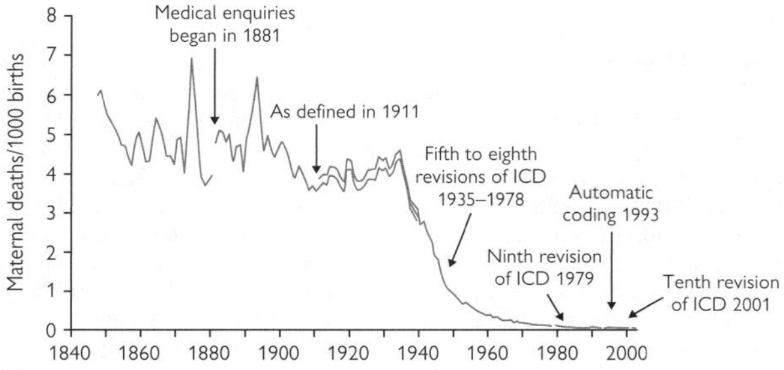

Fig. 2.1 Maternal mortality in England and Wales 1847–2002.

Source: General Register Office, POCS and ONS mortality statistics reproduced in Birth Counts. Table A 10.1.1–A 10.1.4.

CEMACH 2000–2002

- During the triennium 2000–2002, 391 maternal deaths were reported to the enquiry. Of the 391 deaths, 106 were classified as direct and 155 as indirect deaths, representing 27% and 40% of reported cases respectively.
- The overall (direct and indirect) maternal mortality for this triennium was 13.1 compared with the 11.4 deaths per 100 000 maternities in the previous triennium.
- Similarly, the direct maternal mortality of 5.3 in this triennium compared with 5.1 deaths per 100 000 maternities in the previous triennium was also higher, though not statistically significant.

Contributing factors to increased mortality rate

- The increase in numbers of newly arrived refugees or asylum seekers who did not seek care.
- An increase in the numbers of pregnant women who received substandard care.
- The introduction of the CEMACH Regional Managers and a greater awareness among health professionals leading to more comprehensive reporting of deaths.

Risk factors for maternal death

The report identified the following risk factors that may contribute to increased maternal mortality:

- Socially disadvantaged and poor communities.
- Minority ethnic groups are three times more likely to die.
- Late booking/poor attendance at antenatal clinic.
- Obesity—accounts for 35% of women who died.
- Domestic violence.
- Substance abuse.
- Suboptimal care—this was discovered in 67% of women who died.
- Lack of interprofessional communication.
- Age.

CEMACH 2003–2005 findings

Published December 2007

- During this triennium, there were 295 maternal deaths with a rate of 13.95 per 100 000 maternities—a slight but statistically insignificant increase on the previous report.
- For direct comparison with International figures a lower figure of 7 per 100 000 should be noted as this is the number ascertained by examination of death certificates (the method agreed internationally).
- Direct deaths increased slightly (not statistically significant) from the previous report to 6.24 per 100 000. The main causes (thromboembolism, PET/eclampsia and haemorrhage) remained unchanged but there was a large increase in amniotic fluid embolism (17 deaths) for reasons that are unclear.
- Indirect deaths overall changed little; but the reduction in the number of maternal suicides was balanced by an increase cardiac related deaths, particularly from acquired heart disease reflecting poor diet, smoking, alcohol and obesity.

Main recommendations

The report lists 'Top Ten' recommendations, which are summarized as:

- The need for adequate pre-conception counselling and support for women with risk factors for pregnancy e.g. epilepsy, diabetes, mental illness and obesity.
- Improved access to antenatal care, particularly for women who find difficulty in accessing such care with an emphasis on migrant women who often have poorer general health.
- Systolic hypertension (>160mm) requires antihypertensive treatment.
- Women should be advised that CS is not without risk. Women who have had a previous CS should have placental localization in their current pregnancy.
- The need for improved clinical skills by
  - Learning from untoward incidents.
  - Regular skills training and updates in life support, recognition and management of sick mothers.
- Introduction of early warning scoring systems to help identify sick mothers.
- Guidelines for management of obese women, sepsis, and pain and bleeding in early pregnancy.

Anaesthetic deaths

- There were six anaesthetic direct deaths: four were obese and two occurred in early pregnancy (i.e. gynaecology cases).
- Lessons that came out of these deaths were:
  - Problems of managing the obese parturient.
  - Inexperienced trainees working with inadequate supervision.
  - Poor understanding of the risks of anaesthesia in women in early pregnancy.
- In addition, there were 31 deaths where the assessors considered there was sub optimal anaesthetic management. Lessons from these included:
  - Inadequate recognition of degree of haemorrhage and its management.
  - Poor recognition of severity of illness.

Anaesthesia-related deaths

Introduction

- Direct deaths related to anaesthesia remained between 30 and 50 deaths in each triennium until 1981.
- From 1982–1984, this figure dropped to 19 deaths, and the same number of deaths were reported during the years 1985–1996 spanning four triennia.
- In the initial decades, the principal causes of deaths were acid aspiration and lack of the continued presence of the anaesthetist.
- In recent years, anaesthesia-related deaths have been due to failure to intubate and oxygenate the woman adequately. As the number of regional anaesthetics performed in obstetrics has increased, the direct deaths due to anaesthetic causes have steadily decreased.

CEMACH 2000–2002 findings

- There were six direct deaths (plus one late direct death) due to anaesthesia, and all deaths followed general anaesthesia (GA).
- Two deaths and one direct late death resulted from unrecognized oesophageal intubation during anaesthesia.
- Aspiration of gastric contents and anaphylaxis each contributed to one death.
- Working at isolated maternity sites and lack of supervision of junior anaesthetic staff were major contributory factors to the anaesthetic deaths.
- GA was the woman's choice rather than dictated by clinical need in those mothers who underwent CS. One of these women did not speak English. It may have been possible to explain the option of regional anaesthesia if a translator had been requested.
- In the cases of unrecognized oesophageal intubation, senior help was not immediately available and there was a reluctance on the part of anaesthetic staff to consider the possibility of oesophageal intubation. A recommended failed intubation drill was not followed and oxygenation was not maintained while waiting for spontaneous breathing to return.
- Anaesthesia training must concentrate on basic and advanced airway management skills, in particular the recognition and management of oesophageal intubation. The small number of GAs currently administered in obstetrics means that some of this training will have to be delivered in other clinical areas; the use of simulators may be usefully explored.

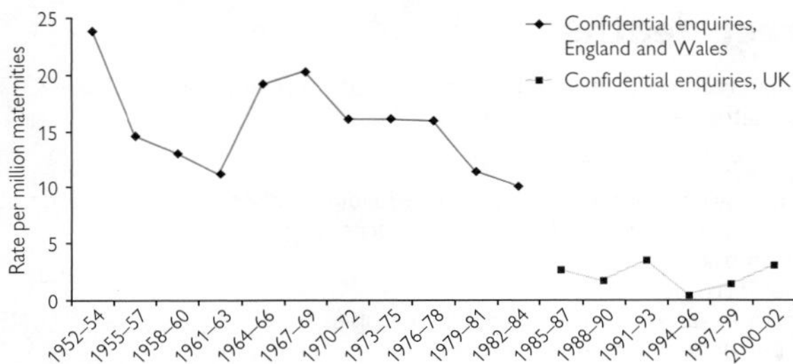

Fig. 2.2 Maternal deaths from anaesthesia in England and Wales 1952–1984 and in the UK 1985–2002.

Reproduced from *Why Mothers Die 2000–2002*, Griselda M Cooper and John H McClure, Anaesthesia, page 125, published 2004, with the permission of Confidential Enquiry into Maternal and Child Health.

Common failings identified

These deaths highlight examples of the following aspects of substandard care, with some deaths falling into several categories:

- Lack of multidisciplinary co-operation.
- Lack of appreciation of the severity of the illness.
- Lack of optimum perioperative care.
- Deficiencies in the management of haemorrhage.

Recommendations for anaesthesia services

- Dedicated obstetric anaesthesia services in all consultant-led units.
- Obstetric anaesthetists should not hesitate to call for assistance, especially in isolated units.
- Training must ensure competence in airway management.
- Early referral of obese women to the anaesthetists.
- Adequate advance notice of high risk cases.
- Women at high risk of, or with, major haemorrhage must involve a consultant obstetric anaesthetist.
- Invasive monitoring via appropriate routes should be used, particularly when the cardiovascular system is compromised by haemorrhage or disease.
- Women who are needle phobic are at greater risk from anaesthesia.

Direct deaths

The maternal mortality rate from direct deaths in the triennium 2000–2002 is 5.3 deaths per 100 000 maternities.

Major causes of direct deaths

The following were identified as the leading causes of direct maternal deaths in the triennium 2000–2002, in decreasing order of frequency:

- Thromboembolism.
- Haemorrhage.
- Death in early pregnancy including ectopics.
- Hypertensive disease of pregnancy.
- Sepsis.
- Anaesthesia.
- Amniotic fluid embolism (AFE).

Thromboembolism

- Deaths from thromboembolism have declined steadily until the triennia 1979–81, following which the rate has remained constant, probably due to greater awareness, increased use of prophylactic therapy and more effective treatment.

Thromboembolism remains the leading cause of direct maternal death.

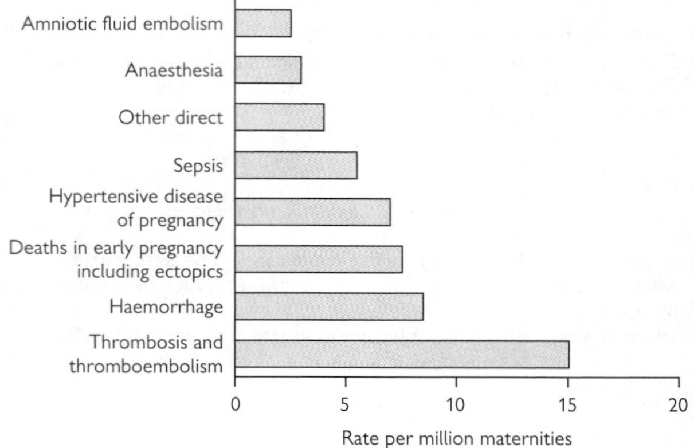

Fig. 2.3 Mortality rate of leading causes of direct deaths.

Reproduced from *Why Mothers Die 2000–2002*, Gwenyth Lewis, Introduction and key findings 2000–2002, page 32, published 2004, with the permission of Confidential Enquiry into Maternal and Child Health.

Risk factors

- Age.
- Travel (long haul flights, even a long car journey).
- Immobility (prolonged bed rest).
- Family history.
- Previous history of thromboembolism.
- Obesity (BMI >30).
- Oral contraceptives (not to be started until 21 days after delivery).

Key recommendations

- Postpartum thromboprophylaxis should be given as soon as possible after delivery, provided there is no postpartum haemorrhage.

Haemorrhage

- There were 17 deaths directly due to haemorrhage, with a striking increase in deaths following PPH, which has more than doubled the mortality rate per million due to haemorrhage since the last triennial report.
- Two mothers did not seek medical care and two mothers refused blood products.
- The quality of resuscitation was considered poor in many that sought medical care, and many high risk women are being booked for delivery in units with no blood bank or Intensive Care Unit (ICU).
- Twelve mothers had hysterectomies and some also had internal iliac artery ligation.
- No deaths were reported in mothers who had B-Lynch sutures or underwent radiological intervention.

Key recommendations

- A multidisciplinary massive haemorrhage protocol must be available on all units and should be updated regularly.
- Regular local 'fire drills' should be performed to rehearse the process of managing massive obstetric haemorrhage, including blood bank and portering services.
- High risk mothers should be delivered in units with on-site facilities for blood bank, intensive care and other interventions; elective procedures should be planned in advance.
- Consultant haematologists should be involved in the care of all mothers with a coagulopathy.
- All available interventions should be considered, e.g. B-Lynch suture, uterine artery embolization or radical surgery in the event of massive haemorrhage, and may require the assistance of additional surgical or radiology staff.

Pre-eclampsia

- 14 direct deaths occurred from eclampsia or pre-eclampsia in the triennium 2000–02, due to intracranial haemorrhage, adult respiratory distress syndrome (ARDS), multiorgan failure or severe disseminated intravascular coagulation (DIC).
- Six mothers had eclamptic fits, and HELLP syndrome was evident in eight mothers who died.
- The deaths associated with intracranial haemorrhage indicate a failure of effective antihypertensive treatment.

Key recommendations

- Protocols to guide management of eclampsia and pre-eclampsia should be in place in all delivery suites.
- Severe, life-threatening hypertension must be treated effectively.
- Magnesium sulphate is the anticonvulsant drug of choice in the treatment of eclampsia.
- Careful monitoring of fluid balance, fluid restriction and central venous pressure monitoring should guide fluid therapy. Early involvement of intensive care specialists in the management of severe pre-eclampsia is recommended.

Indirect deaths

The indirect maternal mortality rate in the triennium 2000–2002 was 7.8 deaths per 100 000 maternities, which is higher than 6.4 deaths per 100 000 maternities in the triennium 1997–1999. Indirect causes for maternal deaths account for ~60% of total maternal deaths in the UK, which contrasts with ~20% of deaths due to indirect causes in the rest of the world. The causes of indirect death are the same throughout the world; however, infectious disease, e.g. HIV/AIDS, is a rising cause of maternal death in most African countries.

Major causes

The causes of indirect death identified in the triennium 2000–2002, in order of decreasing frequency are:

- Cardiac disease, both congenital and acquired.
- Suicide.
- CNS haemorrhage.
- Epilepsy.
- Infection.
- Respiratory disease.
- Gastrointestinal disease.

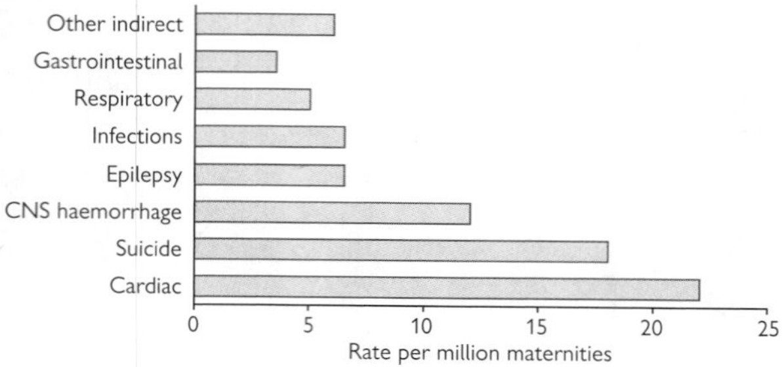

Fig. 2.4 Mortality rate of leading causes of indirect deaths.

Reproduced from *Why Mothers Die 2000–2002*, Gwenyth Lewis, Introduction and key findings 2000–2002, page 32, published 2004, with the permission of Confidential Enquiry into Maternal and Child Health.

The above figures are based on the mortality in the first 42 days after delivery. If mortality after 42 days is considered alone, suicide is the leading cause of death, with 50 known deaths occurring in 2000–2002.

Cardiac disease

The maternal mortality rate due to cardiac disease was two and a half times more in the first triennium compared to 2000–2002.

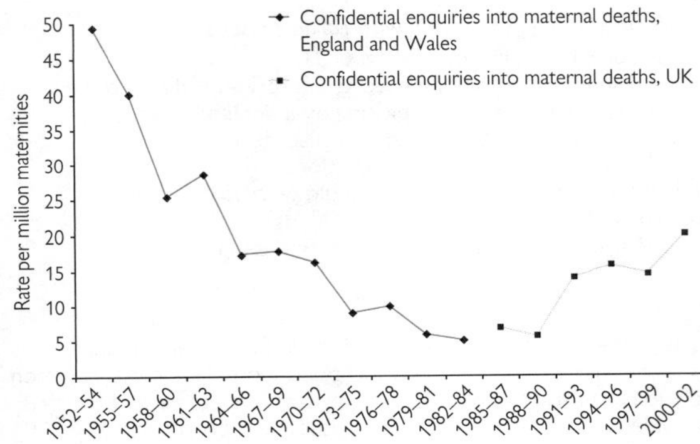

Fig. 2.5 Maternal morality rates from cardiac causes in England and Wales 1952–1984 and in the UK 1985–2002.

Reproduced from *Why Mothers Die 2000–2002*, Michael de Swiet and Catherine Nelson-Piercy, Cardiac disease, page 138, published 2004, with the permission of Confidential Enquiry into Maternal and Child Health.

Table 2.1 Causes of maternal death from heart disease in the UK 1991–2002

Cause of death	2000–2002	Totals 1991–2002
Cardiomyopathy and myocarditis	8	34
Aneurysm of thoracic aorta and its branches	7	28
Myocardial infarction	8	27
Pulmonary hypertension	4	22
All other heart disease	17	39
Valve disease including endocarditis	4	12
Other congenital	2	9
Sudden adult death syndrome	4	6
Myocardial fibrosis	3	4
Other acquired	4	8
All cardiac deaths and totals for 1991–2002	44	150

Reproduced from *Why Mothers Die 2000–2002*, Michael de Swiet and Catherine Nelson-Piercy, Cardiac disease, page 141, published 2004, with the permission of Confidential Enquiry into Maternal and Child Health.

Key recommendations for women with cardiac disease

- Thorough prepregnancy counselling.
- Family members should not be used as interpreters (desire to have a child may prevent them from passing on a detailed history).
- All medical staff should be trained in resuscitation skills.
- Emergency drills for maternal resuscitation.
- Termination of pregnancy services should be readily available
- Units should develop protocols.
- Increased age, obesity and hypertension are risk factors.

Suicide

The profile of the patient who commits suicide in the obstetric population is different from that in the non-obstetric population. The most common profile of women at risk of suicide in late pregnancy and following delivery is:

- White older woman in her second or subsequent pregnancy.
- Married and living in comfortable circumstances.
- Previous history of mental illness and contact with psychiatric services.
- Probably currently being treated.
- Baby is <3 months old.

In addition, mothers are more likely to commit suicide in a violent manner, which highlights the importance of alerting the psychiatric services to the fact that risk factors for maternal suicide may be different from those for women and men in the general population.

Further reading

Why Mothers Die 2000–2002. *Confidential Enquiry into Maternal and Child Health*. RCOG Press 2004.

Lewis, G(ed) 2007. The Confidential Enquiry into Maternal and Child Health (CEMACH). Saving Mother's Lives: reviewing maternal deaths to make motherhood safer-2003–2005. *The seventh report on Confidential Enquiries into Maternal deaths in the United Kingdom*. London: CEMACH

Chapter 3

Maternal physiology

Paul Clyburn, Korede Adekanye
and Shubhranshu Gupta

Cardiovascular system

There are a number of physiological adaptations to pregnancy within the cardiovascular system. It is important to be aware what is considered 'normal' for pregnancy, such that common medical conditions, e.g. hypertension, are recognized and treated promptly.

Blood volume (Fig. 3.1)

- The most striking maternal physiological alteration occurring during pregnancy is the increase in blood volume.
- The magnitude of this increase varies according to the size of the woman, her parity and whether there is one or multiple fetuses.
- The increase in blood volume progresses until term; the average increase in volume at term is 45–50%. The increase is needed for extra blood flow to the uterus, extra metabolic needs of the fetus and increased perfusion of other organs, especially the kidneys.
- The extra volume also compensates for maternal blood loss during delivery. The average blood loss with a vaginal delivery is 500–600mL, and at CS is 700–1000mL.

Red blood cells (Fig. 3.1)

- The increase in red blood cell (RBC) mass is ~33%.
- As plasma volume increases early in pregnancy and at a faster rate than RBC volume, this creates a 'physiological' anaemia.
- The haematocrit falls until the end of the second trimester, when the increase in RBCs starts to equal that of the plasma volume. The haematocrit then stabilizes or may increase slightly near term.

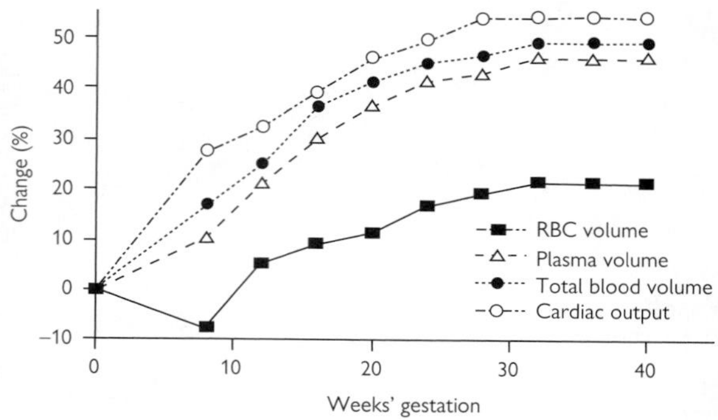

Fig. 3.1 Blood volume and cardiac output changes in pregnancy.

Reproduced with permission from Heidmann BH, McClure JH. Changes in maternal physiology during pregnancy. *BJA CEPOD Reviews* 2003; **3**: 65–68.

Haemodynamic changes in pregnancy

- There is a progressive fall in systemic vascular resistance (SVR) by up to 40%, which creates a maximal decrease in mean arterial pressure by the end of the first trimester.
- The average SVR in pregnancy is two-thirds that of the non-pregnant woman.
- Diastolic BP falls between 5 and 15mmHg, before rising to non-pregnancy levels at term, while systolic BP remains unchanged throughout pregnancy.
- The heart rate increases from ~72 to 85 beats/min (bpm) and stroke volume (SV) increases by up to 30 %. This, combined with the reduction in SVR, increases cardiac output (CO).
- By 24 weeks gestation, CO reaches a maximum of 50% above non-pregnant levels (Fig. 3.1). This is sustained until term, except in the supine position during the third trimester when it falls as a consequence of the gravid uterus compressing the inferior vena cava, reducing venous return (VR).
- CO increases further during labour, even with effective epidural analgesia. It peaks immediately after delivery as a result of uteroplacental transfusion into the maternal intravascular volume. It is during this period, when the preload and afterload of the heart are changing rapidly, that women with impaired cardiac function are at greatest risk.
- Left ventricular wall thickness and left ventricular mass increase progressively throughout pregnancy by up to 30 and 50%, respectively.
- CO returns almost to pre-pregnancy levels within 2 weeks of delivery.

Aorto-caval compression (Fig. 3.2)

- Uteroplacental blood flow is not autoregulated and is therefore dependent upon uterine BP.
- Aorto-caval occlusion occurs when the gravid uterus rests on the aorta and inferior vena cava (IVC). The reduction of VR is in part compensated for by increased distal venous pressure pushing blood through the compressed IVC and collateral venous pathways. This mechanism is in part regulated through autonomic pathways.
- Even in the absence of maternal hypotension, placental blood supply may be compromised in the supine position. After the 20th week of gestation, a left lateral tilt should always be maintained.
- The severity of this effect depends upon:
  - Patient position: in the supine position, 5–8% of pregnant women experience a substantial drop in BP (supine hypotension syndrome).
  - Gestation: IVC compression develops as early as 13 weeks of gestation. The effect becomes maximal at 36–38 weeks.
  - Uterine size: aorto-caval compression is increased in multiple pregnancies and polyhydramnios.

- Systemic BP.
- Presence of a sympathetic block.

- In the unanaesthetized state, most women are capable of compensating for the resultant decrease in SV by increasing SVR and heart rate. There are also alternative venous pathways: the paravertebral and azygos systems.
- During anaesthesia, however, these compensatory mechanisms are reduced or abolished, so that significant hypotension may rapidly develop.

Haemodynamic changes during labour

- CO during labour (between uterine contractions) increases from prelabour values by ~10% during the early first stage, 25% during late first stage and 40% during the second stage.
- These changes result from increased SV with minimal change in heart rate. Systolic and diastolic BPs also rise.
- A progressive rise in sympathetic nervous system activity, which peaks at the time of delivery, accounts for these changes by increasing myocardial contractility, SVR and VR. Central venous pressure (CVP) also rises.
- CO and SVR increase by a further 15 and 25% during contractions, with lesser increases of 15 and 10% with effective analgesia.

Haemodynamic changes during the puerperium

- There is a state of relative hypervolaemia and an increased VR follows vaginal delivery.
- This results from relief of caval compression and a reduction of maternal vascular capacitance.
- CVP rises, and SV and CO increase by as much as 75% above predelivery values.
- Mothers with significant cardiac disease are at increased risk during this period.

Distribution of the increased cardiac output

- There is an increased blood flow to the uterus, kidneys and skin.
- Uterine blood flow is ~10–12% of CO. Mammary artery blood flow increases early in pregnancy; breast tenderness and swelling are among the first symptoms.
- Flow to the liver and brain remains unchanged.

Fluid balance during pregnancy

- Arterial dilatation creates a relatively ‘underfilled’ state, which stimulates the renin–angiotensin–aldosterone system. As a result, sodium and water retention throughout pregnancy leads to a 6–8L rise in total extracellular fluid volume.

- An increase in plasma volume is apparent by 6 weeks gestation and continues until week 32, when it is 40% (~1.2L) above non-pregnant levels.
- Furthermore, shortly after conception, the osmotic threshold for thirst falls and plasma osmolality drops by 10mosmol/kg. A concomitant fall in the threshold for secretion of antidiuretic hormone (arginine vasopressin) prevents a water diuresis and sustains low plasma osmolality until term.
- During the second half of pregnancy, placental production of vasopressinase increases maternal antidiuretic hormone degradation, but plasma antidiuretic hormone levels remain stable as pituitary secretion of antidiuretic hormone increases 4-fold.
- Plasma atrial natriuretic peptide levels are normal until the second trimester, when they rise by ~40%.

Cardiac size/position/ECG

- There are both size and position changes which can lead to changes in the ECG appearance. The heart is enlarged by both chamber dilation and hypertrophy.
- Dilation across the tricuspid valve can initiate mild regurgitant flow, causing a normal grade I or II systolic murmur.
- Upward displacement of the diaphragm by the enlarging uterus causes the heart to shift to the left and anteriorly, so that the apex beat is moved outward and upward.
- These changes lead to common ECG findings of left axis deviation, sagging ST segments and frequently inversion or flattening of the T-wave in lead III.

Clinical implications of cardiovascular changes

- Despite the increased workload of the heart during gestation and labour, the healthy woman has no impairment of cardiac reserve.
- In contrast, for the pregnant women with heart disease and low cardiac reserve, the increase in the work of the heart may cause ventricular failure and pulmonary oedema.
- In these women, further increases in cardiac workload during labour must be prevented by effective pain relief (and sympathetic nervous system blockade), optimally provided by epidural, low dose spinal analgesia or a combination of both in a low dose CSE technique.
- Since CO is highest in the immediate postpartum period, sympathetic blockade should be maintained for several hours after delivery and then weaned off slowly.
- Aorto-caval compression is one of the most important events during pregnancy, especially when the parturient lies supine. Hence, left uterine displacement must always be maintained.
- Downregulation of α and β receptors is an additional important factor, which may necessitate an increased dose of vasopressor.

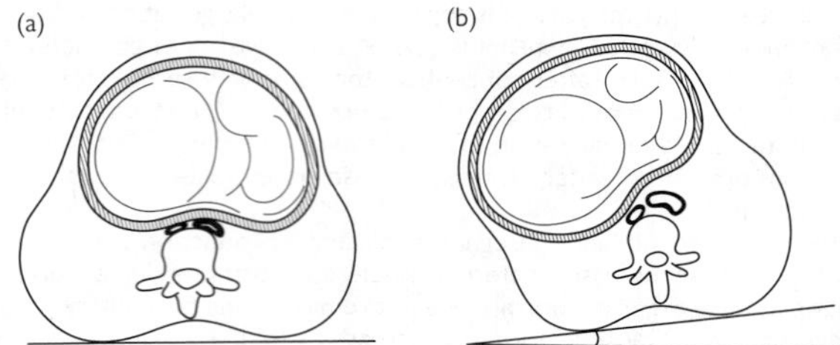

Fig. 3.2 Aorto-caval compression. (a) In the supine position, blood flow through the vena cava and aorta is significantly reduced, causing maternal and fetal compromise. The efficacy of left lateral displacement was demonstrated in 1972. The full left or right lateral position completely relieves aorto-caval compression. (b) Elevating the mother's hip 10–15cm completely relieves aorto-caval compression in 58% of term parturients.

Table 3.1 Summary of cardiovascular changes in pregnancy

Measurement	Change	% Change
Heart rate	Increase	20–30%
Systolic blood pressure	Decrease	10–15% mid-trimester
Stroke volume	Increase	20–50%
Cardiac output	Increase	30–50%
Central venous pressure	No change	—
Systemic vascular resistance	Decrease	20%
Pulmonary artery pressure	Decrease	30%
Pulmonary capillary wedge pressure	No change	—

Respiratory system

Major physiological and anatomical changes occur in the respiratory system during pregnancy due to a combination of both hormonal and mechanical factors. Dyspnoea is a common complaint in pregnancy, affecting over half of women at some stage.

Anatomical changes

- Hormonal changes to the mucosal vasculature of the respiratory tract lead to capillary engorgement and swelling of the lining in the nose, oropharynx, larynx and trachea.
- The thoracic cage increases in both antero-posterior and transverse diameter.
- The enlarging uterus displaces the diaphragm upwards, but the internal volume of the thoracic cage remains unchanged.
- Abdominal muscles have less tone and are less active during pregnancy, causing respiration to be more diaphragmatic.

Ventilatory changes during pregnancy (Fig. 3.3)

- The increased metabolic demands of pregnancy lead to a progressive increase in oxygen consumption, reaching almost 20–30% by term.
- Carbon dioxide production shows similar changes to that of oxygen consumption.
- During labour, oxygen consumption is further increased (up to and over 60%) as a result of the exaggerated cardiac and respiratory workload.
- To compensate, pregnant women breathe more deeply, tidal volume increasing from ~500 to 700mL, while the respiratory rate remains unchanged.
- Effective alveolar ventilation (increased by ~50%) actually surpasses the body's demand for oxygen and carbon dioxide production (increased by ~30–40%), creating a respiratory alkalosis with PCO_2 falling from 5.0 to 4.0kPa.
- Overbreathing is a direct effect of progesterone on the respiratory centre, particularly increasing the sensitivity to CO_2.
- During labour, ventilation may be further accentuated, either voluntarily (Lamaze method of pain control and relaxation) or involuntarily in response to pain and anxiety.

Lung volumes

- Upward displacement by the gravid uterus causes a 4cm elevation of the diaphragm, but total lung capacity decreases only slightly because of compensatory increases in the transverse and antero-posterior diameters of the chest, due to flaring of the ribs.
- These changes are brought about by hormonal effects that loosen ligaments.

- Despite the upward displacement, the diaphragm moves with greater excursions during breathing in the pregnant than in the non-pregnant state. In fact, breathing is more diaphragmatic than thoracic during gestation, an advantage in the supine position and following high regional blockade.
- Lung compliance is relatively unaffected, but chest wall compliance is reduced, especially in the lithotomy position.
- The following changes in lung volumes occur during pregnancy relative to the non-pregnant state (Fig. 3.3):
  - A progressive increase in minute ventilation starts soon after conception and peaks at 50% above normal levels around the second trimester.
  - Tidal volume (TV) increases by 45%.
  - Functional residual capacity (FRC) decreases by 20–30% due to reduction of the expiratory reserve volume by 25% and residual volume by 15%.
  - Closing capacity can encroach on FRC, increasing ventilation/perfusion (V/Q) mismatch and the ready occurrence of hypoxia.
  - Inspiratory capacity increases by 15%.
  - Since dead space remains unchanged, alveolar ventilation is ~70% higher at the end of gestation.

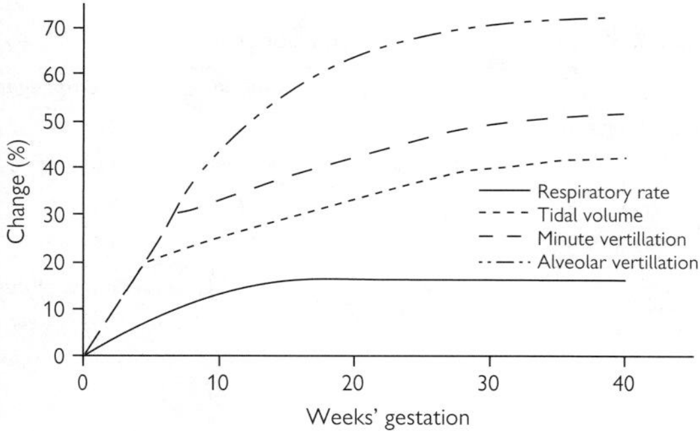

Fig. 3.3 Respiratory changes in pregnancy.

Reproduced with permission from Heidmann BH, McClure JH. Changes in maternal physiology during pregnancy. *BJA CEPOD Reviews* 2003; **3**: 65–68.

Acid–base status (Table 3.2)

- The $PaCO_2$ declines to almost 4kPa by 12 weeks of pregnancy and remains so throughout gestation.
- Although a gradient exists between the end-tidal CO_2 and $PaCO_2$ in non-pregnant individuals, the two are similar during pregnancy.
- The PaO_2 rises due to the decrease in $PaCO_2$. An average PaO_2 of 13.7kPa persists during gestation.
- There is an increased arteriovenous O_2 difference due to increased peripheral oxygen consumption.
- Metabolic compensation for the respiratory alkalosis of pregnancy reduces the serum bicarbonate concentration to ~20mmol/L.
- The development of alkalosis is therefore forestalled by compensatory decreases in serum bicarbonate. Only CO_2 levels <3.7kPa will lead to a respiratory alkalosis.
- Excessive hyperventilation during labour results in marked hypocarbia and severe respiratory alkalosis, which can lead to cerebral and uteroplacental vasoconstriction and a left shift of the oxygen dissociation curve.
- This causes reduced release of oxygen from haemoglobin with consequent decreased maternal tissue oxygenation.

Table 3.2 Ventilation in pregnancy and labour

	Pregnancy	**Labour**	**Non-pregnant**
Respiratory rate (min^{-1})	15	22–70	12
Tidal volume (mL)	480–680	650–2000	450
$PaCO_2$ (kPa)	4.1	2–2.7	5.3
PaO_2 (kPa)	14	13.5–14.4	13.3

Reproduced with permission from Heidmann BH, McClure JH. Changes in maternal physiology during pregnancy. *BJA CEPOD Reviews* 2003; **3**: 65–68.

Clinical implications of respiratory changes

- Symptoms of nasal congestion, voice change and upper respiratory tract infection may be present throughout gestation.
- The changes in respiratory function have clinical relevance for the anaesthetist. Most importantly, increased oxygen consumption and decreased reserve due to the reduced FRC may result in rapid falls in arterial oxygen tension despite careful maternal positioning and preoxygenation.
- Even with short periods of apnoea, whether from obstruction of the airway or inhalation of a hypoxic mixture of gas, the gravida has little defence against the development of hypoxia.
- The increased minute ventilation combined with decreased FRC hastens inhalation induction or changes in depth of anaesthesia when breathing spontaneously.
- Airway management is more challenging. Laryngoscopy may be hindered by weight gain and breast engorgement. Avoid intranasal manipulation as the swollen mucosa is more prone to bleeding.
- In cases of fluid overload or oedema associated with pregnancy-induced hypertension (PIH) or pre-eclampsia, manipulation of the airway can result in profuse bleeding from the nose or oropharynx, and tracheal intubation can be difficult.
- Maintain 'normal' lowered levels of $PaCO_2$ during mechanical ventilation.
- Reduced compliance necessitates higher airway pressures to maintain adequate ventilation.

Table 3.3 Summary of respiratory changes in pregnancy

Measurement	Change	% Change
Rate	No change	—
Tidal volume	Increase	40%
Minute volume	Increase	40%
Alveolar ventilation	Increase	40%
Vital capacity	Increase	100–200mL
Functional residual capacity	Decrease	20%
Total lung capacity	Decrease	5%
Residual volume	Decrease	15%

Renal function

The renal system undergoes marked changes in function during pregnancy due to hormonal effects, the increased metabolic load of the fetus and also due to outflow obstruction of the ureters by the enlarging uterus.

Renal changes during pregnancy

- An 80% increase in renal blood flow and 55% increase in glomerular filtration rate occur by 16 weeks gestation.
- The rise in renal blood flow causes the kidneys to swell so that they appear ~1cm longer on ultrasonography.
- The renal pelvis and ureters dilate, sometimes appearing obstructed to those unaware of these changes.
- Serum levels of creatinine and urea fall, so that levels considered normal outside pregnancy can suggest renal impairment during pregnancy.

Changes in the renal system

Plasma concentration	Non-pregnant	Pregnant
Urea (mmol/L)	2.5–6.7	2.3–4.3
Creatinine (mmol/L)	70–150	50–73
Urate (mmol/L)	0.2–0.35	0.15–0.35
Bicarbonate (mmol/L)	22–26	18–26

- Proteinuria increases slightly during pregnancy, but levels >260mg/24h should be considered abnormal.
- Tubular reabsorption of sodium is increased.
- Aminoaciduria due to reduced absorption is normal in pregnancy.
- Gestational glycosuria reflects reduced tubular glucose reabsorption and does not necessarily indicate abnormal carbohydrate metabolism.
- Furthermore, reduced tubular absorption of bicarbonate creates a metabolic acidosis that compensates for the respiratory alkalosis, maintaining maternal pH at 7.4.
- The production of all three renal hormones—erythropoietin, active vitamin D and renin, increases during healthy pregnancy, but their effects are masked by other physiological changes.
- In early pregnancy, peripheral vasodilatation exceeds the renin–aldosterone-mediated plasma volume expansion, so BP falls by 12 weeks gestation.
- The 40% expansion of plasma volume exceeds the effect of a 2- to 4-fold increase in maternal serum erythropoietin levels, which stimulates only a 25% rise in red cell mass.
- This creates a 'physiological anaemia', which should not normally cause haemoglobin concentration to fall to <9.5g/dL.
- Similarly, active vitamin D circulates at twice non-gravid levels, but concomitant halving of parathyroid hormone (PTH) levels, as well as hypercalcuria and increased fetal requirements, keeps plasma ionized calcium levels unchanged.

Clinical implications of renal changes

- Normal parturients' urea and creatinine values are 40% less than in non-pregnant women. Therefore, the normal range for urea and creatinine should be adjusted for the pregnant state, as values within the normal range for the non-pregnant state may indicate significantly impaired renal function.
- Physiological diuresis during the postpartum period occurs between 2 and 5 days.
- The glomerular filtration rate and urea concentration slowly return to non-pregnant values by the 6th postpartum week.

Haematological changes

- The plasma volume increases up to 50% by term.
- Red cell volume also increases due to increased erythropoietin production, but not enough to prevent the dilutional anaemia of pregnancy. This causes a 15% drop in the measured haemoglobin.
- The blood viscosity is also slightly reduced, causing a slight decrease in cardiac work.
- Normal pregnancy is associated with a demand of 1000mg of additional iron—500mg to increase maternal RBC volume, 300mg transported to the fetus and 200mg for normal iron loss. Serum iron is decreased. There is also an increase in total iron binding capacity (TIBC) and transferrin.
- The platelet count tends to remain normal, although there is an increased turnover of platelets in pregnancy.
- There is an increase in white blood cell count, reaching a peak during labour.
- There is a decreased concentration in plasma protein due to the increase in plasma volume. This results in a drop in colloid oncotic pressure leading to the oedema seen in pregnancy. There is an ~15% drop in total protein and albumin along with a 25% drop in plasma cholinesterase levels.

Coagulation

- In anticipation of haemorrhage at childbirth, normal pregnancy is characterized by low grade, chronic intravascular hypercoagulation within both the maternal and uteroplacental circulation.
- There are increased levels of clotting factors (V, VIII and X), decreased levels of the endogenous anticoagulant protein S and decreased fibrinolytic activity.
- These changes lead to an acquired protein C resistance in up to 38% of pregnant women.
- Therefore, pregnancy is a relatively hypercoagulable state, but during pregnancy neither clotting nor bleeding times are abnormal.

However, postpartum contraction of the uterus by oxytocin is probably more effective at preventing haemorrhage than any changes to the coagulation system.

Clinical implications of haematological changes

- Pharmacokinetics of protein-bound drugs are affected due to reduced protein binding.
- There is a slightly prolonged action of succinylcholine due to reduced levels of plasma cholinesterase.
- Due to the hypercoagulable state of pregnancy, there is an increased incidence of thromboembolic disease, which is the most common cause of maternal mortality in developed countries.

Table 3.4 Summary of haematological changes in pregnancy

Measurement	Change	% Change
Haemoglobin	Decrease	20%
Platelets	Decrease	10–20%
Clotting factors (except XI)	Increase	50–250%
Factor XI	Decrease	

Gastrointestinal system

Anatomical changes

- The stomach is displaced upwards towards the left side of the diaphragm and its axis rotated 45° to the right from its normal vertical position.
- This displaces the intra-abdominal segment of the oesophagus into the thorax in most pregnant women.
- As a result of this, the lower oesophageal high pressure zone (LEHPZ), which normally prevents reflux, is reduced in size.
- The intragastric pressure (IGP) is elevated, especially in the last trimester. Therefore, the barrier pressure is reduced (LEHPZ–IGP).

Physiology of the GIT

- Nausea and vomiting affect ~60% of women during the first trimester.
- Relaxation of intestinal smooth muscle by progesterone creates many of the other pregnancy-induced gastrointestinal changes.
- Gastric motility and small bowel transit are slowed, especially during labour. The gallbladder enlarges and empties slowly in response to meals.
- A decrease in lower oesophageal pressure makes gastro-oesophageal reflux more common.
- Therefore, there is an increased risk of aspiration due to an increase of oesophageal reflux and a decrease in the pH of gastric contents.
- Pulmonary aspiration of gastric contents can occur following either vomiting (active) or regurgitation (passive).

Liver metabolism during pregnancy

- The size of the liver and its blood flow appear not to change during healthy pregnancy; hence liver blood flow accounts for proportionately less of the CO as pregnancy progresses.
- There are, however, changes to hepatic synthetic function and metabolism. Circulating concentrations of fibrinogen, ceruloplasmin, transferrin and binding proteins such as thyroid-binding globulin increase, while serum albumin levels fall by ~20%.
- Serum cholesterol increases by 50% and triglycerides by up to 300%. The normal ranges for aspartate transaminase, alanine transaminase, gamma glutamyl transferase and bilirubin decrease by at least 20% from the first trimester until term.
- After the 5th month, placental production of alkaline phosphatase increases maternal plasma levels by up to 4-fold.
- Telengiectasia and palmar erythema are common signs of healthy pregnancy that resolve postpartum.

Clinical implications

- The pregnant woman should be considered to be a patient with a 'full stomach', with increased risk of aspiration from the start of the second trimester, or earlier if symptomatic.
- During general anaesthesia, airway protection by means of a cuffed tracheal tube is mandatory.
- Special precautions should be heeded, even when induction to intubation time is expected to be brief, to prevent regurgitation.
- Preoxygenation prior to induction and no positive pressure ventilation prior to insertion of the tracheal tube is recommended to prevent distension of the stomach with gas (i.e. rapid sequence induction).
- Cricoid pressure (Sellick's manoeuvre) during induction should be maintained until correct tracheal tube placement has been confirmed. This manoeuvre occludes the oesophagus and obstructs the path for regurgitation (see Chapter 11, page 320).
- Aspiration of solid material causes atelectasis, obstructive pneumonitis or lung abscess, while aspiration of acidic gastric contents results in chemical pneumonitis (Mendelson's syndrome).

Endocrine system

The principle hormone of pregnancy is progesterone. Soon after fertilization, the developing placenta produces human chorionic gonadotrophin (hCG). This sustains the corpus luteum until the 6th–8th week of pregnancy enabling it to produce progesterone. Thereafter, the placenta takes over as the main source of progesterone. The placenta also produces human placental lactogen.

Pituitary function

- Once ovulation has occurred and the uterus is prepared for implantation, the maternal pituitary makes only a small contribution to a successful pregnancy.
- The only pituitary hormone to increase significantly during pregnancy (by ~10-fold) is prolactin, which is responsible for breast development and subsequent milk production.
- Pituitary secretion of growth hormone is mildly suppressed during the second half of pregnancy by placental production of a growth hormone variant.
- Placental production of adrenocorticotrophic hormone (ACTH) leads to an increase in maternal ACTH levels, but not beyond the normal range for non-pregnant subjects.
- Free cortisol levels double and in the second half of pregnancy may contribute to insulin resistance and the appearance of striae gravidarum.
- High oestrogen levels during pregnancy stimulate lactotroph hyperplasia, resulting in pituitary enlargement.
- These high levels, together with those of progesterone, suppress luteinizing hormone (LH) and follicule-stimulating hormone (FSH).
- Plasma FSH levels recover within 2 weeks of delivery, but pulsatile LH release is only resumed in women who do not breastfeed. In suckling mothers, prolactin inhibits gonadotrophin-releasing hormone and hence LH.

Thyroid function

- The normal pregnant women should remain euthyroid.
- There is increased total thyroxine (T_4) and tri-iodothyronine (T_3), but also there is increased production of thyroxine-binding globulin (TBG).
- Free T_4 and T_3 remain unchanged.
- The basal metabolic rate (BMR) increases 15–20% above normal.
- There is lowered T_3 uptake during pregnancy.
- Thyroid-stimulating hormone (TSH) does not cross the placenta.
- During pregnancy, the thyroid faces three challenges:
    - Increased renal clearance of iodide and losses to the fetus create a state of relative iodine deficiency. In geographical areas where dietary iodine intake is low, pregnancy stimulates growth of thyroid goitres.
    - High oestrogen levels induce hepatic synthesis of TBG, but free T_3 and T_4 levels remain within the normal range throughout pregnancy.

- Placental hCG shares structural similarities with TSH and has weak TSH-like activity. Although hCG rarely stimulates free T_4 levels into the thyrotoxic range, trophoblastic disease and hyperemesis gravidarum are often associated with high hCG levels and can lead to hyperthyroxinaemia. In these circumstances, the mother remains clinically euthyroid.

Parathyroid glands

- Pregnancy and lactation are associated with increased calcium demands, and there is an increased loss of urinary calcium in pregnancy. These factors necessitate a 2-fold increase in vitamin D-mediated gut absorption of calcium.
- PTH is reduced in pregnancy, but PTH-related peptide is produced by the placenta and has a compensatory role in maintaining calcium balance.

Pancreas

- The islets of Langerhans and β-cells increase in number during pregnancy, as does the number of receptor sites for insulin. However, there is resistance to the action of insulin due to the presence of human placental lactogen, prolactin and other pregnancy hormones.

Carbohydrate metabolism

- During the first trimester, women are more sensitive to insulin than when non-pregnant.
- From 20 weeks gestation onwards, insulin resistance develops; hence, women in the second half of pregnancy respond to a glucose load by producing more insulin, but with less effect.
- Obese women, who are already insulin resistant, are more likely to develop gestational diabetes.
- Hormones that might mediate this insulin resistance include cortisol, progesterone, oestrogen and human placental lactogen.
- Placental production of human placental lactogen, a growth hormone-like protein, coincides temporally with insulin resistance.

Central nervous system

The central and peripheral nervous system undergo significant changes during pregnancy.

- There are substantial pressure and volume changes in the epidural and subarachnoid spaces, which have important effects on the spread of solutions within these compartments.
- Less LA volume is required to produce the same effect in pregnancy when compared with the non-pregnant state.
- In part, this arises due to engorgement of the epidural veins caused by aorto-caval compression or during the pushing phase of labour.
- This leads to a reduction in the volume available for the spread of LAs within the vertebral canal.
- Therefore, an identical volume of LA will spread more extensively in the pregnant state.
- In addition, the nerve tissue is more sensitive to a specific concentration of LA, an effect mediated via increased oestrogen and progesterone levels.
- Cannulation of an epidural vein when performing epidural catheter insertion (bloody tap) is more common due to engorged epidural veins.
- The constituents of cerebral spinal fluid (CSF) do not change during pregnancy but its pressures are high due to reduced capacitance.
- Between contractions, the CSF pressure may be ~28mmHg but during contractions it may rise to as much as 70mmHg. It is therefore advised not to advance an epidural needle or insert an epidural catheter during contractions for risk of puncturing the dura and subsequent expulsion of CSF at high pressure.
- The increased concentrations of progesterone and endogenous opioids (β-endorphin especially) are the most likely explanation for the observed reduction in minimum alveolar concentration (MAC) for volatile anaesthetic agents.
- There is a similar increase in sensitivity to opioids sedatives and other GA drugs.
- Emotional changes during pregnancy are common. Reduced cognitive ability and memory loss have been demonstrated. Depression, both antenatally and in the postnatal period, is well recognized.

Summary of physiological changes relating to anaesthesia

The hormonal changes that occur from very early on in pregnancy cause a complex series of physiological and anatomical changes that affect every system of the body. To illustrate how all these changes may alter or affect anaesthetic management, it is useful to classify them in terms of general anaesthesia and regional anaesthesia.

General anaesthesia

- Careful attention to the assessment of the airway and any necessary preparation to deal with a potentially difficult airway in the preoperative period.
- Tracheal intubation—increased risk of failed intubation, a smaller tracheal tube required, increased risk of trauma with nasotracheal intubation and increased risk of pulmonary aspiration of gastric contents.
- Maternal oxygenation—increased physiological shunt when supine, increased rate of decline of PaO_2 during apnoea.
- Preoxygenation is essential and should be with a tight-fitting mask for at least 3min.
- When positioning the patient on the operating table, remember to practise left uterine displacement, using either left tilt of between 15 and 30° on the table or a wedge under the right buttock to minimize aorto-caval compression.
- Rapid sequence induction with the application of cricoid pressure is mandatory.
- Intubation may be difficult and so adjuncts for difficult intubation should be available.
- The trained anaesthetic assistant should be careful when applying cricoid pressure if there is a left tilt on the operating table. The temptation to exert cricoid pressure vertically downwards can distort the view at laryngoscopy.
- Once the airway is secured, ventilation should be aimed at keeping the $PaCO_2$ in the normal range for pregnancy.
- There is an increased sensitivity to opioids, sedatives and other GA drugs. The MAC of volatile anaesthetic is slightly reduced.
- Volatile agents cause relaxation of the uterus (uterine atony) and this may result in significant haemorrhage after delivery of the fetus.
- There is decreased sensitivity to endogenous and exogenous catecholamines. Therefore, if vasopressors are required to maintain adequate BP, the necessary dose may be increased.
- Extubation should be done with the patient fully awake in the lateral position, to reduce the risk of aspiration of gastric contents.

Regional anaesthesia

- There is an increased lumbar lordosis and thoracic kyphosis.
- There is a tendency towards a head-down tilt in the lateral position because of greater hip than shoulder dimensions.
- These factors lead to increased rostral subarachnoid spread of LA solution when injected in the lateral position.
- The subarachnoid dose requirement is reduced (~25%).
- There is increased sensitivity to LA agents.

Further reading

Kenneth A. Maternal physiology. In: Chestnut DH, ed. *Obstetric Anaesthesia: Principles and Practice*, 3rd edn. Mosby, 2006, 17–43.

Wilkey AD, Millns JP. Pregnancy and foetal physiology. In: Hutton P, ed. *Fundamentals Principles and Practice of Anaesthesia*. Martin Dunitz, 2002, 563–565.

Chapter 4

Maternal pathophysiology

Paul Clyburn, Korede Adekanye
and Shubhranshu Gupta

Principles of managing cardiac disease

Overview of cardiac disease

Cardiac disease is a major cause of indirect maternal death. It is responsible for more deaths in the UK than haemorrhage and PIH put together.

Cardiac disease affecting pregnancy falls into three categories:

- Known pre-existing cardiac disease before pregnancy.
- Known pre-existing risk factors for developing cardiac disease during pregnancy, e.g. heavy smoker, strong family history for ischaemic heart disease.
- A condition arises during pregnancy when there are no known risk factors, e.g. peripartum cardiomyopathy.

Deaths from pre-existing cardiac disease have remained constant over the last 30yrs, despite an increasing caseload, as women with congenital heart disease survive to childbearing age. In contrast, deaths from acquired cardiac disease have increased during this time.

There are two distinct management challenges:

Women with previously diagnosed cardiac disease

- All women should be risk assessed and receive prepregnancy counselling from an experienced cardiologist or obstetrician.
- All should be seen early in pregnancy and regularly thereafter by an appropriate multidisciplinary team (cardiologist, obstetrician and anaesthetist), who can formulate a management plan for pregnancy and delivery.

Women who develop cardiac disease during pregnancy

- Surveillance should be in place to identify those women with risk factors for developing cardiac disease.
- Surveillance should also identify the early symptoms and signs of the disease process in women who develop a cardiac condition, so that treatment may be promptly instituted.
- When acquired cardiac disease presents, a multidisciplinary approach to management is essential.

Antenatal assessment (see Chapter 5, page 128–131)

- Careful functional assessment and correct classification will help identify women at risk.
- High risk women must have early multidisciplinary care.

New York Heart Association (NYHA) functional classification

- Class I: no breathlessness/uncompromised.
- Class II: breathlessness on severe exertion/slight compromise.
- Class III: breathless on mild extertion/moderate compromise.
- Class IV: breathless at rest/severe compromise.

Further reading

Gamann WR. Cardiovascular disease. In: Chestnut DH, ed. *Obstetric Anaesthesia, Principles and Practice*. 3rd edn. Mosby, 2006, 776–808.

Thorne S. Pregnancy in heart disease. *Heart* 2004; **90**: 450–456.

Principles of analgesia and anaesthesia

- There remains controversy over the preferred mode of delivery for the more high risk cardiac conditions:
  - Elective CS means that delivery occurs at a planned time and also avoids an unplanned, emergency CS, with its consequent higher risks.
  - In general terms, labour is haemodynamically more stable (particularly when low dose epidural techniques are used) than an operative delivery.
  - Therefore, decisions for mode of delivery should be influenced more by obstetric considerations than by the cardiac disease.
  - Regular assessment by an experienced multidisciplinary team is essential. If there is evidence of disease progression during pregnancy, either symptomatically or from echocardiogram findings, delivery of the baby should be expedited.
- If regional anaesthesia is chosen for operative delivery:
  - A rapid onset sympathetic block with greater haemodynamic instability that accompanies a single-shot spinal technique is usually undesirable.
  - Incremental epidural anaesthesia gives greater haemodynamic stability.
  - An alternative is a CSE technique, i.e. low initial spinal dose (5–7.5mg 0.5% heavy bupivacaine + opioid), followed by a gradual incremental epidural extension, titrated against block height and invasive BP monitoring.
- Invasive monitoring should follow a careful risk/benefit analysis in the individual case.
  - Intra-arterial monitoring has a low complication risk and is useful for accurately following changes in BP.
  - Although central venous catheters (and pulmonary artery catheters) may provide useful information in some conditions about cardiac filling pressures and allow infusions of cardioactive drugs, they are difficult to insert in the pregnant woman with cardiac disease who may not tolerate a head-down position. They also increase the risk of infection and air embolus. The information they provide may be difficult to interpret in complex congenital heart conditions.
  - Insertion of an IV long line, e.g. drum-cath, in the antecubital fossa is an alternative method of measuring CVP, is usually better tolerated and is more likely to be easy because of vasodilatation associated with pregnancy.
- Meticulous care should be taken to avoid aorto-caval compression.
- Antibiotic prophylaxis is frequently required.
- Care should be taken with the use of syntocinon as it causes vasodilatation, particularly when given as a rapid bolus.
- Patients may be on heparin. The timing of regional anaesthesia in relation to the administration of heparin is important.
- Patients may be prone to develop complex cardiac dysrhythmias, and cardiology advice should be sort in advance in order to know how best to manage them.

Myocardial disease

CEMACH reports in recent years have demonstrated the increase in deaths resulting from acquired cardiac disease, in particular deaths from ischaemic heart disease. With an increasing median maternal age in the UK and the increasing trend in maternal obesity and other known risk factors, the number of deaths related to ischaemic cardiac disease is set to increase further.

Haemodynamics of ventricular failure

- Understanding ventricular failure is made easier by considering the dynamic relationships between pressure and volume (Fig. 4.1a–e).
- For a normal heart, the end-systolic pressure–volume relationship is relatively steep, while for the failing heart, it is flatter. In addition, the end-diastolic pressure–volume relationship is flatter for the normal heart than for the failing heart.
- Thus, the failing heart responds to changes in resistance by smaller changes in systolic pressure, larger increases in diastolic pressure, and decreases in SV and CO than the normal heart.
- Drugs that impair the inotropic state of the myocardium have more effect in the failing than in the normal heart. The failing heart also has a greater potential for self-perpetuating myocardial depression in the presence of poor coronary perfusion.

Right ventricular failure (RVF)

RVF is associated with enlargement of the liver, peripheral oedema and pleural effusion.

Aetiology

- Right ventricular infarction.
- Pulmonary valvular stenosis.
- Pulmonary hypertension.

Pathophysiology

- Acute RVF may be precipitated by hypoxia and/or hypercapnia. Short episodes of hypoxia associated with difficult intubation, or inadequate ventilation during recovery from anaesthesia can precipitate acute pulmonary arteriolar constriction.
- As the pericardium is relatively non-compliant, acute right ventricular dilatation caused by pulmonary hypertension may precipitate leftward shift of the interventricular septum, so that failure of left ventricular filling complicates the impairment of right ventricular ejection.
- In patients with severe pulmonary hypertension and right ventricular hypertrophy (cor pulmonale), RVF may be acutely disturbed if systemic arterial pressure decreases, causing reduced coronary perfusion pressure to the right ventricle, leading to worsening ischaemia.
- When RVF is associated with a ventricular septal defect (VSD) and pulmonary hypertension, it is important to avoid an anaesthetic technique that causes systemic arteriolar dilatation.
- A decrease in systemic vascular resistance relative to that in the pulmonary arteries will result in a reversal of the shunt through the VSD (Eisenmenger's syndrome), decreasing pulmonary blood flow, causing hypoxia and acutely precipitating RVF.

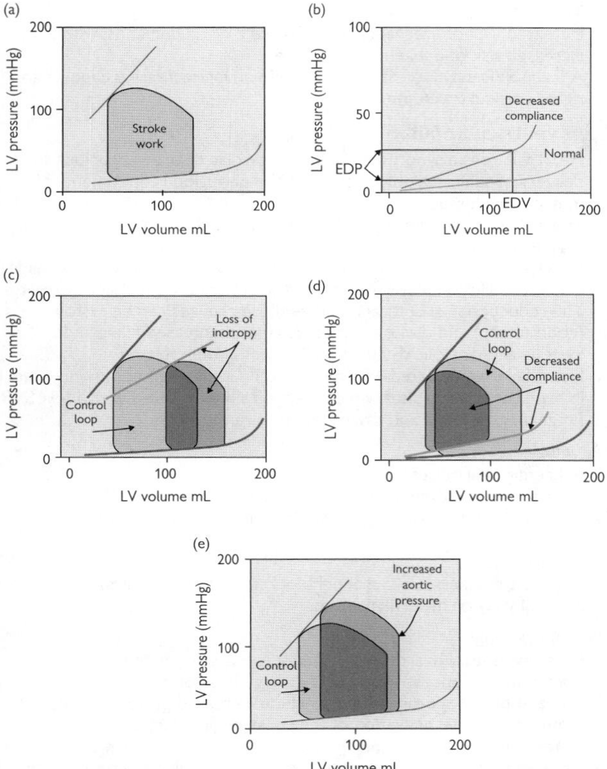

Fig. 4.1 The dynamic pressure and volume relationships in normal and dysfunctional ventricles. (a) SW ≈ SV × MAP. The normal end-diastolic pressure volume relationship (EDPVR) lower curve and end-systolic pressure volume relationship (ESPVR) upper curve. (b) The position of the end-diastolic pressure (EDP) on the EDPVR as compliance decreases, i.e. an upward/leftward shift in the EDPV curve.(c) A downward shift towards the right of the ESPV curve, i.e. a –ve effect of poor contractility on the ESPVR (ventricular systolic dysfunction). (d) Diastolic dysfunction. Pathological conditions such as ischaemic heart disease and ventricular hypertrophy shift the EDPVR up to the left. (e) The effect of increasing afterload on the ventricular EDPVR and ESPVR.

Reproduced with permission from Lippincott Williams & Wilkins. *Cardiovascular Physiology Concepts*, Klabunde RE. 2005.

Interaction with pregnancy

- Increased CO of pregnancy will increase oxygen demands, with an increased risk of ischaemia and failure.
- A fall in SVR may increase a left to right shunt, increasing hypoxia and right ventricular volume load.

Left ventricular failure (LVF)

- Heart failure is a syndrome in which a cardiac disorder prohibits the delivery of sufficient output to meet the perfusion requirements of metabolizing tissues.
- The inability of a failing heart to produce an adequate CO may occur despite a normal filling pressure.
- It is characterized by numerous multisystem adaptive changes, and inadequacy in perfusion may be associated with both low and high CO states.
- The reduction in CO that underlies these changes can be systolic (contractility) and diastolic (in compliance, decreased filling and SV). Systolic and diastolic dysfunctions are commonly related.
- Heart failure associated with an elevated CO is most commonly seen in hypermetabolic states, which are typically associated with a low SVR. Pregnancy, anaemia and thyrotoxicosis are examples.

Aetiology

- Ischaemic heart disease.
- Peripartum cardiomyopathy.
- Non-peripartum cardiomyopathy (idiopathic, alcohol, myocarditis, familial).
- Hypertension.
- Drugs (β-blockers, Ca^{2+} channel blockers, antiarrhythmics).
- Sepsis, hypo- or hyperthyroidism.

Pathophysiology

- In compensatory heart failure, arteriovenous oxygen difference is normal at rest but rapidly widens during stress or exercise. The compensatory mechanisms include increased preload, increased sympathetic tone, activation of the renin–angiotensin–aldosterone system, release of AVP and ventricular hypertrophy (Fig. 4.2).
- Increased preload serves to maximize SV by moving the heart up the Starling curve. Even when the ejection fraction is reduced, an increase in ventricular end-diastolic volume can maintain a normal SV.
- However, worsening venous congestion and excessive ventricular dilatation cause a fall in CO due to downward shift of the ventricular function curve.
- LVF results in pulmonary vascular congestion and progressive transudation of fluids into the pulmonary interstitium and alveoli (pulmonary oedema).
- Increased sympathetic tone can initially maintain CO by increasing heart rate and contractility. However, increased afterload due to vasoconstriction reduces the CO and exacerbates the ventricular failure.
- The renin–angiotensin–aldosterone system causes further increase in peripheral vascular resistance and left ventricular afterload, as well as sodium and water retention (Fig. 4.3).

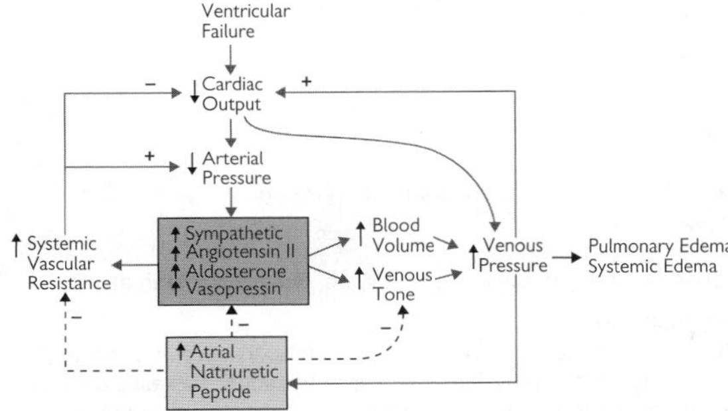

Fig 4.2 Summary of the compensatory mechanisms.

Reproduced with permission from Lippincott & Wilkin. Cardiovascular Physiology Concepts. Klabunde RE 2005.

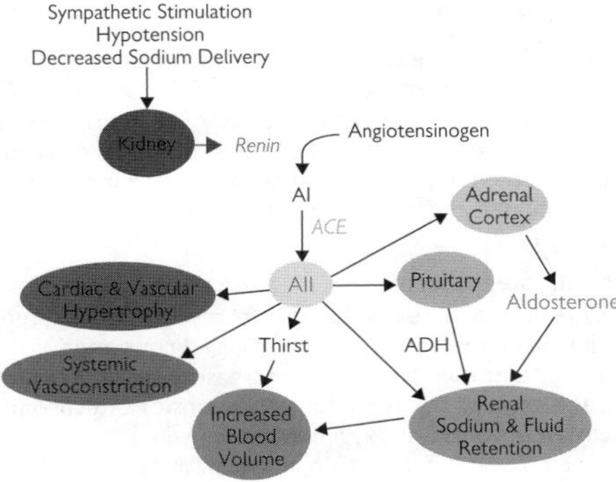

Fig. 4.3 The renin–angiotensin system.

Reproduced with permission from Lippincott & Wilkin. Cardiovascular Physiology Concepts. Klabunde RE 2005.

- Volume overload maintains normal resting SV but the pressure-overloaded ventricle results in progressive diastolic dysfunction.

Interaction with pregnancy

- Pregnancy is associated with increased CO and oxygen consumption, increasing the risk of decompensated LVF.
- The physiological reduction in afterload will counteract this effect to a degree.
- Acute LVF caused by peripartum cardiomyopathy rapidly leads to decompensation with pulmonary oedema.

Ischaemic heart disease (see Chapter 22, p 640)

Aetiology

- Atherosclerosis.
- Anaemia.
- Severe hypotension.
- Cocaine abuse.
- Tachycardia (in association with left ventricular hypertrophy).
- Hypoxaemia.
- Severe hypertension.
- Coronary artery vasospasm, aneurysm, dissection, haematoma.

Pathophysiology

- Myocardial ischaemia is caused by a metabolic oxygen demand that exceeds oxygen supply. The myocardium cannot increase oxygen extraction to compensate for decreased coronary blood flow.
- Coronary blood flow changes in parallel with myocardial oxygen demand. The average resting coronary blood flow is 250mL/min; the myocardium autoregulates blood flow between perfusion pressures of 50 and 120mmHg. Beyond this range, it is pressure dependent.
- Normal coronary perfusion pressure (CPP) is given by the equation:

$$CPP = AoDP - LVEDP$$

- An increase in left ventricular end-diastolic pressure (LVEDP) or decrease in aortic diastolic pressure (AoDP) can reduce CPP.
- Increased heart rate also decreases coronary perfusion because significant tachycardia reduces the duration of the diastolic phase of the cardiac cycle—the period when coronary perfusion occurs.
- The endocardium is most vulnerable to ischaemia as a result of decreased CPP.

Interaction with pregnancy

- Pregnancy results in increased heart rate, myocardial wall tension and contractility, basal metabolic rate and oxygen consumption.
- Labour causes a further progressive increase in oxygen consumption.
- Pain causes increased maternal concentrations of catecholamines, which increase myocardial oxygen demand.
- Each uterine contraction results in an autotransfusion of 300–500mL of blood into the central circulation. Autotransfusion increases preload and may further stress the balance between oxygen supply and demand.
- Oxygen consumption peaks at delivery. Maternal expulsive efforts at delivery may result in a 150% increase in oxygen consumption.
- Even an elective CS can increase the CO by up to 50%. Oxygen consumption can be 25% higher in the postpartum period.

Balance between myocardial oxygen supply and demand during pregnancy.

Parameter	Effect of pregnancy
Supply	
Diastolic time	Decreased
CPP	Decreased
Arterial oxygen content	
Arterial oxygen tension	Increased
Haemoglobin concentration	Decreased
Coronary vessel diameter	Unchanged
Demand	
Basal oxygen requirement	Increased
Heart rate	Increased
Wall tension	
Preload (ventricular radius)	Increased
Afterload	Decreased
Contractility	Increased

Anaesthetic management

Labour

- Epidural anaesthesia is an excellent choice for labour analgesia and vaginal delivery, reducing oxygen requirements and afterload.
- A CSE with intrathecal opioids can establish rapid analgesia without haemodynamic compromise.
- Fluid balance must be meticulously maintained.
- Adequate preload is important avoiding aorto-caval compression and treating haemorrhage early.
- Breathlessness and low oxygen saturation may be an early sign of pulmonary oedema and must be adequately monitored.

Caesarean section

- CSE may be used with a small initial intrathecal dose to establish a good sacral block, with subsequent careful topping up via the epidural.
- Single dose spinal anaesthesia should be avoided because of rapid haemodynamic changes commonly seen.
- GA, if required, should be supplemented with a short-acting opioid (e.g. fentanyl or alfentanil) to obtund the pressor response during induction, laryngoscopy and intubation. Aim to maintain normal HR and BP during delivery.

Postdelivery

- Major fluid shifts and uterine autofusion increase the risk of postdelivery ischaemia and fluid overload.
- The reduction in sympathetic block as regional anaethesia regresses can worsen this effect.
- The mother must be monitored for at least 24h in a high dependency area with BP, heart rate, urine output, oxygen saturation and respiratory rate.

Cardiac shunts

Cardiac shunts may be described as left to right, right to left or bidirectional; or as systemic to pulmonary or pulmonary to systemic. The direction may be controlled by left heart and/or right heart pressures, by a biological or artificial valve, or both. The presence of a shunt can affect left and or right heart pressure either beneficially or detrimentally.

They can also be classified into two groups

- Congenital.
- Acquired.
  - Biological.
  - Mechanical.
- The most common congenital heart defects (CHDs), which cause shunting are atrial septal defect (ASD), VSD, patent ductus arteriosus (PDA) and patent foramen ovale (PFO).
- In isolation, these defects may be asymptomatic or may produce symptoms which can be mild to severe.
- Shunts are often present in combination with other defects, which can also be asymptomatic, mild to severe.
- Some acquired shunts are modifications of congenital ones: a balloon septostomy can enlarge a foramen ovale, PFO or ASD.
- Mechanical shunts are used in some cases of CHD to control blood flow or BP. One example is the modern version of the Blalock–Tausig shunt. These women may be asymptomatic and may have relatively normal intracardiac pressures and blood flow pattern.
- Antibiotic prophylaxis may be recommended.
- The presence of a paediatrician at delivery is warranted because of the high incidence of congenital cardiac lesions in the offspring of these women.

Left to right shunts

A left to right shunt is a cardiac shunt, which allows, or is designed to cause, blood to flow from the left to the right heart.

- This occurs when:
  - There is an opening or passage between the atria, ventricle and/or great vessels, and the pressure in the left heart is higher than in the right heart.
  - Or the shunt has a one-way valvular opening.

Aetiology

- ASD.
- VSD.
- PDA.
- Aortic coarctation is frequently associated with atrial and ventricular septal defects.

Pathophysiology

- Pulmonary blood flow is increased; the magnitude of this increase is dependent upon both the size of the defect and the pressure on either side. It also depends upon the impedance of systemic and pulmonary circulations, which are the systemic and pulmonary vascular resistance (SVR and PVR) respectively.

- Drugs that increase SVR or decrease PVR will increase the shunt.
- If flow is high enough over a period of time, right ventricular hypertrophy occurs and reversal of the shunt takes place (Eisenmenger syndrome).

Atrial septal defect (ASD)

Atrial septal defects account for ~10% of congenital heart disease. There are four types of ASD:

- Ostium secundum defects (70–80%).
- Ostium primum defects (20%).
- Sinus venosus defects (10%).
- Coronary sinus defects (<1%).

Pathophysiology

- Left to right shunt—the size of which depends upon the ventricular compliance and the size of the defect.
- The shunt results in right ventricular (RV) diastolic overload and increased pulmonary blood flow.
- The left to right shunt worsens after the first few weeks of life, due to the fall in PVR and increase in SVR.
- Chronic volume overload eventually results in increased left atrial, right atrial and RV sizes, atrial arrhythmias and RV dysfunction. Rarely, it may cause congestive cardiac failure.
- An age-related reduction in LV compliance augments the left to right shunt and is one of the causes of the progression of symptoms with age. In addition, modest pulmonary arterial hypertension increases with age, so the RV is exposed to pressure as well as volume overload, and may eventually fail.
- LV dysfunction due to coronary artery disease and systemic hypertension may increase the left to right interatrial shunt, resulting in a more rapid clinical deterioration than would be expected.
- Eventually ~10% of ASDs develop a right to left shunt secondary to pulmonary vascular disease.

Interaction with pregnancy

- An ASD is usually well tolerated in pregnancy; the major risk is of paradoxical embolism causing embolic stroke.
- Increased shunting in pregnancy is counterbalanced by the decreased SVR. However, patients with ostium primum ASD associated with cleft mitral or tricuspid valves with insufficiency are at increased risk of left or RVF.
- Haemorrhage may cause a significant increase in left to right shunting by reducing systemic venous return and increasing SVR.
- Women older than 30 years are at higher risk of developing atrial arrhythmias and right ventricular dysfunction as a result of the increased blood volume of pregnancy.
- Any degree of pulmonary hypertension may worsen due to an increase in CO and associated shunt.

Ventricular septal defect (VSD)

With the exceptions of bicuspid aortic valve and mitral valve prolapse, VSD is the most common congenital cardiac malformation, occurring in ~3 per 1000 liveborn babies. Defects may exist in isolation, in association with other lesions such as coarctation of the aorta, or as an integral part of lesions such as tetralogy of Fallot.

Pathophysiology

- Depends upon the size of the VSD and PVR. 50–70% of small defects close spontaneously.
- A large VSD permits a large left to right shunt if there is no pulmonary stenosis or increased PVR. Large defects allow the ventricle to function as a single chamber with two outlets.
- Resistance to LV emptying will increase the size of any left to right shunt.
- There is a high risk of endocarditis in small VSDs due to the high velocity jet from the left to right ventricle, particularly if the jet is directed on to the tricuspid valve.
- The adult with an isolated uncorrected restrictive VSD is acyanotic with normal arterial and jugular venous pulses.

Interaction with pregnancy

- In small to moderate sized defects, pregnancy is usually tolerated well but there is a risk of developing infectious endocarditis and heart failure.
- Any degree of pulmonary hypertension may worsen due to an increase in CO and associated shunt.
- Pulmonary hypertension may worsen in subsequent pregnancies, so every pregnancy must be monitored, even if previously asymptomatic.
- With larger defects, there is a risk of developing Eisenmenger syndrome (reverse shunt), ventricular arrhythmias and aortic insufficiency.

Patent ductus arteriosus (PDA)

The ductus venosus is a vessel leading from the bifurcation of the pulmonary artery to the aorta distal to the left subclavian artery. Normally, this vascular channel is open in the fetus but closes immediately after birth.

Pathophysiology

- Consequences of a patent arterial duct in adulthood depend on the size of the shunt and the pressure relationship between the pulmonary and systemic circulation.
- Small ducts are of no haemodynamic significance and are associated with a low risk of infective endocarditis.
- Moderate sized ducts may cause left heart volume overload. The size of the shunt is proportional to the size of the PDA, and left ventricular hypertrophy compensates. This may lead to late atrial fibrillation and ventricular dysfunction.
- A large non-restrictive duct may cause pulmonary vascular disease (see Eisenmengee syndrome, p 84–5). If a duct is clinically detectable, i.e. there is a machinery murmur in the left subclavicular area, then closure is usually recommended to avoid long-term haemodynamic complications.
- Severe pulmonary vascular disease results in reversal of flow through the ductus, deoxygenated blood is shunted to the descending aorta, and toes (but not fingers) become cyanosed and clubbed, leading to differential cyanosis.

Interaction with pregnancy

- In small to moderate sized defects, pregnancy is usually tolerated well.
- Any degree of pulmonary hypertension may worsen due to an increase in CO and associated shunt.

Anaesthetic management

General principles

- If there is no RVF, there are few problems.
- Women with small defects can be treated as normal except for antibiotic prophylaxis.
- IV equipment should have filters as there is a risk of paradoxical embolus.
- It is important to avoid hypercarbia and acidosis which may increase PVR.
- Avoid tachycardia and increases in SVR that result in increased left to right shunt.
- Antibiotic prophylaxis is usually required.

Labour analgesia

- For large or symptomatic defects, early administration of epidural anaesthesia is indicated, as effective analgesia will reduce sympathetic stimulation and a rise in SVR.
- A slow onset of epidural anaesthesia is preferred. A rapid decrease in SVR could result in a reversal of shunt flow, and an asymptomatic left to right shunt may become a right to left shunt with maternal hypoxaemia.
- Patients with a large defect should receive supplemental oxygen, and haemoglobin oxygen saturation should be monitored during labour. Even mild hypoxaemia can result in increased PVR and reversal of shunt flow.

Caesarean section: regional

- Women with small asymptomatic shunts can be treated as normal.
- A low dose incremental CSE is a good choice to provide a dense sacral block with a gradual onset of sympathetic block.

Caesarean section: general

- Rapid uptake of anaesthetic gases due to increased pulmonary blood flow leads to slow onset of GA.
- A fall in SVR, caused by volatile agents, reduces the shunt.

Right to left shunt (see Chapter 22, p 606)

A right to left shunt is a cardiac shunt which allows, or is designed to cause, blood to flow from the right heart to the left heart. This occurs when:

- There is an opening or passage between the atria, ventricles and/or great vessels.
- Right heart pressure is higher than left heart pressure, and/or the shunt has a one-way valvular opening.

Aetiology

Right to left shunts can be broadly classified as:

- Increased pulmonary blood flow.
  - Truncus arteriosus.
  - Single ventricle.
  - Transposition of great arteries.
  - Total anomalous pulmonary venous drainage.
  - Hypoplastic left ventricle.
- Decreased pulmonary blood flow.
  - Tetralogy of Fallot.
  - Pulmonary atresia.
  - Ebstein anomaly.
  - Hypoplastic right ventricle.
  - Truncus arteriosus.
- The most common of these abnormalities are tetralogy of Fallot, tricuspid atresia, pulmonary atresia, transposition of great arteries with large ASD, and Ebstein's anomaly.
- Patients with these congenital abnormalities are strongly advised against pregnancy. However, if pregnancy does occur, specialist care and further counselling from an experienced cardiologist is essential.
- Termination of pregnancy may be advised, although this also carries significant risks.

Eisenmenger syndrome (see Chapter 22, p 612)

Pathophysiology

A chronic, uncorrected, left to right shunt may produce right ventricular hypertrophy, elevated pulmonary artery pressures, right ventricular dysfunction and ultimately, as right- exceeds left-sided pressures, the syndrome first described by Eisenmenger in 1897.

- The primary lesion may be an atrial or ventricular septal defect or an aorto-pulmonary communication, such as PDA or truncus arteriosus.
- The pulmonary and RV musculatures undergo remodelling in response to chronic pulmonary volume overload. High, fixed pulmonary arterial pressure gradually limits flow through the pulmonary vessels.
- A reversal of shunt flow occurs when pulmonary arterial pressure exceeds the level of systemic pressure. The primary left to right shunt becomes a right to left shunt.
- Initially, the shunt may be bidirectional; acute changes in the PVR or SVR may influence the primary direction of blood flow. However, pulmonary vessel occlusive disease ultimately leads to irreversible pulmonary hypertension. Therefore, the correction of the primary intracardiac lesion is not helpful.

Interaction with pregnancy

- These women are often unable to respond to increased demands for oxygen during pregnancy.
- Maintenance of satisfactory oxygenation requires adequate pulmonary blood flow. The decrease in PVR seen in normal pregnancy does not occur because the PVR is fixed.
- The decrease in SVR in pregnancy tends to exacerbate the severity of right to left shunt.

- The pregnancy-associated decrease in functional residual capacity of the lung also predisposes to maternal hypoxaemia.
- There is an increased risk of thromboembolic episodes leading to increased maternal mortality.

Anaesthetic implications

General principles

- A multidisciplinary approach with close communication between obstetrician, cardiologist and anaesthetist is required early.
- A senior anaesthetist should be involved at an early stage in delivering any form of anaesthesia.
- Operative delivery is frequently required because of maternal decompensation in the third trimester.
- SVR must be maintained.
- Aorto-caval compression must be avoided, optimizing intravacular volume and VR.
- Blood loss must be treated promptly.
- Prevent pain, hypoxia, hypercarbia and acidosis, which may increase PVR, thereby increasing the shunt and causing further maternal hypoxaemia.
- Supplemental oxygen must be provided at all times during labour, CS and postdelivery.
- Pulse oximetry is very useful in detecting early acute changes in shunt flow.

Labour

- Epidural for pain relief to prevent sympathetic stimulation can be considered if not contraindicated due to anticoagulation.
- There should be a very slow induction of epidural anaesthesia minimizing any fall in SVR.

Caesarean section

- GA can be very challenging. Rapid sequence induction causes decreased CO and reduced SVR, which increases the right to left shunt flow and should be avoided under all circumstances.
- Avoid myocardial depression during a GA.
- Slow controlled induction of GA, whilst being associated with an increased risk of aspiration, is the preferred option. Intermittent positive pressure ventilation (IPPV) results in reduced VR, causing reduced CO.
- Regional anaesthesia has been described, but the fall in SVR-associated extensive regional anaesthesia will increase the shunt.
- Very low dose CSE or small incremental epidural technique should be used.
- Phenylephrine infusion should be used to control the SVR.

Further reading

Uebing A *et al.* Pregnancy and congenital heart disease. *British Medical Journal* 2006; **332**: 401–406.

Stenotic cardiac lesions

Mitral stenosis

Aetiology

Chronic rheumatic heart disease is the most common aetiology of mitral stenosis, which causes limited blood flow across the mitral valve to a variable extent.

Incidence

It is more common, and presents earlier, in the Middle East, the Indian subcontinent and the Far East than in the West, and is twice as common in females as in males.

Pathophysiology

- The cross-sectional area of a normal mitral valve is 4–5cm^2. When mitral valve area falls to ~2.5cm^2, peak early diastolic ventricular filling rate falls and diastasis is lost.
- The main disturbance in mitral stenosis is of LV filling. This has little impact when the heart rate is slow and the filling period relatively long, but during exercise as the heart rate increases, flow is maintained only by a pressure drop between atrium and ventricle.
- As stenosis increases, a pressure drop is present at rest and mean left atrial pressure (LAP) rises. Patients with symptomatic mitral stenosis have a valve area of 0.75–1.25cm^2, and a pressure drop as high as 20–30mmHg across the valve during diastole.
- CO falls and PVR usually increases.
- The subvalvular apparatus may interfere with LV filling by restricting wall movement, so reducing stroke volume and increasing LAP in the absence of any diastolic pressure drop across the valve itself.
- LV cavity size is usually normal in young patients, but increases with age, and end-diastolic pressure may rise.
- A number of factors contribute to left ventricular disease, including restriction of filling, coronary emboli, and distortion of the septum by right ventricular hypertrophy and overload.

Classification

According to the valve orifice assessed by echocardiography.

- Mild >2cm^2.
- Moderate 1–2cm^2.
- Severe <1cm^2.

Interaction with pregnancy

- Mitral stenosis limits the patient's ability to increase CO during pregnancy and can be poorly tolerated if the woman is symptomatic prior to pregnancy.
- Women who are asymptomatic tolerate pregnancy well.
- The increased heart rate of pregnancy limits the time for the filling of the left ventricle and results in increased left atrial and pulmonary arterial pressures, leading to increased likelihood of pulmonary oedema.

- Atrial fibrillation (AF) leads to increased risk of maternal morbidity and mortality in mitral stenosis. Both the loss of atrial systole and increased ventricular rate result in decreased CO and increased risk of pulmonary oedema.
- There is an increased risk of systemic embolization.
- Women with previous pulmonary congestion have an increased risk of mortality during and after pregnancy.
- The risk of maternal death is greatest during labour and the postpartum period. The sudden increase in preload after delivery may cause severe pulmonary oedema.
- Hypovolaemia and sudden decrease in venous return (VR) secondary to haemorrhage or supine position are poorly tolerated and should be avoided.

Anaesthetic implications

General principles

- Antibiotic prophylaxis is essential.
- Anticoagulants should be discussed with the obstetricians and cardiologist.
- Perioperative complications include:
    - Acute pulmonary oedema.
    - RVF.
    - AF.
    - Systemic embolization.
    - Subacute bacterial endocarditis.
    - Pneumonia.

The main areas for consideration are HR, rhythm and preload:

- Tachycardia decreases ventricular filling time and thus CO. It also increases LAP, causing pulmonary oedema.
- Bradycardia tends to causes a decrease in CO due to fixed SV. AF, which may be induced by anaesthesia, will further decrease the ventricular filling by ~30%.
- Preload: hypovolaemia may result in reduced LAP and reduction in left ventricular filling. Excessive fluid, on the other hand, will cause pulmonary oedema.
- Afterload: a large decrease in SVR may cause severe hypotension as a result of a relatively fixed CO.
- Patients with mitral stenosis have decreased lung compliance, increased airway resistance, an elevated alveolar–arterial oxygen (A-a O_2) gradient and an increased work of breathing. Give supplemental oxygen during labour and delivery.
- Invasive BP monitoring during delivery is essential in mothers with moderate to severe mitral stenosis.
- Regardless of the method of delivery or anaesthetic technique, the patient is at risk of developing pulmonary oedema during the post-partum period. These patients require high dependency care during the immediate postpartum period.

Labour

- It is important to provide adequate analgesia with the onset of painful contractions. Give epidural analgesia during active labour and maintain it during the immediate postpartum period to reduce preload and prevent pulmonary oedema.

Caesarean section: regional

- Regional technique is preferred for CS. Epidural has traditionally been the preferred method because it is easier to maintain haemodynamic stability with a slow induction of anaesthesia.
- Good haemodynamic stability can be achieved with a low dose incremental CSE.

Caesarean section: general

- If GA is required, avoid drugs that produce tachycardia (e.g. atropine, ketamine). A β-adrenergic receptor blocker and a modest dose of opioid should be administered before or during the induction of anaesthesia.
- Small doses of phenylephrine ensure haemodynamic stability.

Aortic stenosis (see Chapter 22, p 591)

Aortic stenosis (AS) represents a fixed obstruction to LV ejection into the aorta. The obstruction is most commonly at the level of the valve itself—aortic valvar stenosis, but may also be immediately above the sinuses—supravalvar stenosis, or within the left ventricle—subvalvar stenosis.

Aetiology

- Congenital AS, due to a valve with a single commissure, most frequently presents in infancy or childhood. A congenital bicuspid valve, consisting of fusion of one of the three commissures, is a much more common abnormality.
- Rheumatic AS develops as the result of commissural fusion in a tricuspid valve and may subsequently become calcified.
- Very rarely, vegetations in infective endocarditis cause significant LV outflow tract obstruction.

Structural and functional changes

- The normal aortic valve area (AVA) is 2.6–3.5cm^2 in adults. Haemodynamically significant obstruction occurs as the AVA approaches 1.0cm^2.
- Blood flow across a stenotic aortic valve causes a pressure drop between the LV cavity and the aorta, which in symptomatic cases may be >60mmHg at rest, and reach >200mmHg on exertion.
- Stroke work is increased and LV hypertrophy develops. Wall thickness increases, although cavity size remains normal or even falls (concentric hypertrophy).
- Initially, hypertrophy allows generation of the high interventricular pressures required to maintain CO through the stenosis, without dysfunction (compensated AS).

Classification

- Grade 1 AVA—1.2–1.8cm^2 and mean gradient 12–25mmHg.
- Grade 2 AVA—0.8–1.2cm^2 and mean gradient 25–40mmHg.
- Grade 3 AVA—0.6–0.8cm^2 and mean gradient 40–50mmHg.
- Grade 4 AVA—<0.6cm^2 and mean gradient >50mmHg.

It should be remembered that classification of AS by gradient rather than area will underestimate disease severity once the LV starts to fail.

Interaction with pregnancy

- Women with severe aortic disease should undergo corrective surgery before pregnancy.
- Symptoms early in pregnancy may warrant termination, although valvotomy has been described.
- The increased blood volume of pregnancy allows women with mild AS to tolerate pregnancy well, although they are at risk of developing infective endocarditis after delivery.
- AS is well tolerated if the following conditions apply:
  - Peak gradient <80 and mean <50mmHg before pregnancy.
  - Normal LV function.
  - Absence of symptoms.
- The increased CO associated with pregnancy will increase the apparent gradient across the value. The severity and progression of AS in pregnancy should be determined by AVA.
- Women with severe AS have a limited ability to compensate for the cardiovascular demands of pregnancy. These patients develop angina, dyspnoea or syncope.
- As AS becomes more severe, dilation of the aortic root immediately distal to the aortic valve may result. This may be associated with pregnancy and should be monitored regularly.
- The lesion may develop after pregnancy when infective endocarditis causes persistent fever or results in the sudden appearance of aortic insufficiency.

Anaesthetic implications

General principles

- The physiological objective is to maintain the basic haemodynamic state by carefully managing heart rate, filling pressure and systemic BP.
- Tachycardia: reduces CO by increasing the dynamic impedance of stenosis. It also causes myocardial ischaemia (sometimes LVF).
  - Treat the cause (light anaesthesia, hypovolaemia, etc.).
  - DO NOT GIVE β-adrenoceptor blockers.
- Bradycardia: moderate degrees are tolerated. It reduces the dynamic impedance of stenosis. If severe, use tiny doses of glycopyrrolate and avoid overcorrection.
- Preload: must be maintained to ensure adequate filling of the hypertrophied ventricle. CVP or pulmonary capillary wedge pressure (PCWP) should be maintained at high normal levels.
- Afterload: effect of systemic pressure significantly changes coronary perfusion.

Labour

- Careful titration of a low dose epidural is beneficial, reducing maternal tachycardia and avoiding excessive straining in the second stage of labour by facilitating instrumental delivery.
- Any mother with symptomatic, moderate or severe AS should have an arterial line and very close attention to preload, avoiding aorto-caval compression, dehydration and haemorrhage.

Caesarean section: regional

- Moderate to severe aortic stenosis is a contraindication to single-shot spinal anaesthesia for CS.
- Slow induction with an epidural allows titration of appropriate IV infusions and allows the patient to develop compensatory vasoconstriction above the block.
- A low dose CSE with small incremental epidural top-ups gives good haemodynamic stability and a more predictable block.
- Invasive BP monitoring is essential when managing the mother with moderate to severe AS, and a CVP or long line is useful.
- BP should be controlled with a phenylephrine infusion.

Caesarean: general

- Thiopental may result in unwanted myocardial depression and so should be avoided. Etomidate and a modest dose of opioid is the preferred choice for induction of anaesthesia.

Pulmonary stenosis

- This is generally well tolerated, although in severe cases it may precipitate right heart failure, tricuspid regurgitation or atrial arrhythmias.
- Although women with severe disease may be asymptomatic, the increased haemodynamic load of pregnancy may precipitate heart failure.
- Women with a prepregnancy peak catheter gradient of >50mmHg should be considered for balloon valvuloplasty or surgery preconception.
- Even during pregnancy, balloon valvuloplasty may be feasible if symptoms of pulmonary stenosis progress.
- Anaesthetic management of delivery follows the same principles as that for other stenotic valve lesions.

Tricuspid stenosis

- Although functional tricuspid stenosis may occur with a large flow through the right heart such as occurs in an ASD, organic tricuspid stenosis is nearly always the result of chronic rheumatic heart disease.
- Rheumatic tricuspid stenosis nearly always co-exists with rheumatic mitral valve disease, although its incidence is about 1/10. The two conditions are similar, with respect to both their pathology and the functional disturbance that they cause.

- The primary functional abnormality is obstruction to RV filling associated with a diastolic pressure drop across the valve. In clinically severe tricuspid stenosis, however, this drop is smaller than it would be with clinically severe mitral stenosis, and is usually within the range of 3–10mmHg.
- This causes a corresponding increase in right atrial pressure, which leads to ascites and peripheral oedema.

Anaesthetic implications

- Considerations are similar to those for mitral stenosis.
- Fluid overload in right-sided stenotic lesions does not lead to early pulmonary oedema.

Regurgitant cardiac lesions

Mitral regurgitation (MR)

Aetiology

- There are many causes of MR. Any of the components of the mitral valve apparatus may be involved.
- Infective endocarditis is a major cause of mitral regurgitation.
- Systemic lupus erythematosus (SLE) can affect both mitral and aortic valves, causing thickening of the cusps and the appearance of sterile vegetations (Libman–Sachs endocarditis). They rarely give rise to significant haemodynamic disturbance, but may predispose to emboli and to infective endocarditis.

Pathophysiology

- MR results in volume overload of the LV at the end of diastole, i.e. increased preload as well as a reduction in afterload due to the regurgitation of blood into the left atrium.
- Pure MR increases LV output. Since the pressure in the left atrium is lower than that in the aorta, the net force opposing LV ejection is reduced, and SV may be up to 3 times normal.
- Ejection begins almost immediately after the start of LV contraction and, by the time the aortic valve opens, up to a quarter of the SV may already have entered the left atrium. CO is therefore decreased despite increased SV.
- Left atrial pressures are increased, with the V or systolic wave sometimes reaching 50–60mmHg. These high pressures shorten the phase of isovolumetric relaxation and greatly increase the velocity of early diastolic LV filling, thus causing the third heart sound.
- Resting LV output is maintained by a sinus tachycardia that is always present when MR is severe.
- Chronic decompensated MR results when systolic dysfunction prevents effective ventricular contraction.
- Untreated decompensated MR rapidly progresses to pulmonary oedema and congestive cardiac failure.

Interaction with pregnancy

- MR is typically well tolerated in pregnancy. Pregnant women with rheumatic MR tolerate the increased blood volume and heart rate if the rhythm is sinus. The physiological offloading of the LV due to systemic vasodilation is beneficial.
- There is an increased risk of AF during pregnancy which may cause acute decompensation.
- The hypercoagulability of pregnancy increases the risk of systemic embolization.
- A raised SVR is poorly tolerated by parturients with regurgitant valvular lesions. During labour, an increase in SVR is caused by labour pain, expulsive efforts (Valsalva manoeuvre) and aortic compression by the uterus.

Anaesthetic management

General principles

- These women are at increased risk of infective endocarditis, and antibiotic prophylaxis is indicated.
- The aim of management is as follows:
  - Prevent an increase in SVR (pain).
  - Maintain a heart rate that is normal or slightly increased.
  - Maintain sinus rhythm and treat acute AF aggressively. Haemodynamic instability should be treated with prompt cardioversion.
  - Avoid aorto-caval compression and maintain VR, but prevent an increase in central venous volume.
- In contrast to patients with mitral stenosis, patients with MR may benefit from the chronotropic effects of ephedrine if a vasopressor is required.

Labour

- Low dose epidural analgesia is preferred. Epidural anaesthesia prevents the increase in SVR that is associated with pain. It also decreases SVR, which assists the forward flow of blood and helps prevent pulmonary congestion.
- Careful administration of crystalloid and left uterine tilt are necessary to maintain VR and LV filling as an epidural may cause decreased VR.

Caesarean section: regional

- Regional technique is preferred for CS. Epidural has traditionally been the preferred method because it is easier to maintain haemodynamic stability with a slow induction of anaesthesia.
- Good haemodynamic stability can be achieved with a low dose incremental CSE.

Caesarean section: general

- A careful IV induction of thiopental with opioids should be administered to minimize myocardial depression and maintain heart rate and SVR.

Mitral valve prolapse (MVP)

- The MVP syndrome is also called floppy valve syndrome, the systolic click–murmur syndrome and Barlow's syndrome. Myxomatous degeneration of the mitral valve affects the cusps, chordae tendinae and the annulus, and may cause the valve to bellow into the left atrium during systole. Involvement of the chordae tendinae can lead to chordal rupture and subsequent MR.
- MVP is also associated with many medical conditions including von Willebrand's disease, Ehlers–Danlos syndrome, kyphoscoliosis, pectus excavatum, osteogenesis imperfecta, myotonic dystrophy and Marfan's syndrome, all of which can have implications in pregnancy. See Chapter 22 for further details.

Aortic regurgitation (AR)

AR increases SV and, when severe and uncorrected, causes irreversible LV disease.

Aetiology

- Pathology of any components of the aortic valve can lead to AR. These include reduction in leaflet mobility, shortening of free leaflet edges, perforation of leaflets and annular dilatation.
- Chronic rheumatic involvement leads to an aortic valve whose cusps are thickened, with rolled edges and fused commissures. There may be superimposed calcification or thrombosis.
- Infective endocarditis may lead to cusp destruction or perforation.
- Marfan's syndrome, syphilitic aortitis, ankylosing spondylitis, rheumatoid arthritis, Reiter's syndrome or relapsing polychondritis all cause dilatation of the aortic ring, which can lead to AR. These conditions are associated with other problems in pregnancy (see Chapter 22).
- Dissecting aneurysm involving the aortic root may separate the cusps from the valve ring; and the presence of a high ventricular septal defect or Fallot tetralogy may leave the cusps unsupported from below.

Pathophysiology

- AR is associated with an increase in LV stroke volume. Volume overload results in eccentric hypertrophy and ventricular dilatation.
- Due to the increased volume of blood ejected, there is pressure overload as well. This results in concentric hypertrophy.
- Ventricular mass is therefore increased, but wall thickness is usually within normal limits.
- In moderately severe AR, the SV is twice normal and, in severe cases, up to 3 or even 4 times normal.
- The characteristics of ejection are altered in that the end-diastolic pressure in the aorta is low, so that the resistance to ejection of blood by the LV is reduced and ventricular systole is prolonged.
- These factors, together with the large SV, explain the characteristic rapid upstroke and large volume pulse. Peripheral vasodilatation also contributes to the large forward SV. All these are features of compensated AR.
- In long-standing cases, LV cavity size increases out of proportion to the SV, with loss of the normal myocardial architecture, so that the cavity becomes more spherical in shape; the walls become stiffer and the end-diastolic pressure increases.
- Eventually, LVEDP and left atrial pressures begin to increase. Pulmonary hypertension and congestive cardiac failure are features of decompensated AR.

Interaction with pregnancy

Aortic insufficiency is tolerated well during pregnancy for three reasons:

- Increase in maternal heart rate decreases the time for regurgitant blood flow during diastole.
- The fall in SVR favours the forward flow of blood and decreases the amount of regurgitant blood flow.
- Increased blood volume in pregnancy helps maintain adequate filling pressures.

Anaesthetic management

General principles

- The goals of anaesthetic management are as follows:
  - Maintain normal or slightly raised heart rate.
  - Bradycardia should be treated promptly.
  - Prevent any increase in SVR.
  - Avoid aortocaval compression.
  - Avoid myocardial depression during GA.
- Epidural or low dose CSE anaesthesia decreases the afterload and therefore the degree of regurgitant flow. It is preferable early in labour if a vaginal delivery is planned or for CS.
- The analgesic effects of an epidural during labour prevent undue sympathetic stimulation. This helps in reducing afterload and hence prevents LV fluid overload.

Tricuspid regurgitation

- Isolated tricuspid regurgitation is well tolerated in pregnancy.
- The degree of toleration when associated with other cardiac lesions depends on the pathological process involved.
- The tricuspid valve is much more liable to develop functional regurgitation than the mitral valve, often occurring in association with dilatation of the right ventricular cavity.
- It is particularly common in patients with pulmonary hypertensive mitral valve disease, but may also occur with primary pulmonary hypertension, or in the terminal stages of many types of congenital heart disease, particularly those with a significant left to right shunt.
- Severe, non-rheumatic tricuspid regurgitation is being increasingly recognized as occurring late after mitral valve replacement, in the absence of significant left-sided disease or pulmonary hypertension.
- Organic tricuspid regurgitation may be congenital, as an isolated abnormality or associated with the Ebstein anomaly.
- Acquired tricuspid regurgitation may be rheumatic in origin, or result from infective endocarditis of a previously normal valve, which occurs commonly in IV drug users.
- Mid-systolic prolapse of the tricuspid valve can occur in exactly the same way as that of the mitral valve, and is common in Marfan's syndrome.
- The anaesthetic management of the mother with tricuspid regurgitation is the same as for MR.

Further reading

Stout KK *et al.* Pregnancy in women with valvular heart disease. *Heart* 2007; **93**: 552–558.

Pulmonary hypertension (see Chapter 22, p 651)

Pulmonary circulation

- The pulmonary circulation is unique because of its high blood flow, low pressure (normally 25/8, mean 12mmHg) and low resistance (normally 200–250dynes/s/cm^5).
- It can accommodate large increases in blood flow with only modest increases in pressure because of its ability to recruit and distend lung blood vessels.
- The normal pulmonary circulation is largely passive, since its pressures are determined mainly by the function of the right and left ventricles.
- The precapillary arteries of the lungs are sensitive to falls in both alveolar and capillary oxygen partial pressure. At values of oxygen partial pressure <7.2kPa, their vascular smooth muscle cells contract, due to the activity of voltage-dependent potassium channels, ensuring a matching of the distribution of perfusion of the capillaries to ventilation of the alveoli.

Aetiology

- Primary pulmonary hypertension is a rare disease affecting young women of child-bearing age.
- Secondary pulmonary hypertension:
    - Cardiac diseases: left to right shunt (ASD, VSD, PDA), LVF, mitral valve disease.
    - Respiratory disease: chronic obstructive, chronic parenchymal.
    - Pulmonary thromboembolism.
    - Pulmonary vasculitides: SLE, rheumatoid.
    - Infection: HIV, schistosomiasis.
    - Hyperviscosity syndrome: myeloma.
    - Drugs: oral contraceptives, amphetamines, crotalaria teas.

Pathophysiology

- Pulmonary hypertension is present when pulmonary artery pressure rises to a level inappropriate for a given CO.
- The hallmark of pulmonary hypertension is increased PVR with increased work placed on the right side of the heart.
- Pulmonary hypertension is defined as a mean pulmonary artery pressure (MPAP) ≥25mmHg at rest or 30mmHg on exercise.
- Once present, pulmonary hypertension is self-perpetuating. It induces secondary structural abnormalities in the pulmonary vessels, including smooth muscle hypertrophy and intimal proliferation, and these may eventually stimulate atheromatous change and *in situ* thrombosis, leading to further narrowing of the arterial bed.
- Up to 60% of the pulmonary vascular bed can be obstructed before the symptoms of pulmonary hypertension develop.

- The progressive reduction in number and narrowing of the lumen of precapillary arteries initially cause a loss of capacity of the pulmonary circulation to accommodate the increased pulmonary blood flow of exercise. Whilst the resting pulmonary artery pressure may not be raised initially, with exercise the pressure rises rapidly.
- RVF, defined as an inability to sustain the required CO, contributes to the exercise intolerance, and the patient experiences breathlessness.
- With disease progression, the PVR increases and so too does the load on the right ventricle. CO subsequently falls and RVF ensues.
- With RVF at rest, the right atrial pressure rises and reduced VR results in the development of peripheral oedema and ascites.

Clinical features

- Unexplained breathlessness, with no obvious heart or lung disease.
- Symptoms of RVF including: syncope, angina-like chest pain and peripheral oedema.
- General malaise and cachexia of cardiac failure are end-stage symptoms.
- In 85 % of patients, a loud second heart sound is heard.
- The ECG shows RV strain and right bundle branch block (RBBB) pattern.
- Chest radiography shows large pulmonary arteries.
- The screening test is transthoracic echocardiography with Doppler estimation of the tricuspid valve regurgitant flow velocity, which estimates the systolic pulmonary artery pressure.
- Echocardiographic evidence of decompensated right heart failure including hypertrophic and dilated RV, tricuspid regurgitation and right to left septal shift can be seen.

World Health Organization classification of pulmonary hypertension

- Pulmonary artery hypertension.
- Pulmonary hypertension with left heart disease.
- Pulmonary hypertension associated with lung diseases and/or hypoxaemia.
- Pulmonary hypertension associated with thrombotic and/or embolic disease.
- Miscellaneous group.

Interaction with pregnancy

- Pulmonary hypertension is tolerated badly during pregnancy because of insufficient adaptation of the RV to increases in CO, together with a poorly compliant pulmonary vasculature.
- Pregnancy causes an increase in CO of 30–50%, an increase in blood volume of 40–50% and an increase in oxygen consumption of 20%. An impaired RV can be pushed into failure by these increased gestational demands, and by increases in CO and potential volume injections of up to 500mL with each uterine contraction in labour.
- Postpartum intravascular volume shifts resulting from haemorrhage or diuresis are poorly tolerated. The greatest risk occurs in the peripartum period, and most deaths occur between 2 and 9 days postpartum.
- Mortality remains at 30–50% and pregnancy is not recommended. Death results from irreversible RVF or arrhythmias.

Anaesthetic management

General principles

- The primary goals of anaesthetic management are similar to those for patients with Eisenmenger syndrome.
- Prevent pain, hypoxia, acidosis and hypercapnia, which are the predisposing factors for increase in PVR.
- Maintain intravascular volume and VR.
- Avoid aorto-caval compression.
- Maintain SVR as close to normal as possible. These patients are not able to increase CO with a decrease in SVR.
- Avoid myocardial depression during GA in women with fixed pulmonary hypertension.
- Provide supplemental oxygen throughout labour and delivery.
- Oxytocin can lower SVR and elevate PVR, resulting in a drop in CO. Care must be taken during administration.
- Pulmonary vascular dilators [e.g. epoprostenol (prostacyclin)] have been successfully used in pregnancy, but their use should be restricted to centres with experience in using these drugs.

Labour

- Low dose epidural anaesthesia can be considered, but slow induction is of prime importance. Hypotension should be actively managed.

Caearean section: regional

- A single-shot spinal is usually contraindicated; a low dose CSE may be an alternative where a subarachnoid block is desired. This will still avoid the rapid onset ↓ in SVR that follows single-shot spinal-induced sympathectomy.

Caesarean section: general

- GA causes an increase in pulmonary artery pressure during laryngoscopy and intubation. Opioids can help minimize these effects.
- Inhalation of nitric oxide (NO) might be considered as it causes pulmonary vasodilatation.
- Intensive postoperative management is important because there is an increased incidence of sudden death during this period.

Further reading

Weiss, BM *et al.* Pulmonary vascular disease and pregnancy: current controversies, management strategies, and perspectives. *European Heart Journal* 2000; **21**: 104–115.

Respiratory disease

General considerations

- Although minute ventilation does increase by 40% during pregnancy, this is trivial in comparison with the marked increase (perhaps 10-fold) that is possible during exercise.
- This considerable reserve of ventilatory capacity is not greatly challenged by pregnancy, and respiratory failure due to chronic respiratory disease is uncommon in pregnancy.
- The major problem for women with chronic conditions such as asthma or tuberculosis (TB) is the effect of therapy on pregnancy.
- Breathlessness is a common symptom in pregnancy, presumably associated with the 40% increase in ventilation that occurs in normal women. However, this cannot be the entire explanation because ventilation increases from before 4 weeks gestation, whereas the maximum incidence of onset of breathlessness is at 28–31 weeks gestation.
- Acute respiratory failure is a major cause of maternal mortality; adult respiratory distress syndrome (ARDS) carrying a mortality of ~70%. Indeed, much of the practice of modern obstetrics is directed towards the avoidance of ARDS. For example, the trend towards regional rather than GA reduces the risk of inhalation of stomach contents.
- Regional, rather than GA, is specifically indicated in all patients with significant respiratory disease.

Upper airway obstruction

- The upper airway includes the nose, mouth, pharynx, larynx and external thoracic trachea.
- Signs and symptoms of upper airway obstruction may present acutely (e.g. foreign body), insidiously (e.g. decline in conscious state) or progressively (e.g. laryngeal oedema).

Aetiology

Acute

- Infection (e.g. epiglottitis, tetanus, abscess, diphtheria).
- Trauma (e.g. maxillofacial injury, airway burns).
- Foreign body (e.g. food bolus).
- Loss of airway tone (e.g. residual muscle relaxation, myasthenia gravis, depressant drugs, decreased level of consciousness).
- Equipment related (e.g. occlusion of tracheal tube).
- Allergic reactions.
- Laryngospasm (e.g. postextubation, hypocalcaemia).

Chronic

- Tumour (e.g. pharynx, larynx).
- Scarring.

Acute on chronic conditions

- Infection.
- Haemorrhage.

- Trauma.
- Inflammation.

Any of the above may present acutely, insidiously or progressively.

Interaction with pregnancy

- Anatomical changes in pregnancy include capillary engorgement and mucosal oedema of the upper airway from the nasal passages down to the pharynx, false cords, glottis and arytenoids. The presence of pre-eclampsia may make the symptoms much worse.
- Increase in minute ventilation and airway oedema will make stridor worse.
- Increasing audible stridor must be differentiated from wheeze associated with asthma. If the diagnosis is in doubt, formal flow/volume loop respiratory function tests will help.

Anaesthetic implications

- Oedema of the airway makes upper airway obstruction and bleeding more likely during mask anaesthesia and may make tracheal intubation more difficult.
- A smaller diameter tracheal tube is recommended.
- The increase in chest diameter and enlarged breasts can make laryngoscopy with a standard Macintosh laryngoscope more difficult (a short-handled laryngoscope is often easier to use).
- Failure to intubate the trachea is 7 times more common in the term parturient compared with non-pregnant patients.

Asthma

- Asthma is defined by the presence of three characteristic findings:
  - Reversible airway obstruction.
  - Airway inflammation.
  - Hyper-responsive airway.
- Airway obstruction produces symptoms of cough, wheeze and dyspnoea. Inflammation produces airway obstruction.
- A hyper-responsive airway is marked by an exaggerated response to a variety of bronchoconstricting stimuli such as cold, histamine, prostaglandin $F_{2\alpha}$, etc.
- Bronchial asthma is one of the most common co-existing medical conditions affecting women in the reproductive age group, with a prevalence of 3–5%.
- Asthma occurs in ~1% of pregnant women; 10% of these will need hospital admission for an acute exacerbation.

Pathophysiology

- Neural imbalance:
  - The parasympathetic nervous system provides the dominant constrictor input to the airways.
  - Postganglionic fibres release acetylcholine to activate muscarinic receptors and thus stimulate smooth muscle contraction of airways.
  - The sympathetic nervous system, on the other hand, acts to decrease airway tone but the sympathetic innervation of the airway is sparse.

- Airway inflammation: the process of inflammation involves the production of airway wall oedema and infiltration of the mucosa by a variety of inflammatory cells such as neutrophils, mast cells, macrophages and eosinophils. These cells produce and release mediators of inflammation including histamine, leokotriene, prostaglandin, thromboxanes and platelet-activating factor. Inflammation is one of the factors modulating the course of asthma.
- Airway epithelium: the loss of airway epithelium leads to increased exposure to constricting stimuli and enhanced airway responsiveness.

Interaction with pregnancy

- There has always been concern about a possible effect of asthma on the outcome of pregnancy.
- Pregnancy generally has a positive affect on asthma, although in a small number of patients asthma may worsen.
- Deterioration in symptom control is most frequently associated with failure to take usual preventative medication because of the mistaken belief that the treatment will be harmful to the fetus.
- It is recommended that long- and short-acting β_2 agonists and inhaled steroids should be continued, and acute exacerbations treated with oral prednisolone.
- At the present time, there are limited data on the new leukotriene antagonists, and it is recommended that this therapy is stopped during pregnancy and whilst breastfeeding.
- It is unusual for patients to have acute attacks of asthma in labour, probably because of increased production of endogenous steroids.
- Prostaglandins given at delivery can precipitate an asthma attack and should be given with caution.
- Wheeze in the peridelivery period must be differentiated from other causes such as pulmonary oedema and upper airway obstruction.

Factors improving asthma are

- Progesterone-induced relaxation of airway smooth muscle.
- Increased production of bronchodilating prostaglandin.
- Increased circulating cortisol.

Factors worsening asthma are

- Decreased sensitivity to β-adrenergic agonists.
- Increased production of bronchoconstricting prostaglandin.
- Reduced sensitivity to circulating cortisol because of binding of steroid hormone (e.g. progesterone) to cortisol receptors.

Anaesthetic management

- Good preoperative assessment with details of the course of asthma in each individual is very important.
- The medical history should include information about the symptoms of wheeze, dyspnoea and cough.
- Further information should include the frequency and severity of symptoms, the course of these symptoms during pregnancy and the date of the most recent flare-up.
- Patients who suffer frequent, severe exacerbations are at increased risk of morbidity. Look for signs of an acute exacerbation of asthma including tachypnoea, exaggerated pulsus paradoxus and use of accessory muscles of respiration. Chest X-ray, ABG and pulmonary function tests should be done routinely.
- The goals of analgesia for labour and delivery in asthmatic women include provision of pain relief, a reduction in the stimulus to hyperpnoea and prevention of maternal stress.
- It is more important in patients who report exacerbations due to stress and exercise. Epidural for labour during the first stage provides continuous pain relief and reduces the stimulation for hyperventilation. It can also be topped up for a CS.
- Regional anaesthesia has a definite advantage over a GA technique as it avoids the initiation or exacerbation of a reactive airway during airway instrumentation, thereby reducing the incidence of bronchospasm.
- GA for asthmatic patients undergoing CS requires considerations for preventing aspiration and intraoperative or postoperative bronchospasm during emergence.
- Rapid sequence induction may be accomplished using thiopental or propofol. The latter provides better protection against bronchospasm associated with tracheal intubation in asthmatic patients.
- Bronchodilators can be used prophylactically prior to induction or in the event of bronchospasm.
- The management of patients with asthma requires little modification in pregnancy. In the unlikely event of an attack severe enough to require ventilation, maternal hypoxaemia should be avoided because of the associated severe fetal hypoxaemia; so also should hypocapnia (PCO_2 <2.3kPa) and alkalosis (pH >7.6) since these have been associated with fetal hypoxaemia, probably due to impaired placental transport.

Chronic bronchitis, bronchiectasis, emphysema

- These conditions are now very uncommon in pregnancy.
- As pulmonary hypertension is poorly tolerated in pregnancy, cor pulmonale is likely to be the factor limiting maternal safety.
- The presence of arterial hypoxaemia puts the fetus at risk from intrauterine growth restriction (IUGR).

Restrictive lung disease

Restrictive lung disease is characterized by a reduced vital capacity, usually with a small resting volume and normal airway resistance. The reduced lung volume is due either to alteration in lung parenchyma or to disease of the pleura, chest wall or neuromuscular apparatus.

Aetiology

- *Intrinsic lung disease or disease of the lung parenchyma.* This is due to infiltration or scarring of the lung tissue (interstitial lung disease) or filling of the air spaces with exudates and debris (pneumonitis). Pulmonary infiltration can be due to:
  - Known causes such as asbestosis, radiation, drugs (chemotherapy).
  - Unknown causes such as amyloidosis, sarcoidosis, collagen vascular disease.
- *Extrinsic or extraparenchymal lung disease.* Examples include:
  - Chest wall or respiratory muscle disease: kyphoscoliosis, myasthenia gravis, Guillan–Barré syndrome, poliomyelitis.
  - Pleural thickening: tumour, inflammation.
  - Space-occupying lesion: tumour, pleural effusion, pneumothorax.
  - Lung resection.

Pathophysiology

- With intrinsic lung disease, the main pathophysiological effect of diffuse parenchymal disorders is a reduction in all lung volumes due to the excessive recoil of the lungs, in comparison with the outward recoil forces of the chest wall. Expiratory airflow is reduced in proportion to the lung volume.
- Arterial hypoxaemia in these conditions is primarily due to ventilation–perfusion mismatch, with further contribution from intrapulmonary shunt. The diffusion of oxygen is impaired, which contributes a little towards hypoxaemia at rest but is primarily the mechanism of exercise-induced desaturation.
- Hyperventilation at rest and during exercise is caused by the reflexes arising from the lungs and the need to maintain minute ventilation by reducing tidal volume and increasing respiratory frequency.
- In extrinsic lung disorders of the pleura and thoracic cage, the total compliance by the respiratory system is reduced and hence lung volumes are reduced. Atelectasis results in ventilation–perfusion mismatch. In kyphoscoliosis, a Cobb angle >100° is usually associated with respiratory failure.
- Neuromuscular disorders affect an integral part of the respiratory system, i.e. ventilation. This can be impaired at the level of the CNS, spinal cord, peripheral nervous system, neuromuscular junction or respiratory muscles.

Kyphoscoliosis—interaction with pregnancy (see Chapter 22, p 655)

- Mild degrees of kyphoscoliosis have no effect on pregnancy, and successful pregnancy is possible in patients with severe disease and a vital capacity of as little as 1000mL.

- As in the other chest diseases, hypoxaemia and pulmonary hypertension are the limiting factors, and some women with severe kyphoscoliosis become exhausted and then hypoxaemic in the last trimester.
- Pulmonary function tests should be performed during pregnancy.
- Any suggestion of excessive fatigue or deterioration in serial lung function tests is an indication for hospital admission for rest and nasal IPPV if this is not available at home.
- Progressive hypoxaemia, with or without evidence of fetal compromise, is an indication for delivery.
- Labour and/or CS are best managed with the assistance of regional anaesthesia if possible, which reduces the risk of atelectasis. If regional anaesthesia is not possible due to spinal deformity, GA must be performed with the back-up of critical care facilities for postoperative ventilation if required.

Cystic fibrosis (see Chapter 22, p 607)

- Better management in childhood means that more women with cystic fibrosis are surviving and are having children.
- Pregnancy does not affect mortality when pregnant women with cystic fibrosis are compared with non-pregnant women with cystic fibrosis. However, 24% of all deliveries are preterm.

Pathophysiology

- Cystic fibrosis is an autosomal recessive disorder where there is an abnormality in the epithelial tissues, especially in the respiratory, digestive and reproductive tracts. The defect is thought to lie in the epithelium's cAMP-mediated activation of chloride conductance.
- The viscosity of airway secretions is increased, causing widespread obstruction of small airways with a resultant reduction in lung volumes. This causes ventilation–perfusion mismatch and arterial hypoxaemia.
- Chronic airway obstruction leads to impaired mucus clearance, increasing the episodes of pulmonary infection. Recurrent infection leads to inflammatory changes and cyst formation.
- Spontaneous pneumothorax may occur. Chronic hypoxaemia and lung destruction may produce pulmonary hypertension and cor pulmonale.

Interaction with pregnancy

Factors leading to the deterioration of pulmonary function during pregnancy are:

- Increased airway responsiveness and obstruction.
- Increased work of breathing.
- Cardiovascular changes such as congestive heart failure and pulmonary hypertension associated with the increased blood volume of pregnancy.
- Poor outcomes were associated with a pregnancy weight gain of <4.5kg and a prepregnancy forced vital capacity of <50% of the predicted value. This group is likely to produce a preterm infant and to suffer increased loss of pulmonary function and increased maternal mortality.
- High quality multidisciplinary medical and obstetric care is essential.
- The deterioration of pulmonary function is dependent upon the severity of the disease before pregnancy.

Anaesthetic management

- There should be continuous monitoring of maternal oxygen saturation as there is an increased incidence of hypoxaemia.
- Adequate analgesia should be provided to prevent maternal hyperventilation.
- Continuous lumbar epidural analgesia with a sensory block maintained at the level of 10th thoracic dermatome can provide excellent pain relief and reduce the stimulus for hyperventilation.
- High thoracic motor block should be prevented as this will cause respiratory depression that will further increase hypoxaemia.
- Regional anaesthesia is indicated for surgery, but non-invasive positive pressure ventilation (NIPPV) has been described with very poor respiratory function.
- Regional anaesthesia for surgery avoids tracheal intubation and positive pressure ventilation. This technique reduces the incidence of bronchospasm and pneumothorax.
- Considerations for a GA for CS include:
  - Humidification of gases to prevent inspissation of mucus.
  - Frequent suctioning to prevent tracheal tube obstruction.
  - Allow a long expiratory pause to prevent air trapping; this would help reduce pneumothorax secondary to volu-trauma.
  - Nitrous oxide should be avoided to prevent worsening of any pre-existing pneumothorax.
  - Active chest physiotherapy should commence as early as possible postoperatively.
  - Antibiotic prophylaxis as per the sputum sensitivity.

Tuberculosis

- Before the advent of antituberculous therapy, TB was the cause of many maternal deaths, particularly in the puerperium.
- A high index of suspicion is necessary to make the diagnosis in pregnancy.
- Most centres in the UK do not screen for TB in pregnancy (Mantoux testing and or chest radiographs).
- Recent evidence from infectious disease surveillance suggests an upsurge in TB prevalence; there is a very strong association between TB and HIV/AIDS in poorer nations where the vulnerable women of child-bearing age are still highly susceptible to contracting the disease.

Further reading

Linderman KS. Respiratory disease. In: Chestnut DH. *Obstetric Anaesthesia, Principles and Practice*, 3rd edn. Mosby, 2006, 1011–1026.

Edenborough FP *et al.* Pregnancy in women with cystic fibrosis. *British Medical Journal* 1995; **311**: 822–823.

Renal disease

Renal disease in pregnancy can be broadly classified as:

- Renal disease occurring during pregnancy.
  - Urinary tract infection.
  - Urolithiasis.
  - Hypertensive disorders of pregnancy.
  - Acute renal failure.
- Pre-existing renal disease in pregnancy.
  - Chronic hypertension.
  - Chronic renal failure.

Important physiological changes take place in the renal system during pregnancy:

- Increased vascular volume leading to renal enlargement.
- Dilatation of the renal pelvis and ureters due to hormonal changes leads to decreased peristalsis.
- Obstruction to the ureteric drainage at the pelvic brim occurs due to pressure effects by dilated uterine and ovarian veins and the gravid uterus.

Together, these changes predispose pregnant women to vescicoureteric reflux and ascending infection. Increased CO and decreased intrarenal resistance cause an 80% increase in renal blood flow and a 50% increase in glomerular filtration rate (GFR). Plasma creatinine concentration >73mcmol/L and urea concentration >4.3mmol/L (normal values for non-pregnant women) are considered abnormal as a consequence of increased GFR. Tubular sodium reabsorption and osmoregulation are reset, allowing a physiological hypervolaemia of pregnancy.

Urinary tract infection (UTI)

- Urinary stasis and increased vesicoureteric reflux lead to increased risk of infection. Untreated UTI will develop into acute pyelonephritis in ~20% of cases.
- Symptoms of acute pyelonephrits include fever, chills, flank pain and other symptoms of lower UTI. The most common causative organisms found are *E. coli*, *Klebsiella* and *Proteus*.
- Useful antibiotics are nitrofurantoin (not in first trimester), trimethoprim, ampicillin and the cephalosporins.
- Once the mother has been identified as susceptible, she should be screened during pregnancy.

Anaesthetic management

Regional anaesthesia—spinal or epidural—can be considered, provided the patients are receiving antibiotic cover and not frankly septic. Epidural analgesia may produce a modest increase in maternal temperature in an already febrile patient. Local guidelines should be followed.

Urolithiasis

- Urolithiasis is characterized by the abnormal formation of calculi within the renal calyces or pelvis.
- Supersaturation of minerals involved in calyx formation due to stasis and acidic urine cause stone formation. Most stones are calcium oxalate (70%) or calcium phosphate (10%).
- Pregnancy seems to predispose some susceptible women to multiple, recurrent stone formation.
- Pain can be severe and difficult to manage.

Anaesthetic management/pain management

- The ureters receive sensory innervation through the renal, ovarian and hypogastric plexus (T11 to L1 spinal segments).
- NSAIDs are generally contraindicated in pregnancy and although affective in the non-pregnant population should not be used.
- Intravenous paracetamol is safe in pregnancy and can be beneficial.
- Opioids may be required.
- Epidural analgesia provides pain relief and facilitates passage of the stone due to decreased ureteric spasm.

Acute renal failure (ARF)

- ARF is characterized by a rapid rise in serum creatinine levels (>73mcmol/L) and urea (>4.3mmol/L), and is confirmed by decreased GFR.
- Plasma creatinine levels roughly double for every 50% reduction in GFR.
- Urine output may fall to <400mL/day.

Causes of ARF

- Prerenal: include hypovolaemic states such as haemorrhage, hyperemesis gravidarum and low CO states such as heart failure, arrhythmias and other diseases of the myocardium.
- Renal: e.g. acute tubular necrosis, septic abortion, amniotic fluid embolism, acute glomerulonephritis, pyelonephritis, HELLP syndrome and eclampsia/pre-eclampsia.
- Postrenal: e.g. urolithiasis, ureteral obstruction by the gravid uterus.

ARF is unusual in pregnancy and reflects severe underlying disease that requires urgent diagnosis and treatment. Many mothers will require urgent referral and transfer to a Critical Care Unit for further management.

Chronic renal disease

- Many women with chronic renal disease now become pregnant. This is especially true with more effective treatments for associated chronic anaemia and better nutrition.
- The pregnancy outcome depends on prepregnancy:
  - Renal dysfunction.
  - Hypertension.
  - Proteinuria.
  - Underlying renal condition.

- A normal creatinine can indicate significantly impaired renal function in the pregnant woman.

Pregnancy is associated with

- Increased rate of decline of renal function.
- Increased risk of significant proteinuria.
- Worsening hypertension.
- Increased risk of pre-eclampsia.
- Increased risk to fetus (IUGR and premature delivery).

Management is complex and depends on the severity and underlying cause of the renal impairment. A multidisciplinary approach is required, with significant input from renal physicians and dieticians.

Renal transplant recipients

- Pregnancy is increasingly common after renal transplantation.
- Outcome is generally good if pregnancy is deferred until 1yr post-transplant.
- The new immunosuppressive drugs are well tolerated and most are thought to be safe in pregnancy.
- If the graft is not functioning well prior to pregnancy, the result tends to be the same as for chronic renal impairment, with increased renal functional decline and increased risk of complications.

Anaesthetic management

This is influenced by the extent of renal dysfunction and hypertension. Uraemic patients may be hypovolaemic or hypervolaemic, depending on the time of last dialysis. Close observation of fluid balance must be undertaken.

Regional anaesthesia

- Hypovolaemia and autonomic neuropathy may cause profound hypotension following regional blockade.
- Proper rehydration and slowly established epidural anaesthesia will minimize the impact of the autonomic neuropathy.
- Coagulation should be checked before regional anaesthesia is considered.
- Ephedrine and other vasopressors may have an increased effect.
- Care should be continued on an HDU/ITU.

General anaesthesia

- If required, the patient should be medically optimized if possible.
- Airway assessment is important due to facial oedema.
- Fibreoptic intubation should be considered in severe pre-eclampsia.
- Obtund the hypertensive response to laryngoscopy using opioids, and the paediatricians should be informed of the potential for fetal respiratory depression.
- An arterial line should be considered for close monitoring to avoid wide swings of BP.
- Delayed gastric emptying and increased gastric acidity increase the risk of aspiration pneumonitis. H_2 receptor blockers should be administered routinely along with sodium citrate.

- Suxamethonium causes an increase in potassium levels in an already hyperkalaemic patient. Potassium levels should be checked prior to any elective procedure.
- Assess neuromuscular function with a nerve stimulator if magnesium has been used in patients as this may prolong the duration of action of muscle relaxants.
- The sleep dose of thiopental required may be reduced due to decreased protein binding in this group of patients.

Further reading

Gambling DR. Hypertensive disorders in pregnancy. In: Chestnut DH. *Obstetric Anaesthesia, Principles and Practice*, 3rd edn. Mosby, 2006, 875–920.

Epstein FH. Pregnancy and renal disease. *New England Journal of Medicine* 1996; **335**: 277–278.

Diabetes

Aetiological classification of diabetes mellitus

- *Type 1*: autoimmune/non-immune forms, early onset β-cell destruction, genetic susceptibility and environmental factors implicated. Ketosis occurs with absolute lack of insulin, previously known as 'insulin-dependent diabetes mellitus (IDDM)'.
- *Type 2*: previously known as 'non-insulin-dependent diabetes (NIDDM)' or 'maturity-onset'. Encompasses a spectrum of insulin hyposecretion and insulin resistance. Ketosis is rare. Risk factors include obesity, reduced exercise and racial origin.
- *Others*: where the cause is known, such as gestational diabetes, drug-induced diabetes, pancreatic disease, endocrinopathies such as acromegaly/Cushing's disease.

Metabolic changes in pregnancy

- Pregnancy induces substantial alterations in carbohydrate, lipid and amino acid metabolism, which have been described as a combination of 'facilitated anabolism' and 'accelerated starvation'.
- These changes appear to ensure the optimal availability of nutrients for both fetus and mother.

Carbohydrate metabolism

- Fasting plasma glucose concentrations gradually decline during pregnancy by ~0.5mmol/L, reaching a nadir in the third trimester.
- Postprandial glucose concentrations increase, despite a rise in both basal and stimulated insulin secretion. This appears to be due to peripheral insulin resistance induced by placental hormones, and to the effects of oestrogen and progesterone on the maternal pancreas.

Lipid metabolism

- Plasma concentrations of triglycerides, cholesterol, phospholipids and free fatty acids all increase during pregnancy.
- The increase in circulating free fatty acid concentrations is thought to have an important influence on maternal metabolism, providing an alternative source of maternal fuel at a time in pregnancy when fetal and maternal glucose needs are maximal.

Gestational diabetes

- Gestational diabetes may be defined as '...carbohydrate intolerance of variable severity with onset or first recognition during the present pregnancy...'.
- This definition includes not only those women in whom diabetes occurs transiently during pregnancy and regresses after delivery, but also those in whom type 2 diabetes arises *de novo* during pregnancy and persists long term. Some of these women may have had undiagnosed diabetes for some time and are at high risk of fetal and maternal complications.

Obstetric complications of diabetes in pregnancy

- Early fetal loss and congenital abnormalities occur 3–5 times more commonly than in the background population.
- Proteinuric hypertension occurs approximately twice as often in diabetics compared with normal women.
  - Serum urate and creatinine concentrations should therefore be measured at every antenatal visit, and 24h urine protein concentrations from 24 weeks gestation.
  - These provide the earliest biochemical evidence of proteinuric pre-eclampsia and also serve to clarify those BP changes in late pregnancy which are due to pre-existing essential hypertension.
  - Although the reason for the increased incidence of pre-eclampsia in diabetics is unknown, a link with glycaemic control has been established, and the incidence of this complication is reduced with optimal diabetic control.
- Diabetic nephropathy is associated with rapid decline of renal function.
- Cardiovascular disease must be investigated.
- Retinopathy can rapidly deteriorate.
- Type 1 diabetes is associated with other autoimmune problems, e.g. hypothyroidism, and should be screened for.
- Diabetics are at increased risk of wound infection following surgery, and prophylactic antibiotics are therefore advised following CS (elective and emergency) or operative vaginal delivery.
- Diabetic mothers are at an increased risk of operative delivery because of a large baby and other obstetric complications such as pre-eclampsia.

Treatment of diabetes

- Tight glycaemic control is recommended to reduce the risk of macrosomia and other complications.
- Insulin therapy is recommended for all but the mildest gestational diabetic where diet control may be adequate.
- Insulin requirements increase in pregnancy although in the last few weeks of pregnancy this may decline.
- It is recommended that fasting glucose should be between 3.5 and 5.5mmol/L, and a 2h postprandial level of not more than 7mmol/L.
- Hypoglycaemia is a common problem because of fluctuating insulin requirements and aiming for tight glyaemic control.
- Insulin requirements can drop dramatically in the postpartum period, and blood glucose levels must be very carefully monitored.

Anaesthetic management

- Clinical decisions must be guided by logical extensions of studies of non-pregnant diabetic patients and non-diabetic pregnant patients.
- A good preoperative multisystem evaluation should be done.
- Autonomic cardiovascular dysfunction should be ruled out and, if present, should be treated with vasopressers. BP should be monitored more frequently during labour and delivery.
- Autonomic neuropathy, if present, increases gastroparesis and hence increases the risk of aspiration. There is also a decreased cough reflex threshold and obstructive sleep apnoea. The anaesthetist should ensure proper perioperative positioning and padding of the extremities during administration of anaesthesia.
- Epidural anaesthesia is preferred over a single-shot spinal for CS because of slower onset of sympathetic block and therefore more time to treat hypotension aggressively. Alternatively, a low dose CSE is a good option.
- Epidural analgesia during labour also reduces sympathetic stimulation. This prevents hyperglycaemia and increased insulin requirements.
- The diabetic stiff joint syndrome is common in prolonged type 1 diabetics. Limited atlanto-occipital joint movement may predispose to difficult intubation. Look for the prayer sign as one of the screens for a difficult intubation.
- The stiff joint syndrome is also associated with a non-compliant epidural space. As a result, smaller volumes of LA might be sufficient.
- Strict aseptic technique should be followed during administration of central neuraxial blockade as these patients are more prone to infections.

Further reading

Wissner RN. Endocrine disorders. In: Chestnut DH. *Obstetric Anaesthesia, Principles and Practice*, 3rd edn. Mosby, 2006, 809–841.

Coagulation disorders

- Normal pregnancy is accompanied by major changes in the coagulation and fibrinolytic systems. There are significant increases in the procoagulant factors (V, VIII and X) and a very marked increase in plasma fibrinogen.
- In uncomplicated pregnancy, there is no change in antithrombin concentrations during the antenatal period, a fall during delivery, and then an increase 1 week postpartum. Protein C levels appear to remain constant or increase slightly, but protein S activity falls significantly during normal pregnancy.
- These physiological changes alter the usual balance between the procoagulants and anticoagulants in favour of the factors promoting blood clotting.
- In addition, fibrinolytic activity appears to be reduced during healthy pregnancy but returns to normal rapidly after separation of the placenta and completion of the third stage of delivery. This effect is mediated by placentally derived plasminogen activator inhibitor type II.
- These changes in the haemostatic systems, together with the increase in blood volume, help to reduce the chances of abnormal haemorrhage at delivery, but they also convert pregnancy into a hypercoaguable state that may carry special hazards for both the mother and fetus.
- These hazards include a spectrum of haemostatic disorders, from thromboembolism through to the many conditions associated with disseminated intravascular coagulation (DIC).

The coagulation disorders can be broadly classified into
- Thrombocytopenic coagulopathies.
- Congenital coagulopathies.
- Acquired coagulopathies.
- Hypercoaguable disease.

Thrombocytopenic coagulopathies

Incidental/gestational thrombocytopenia

- As pregnancy advances, there is a progressively small, but significant, fall in the platelet count in individual patients, probably due to haemodilution.
- Approximately 8% of healthy pregnant women have thrombocytopenia at term, with platelet counts between 90 and 150×10^9/L.
- These women have no history of pre-eclampsia or immune thrombocytopenia, and there is no increased incidence of thrombocytopenia in their offspring.

Autoimmune thrombocytopenic purpura (AITP) (see Chapter 22, p 664)

- Antibodies directed against platelet antigens are produced primarily in the spleen, where phagocytosis by macrophages also occurs. Antibody production can also take place in the liver and bone marrow.

- The binding of complement to platelets can facilitate their clearance, and antibody binding to megakaryocytes can lead to ineffective production of platelets.
- Antiplatelet antibodies (immunoglobulin G) attack platelet membrane glycoproteins and destroy platelets at a rate that cannot be compensated for by bone marrow.

Interaction with pregnancy

- If AITP is diagnosed during pregnancy, conservative management is usually sufficient.
- Corticosteroids are administered if the platelet count falls below 20×10^9/L before the onset of labour or $<50 \times 10^9$/L at the time of delivery.
- Immunoglobulin can be administered if the patient fails to respond to corticosteroid therapy.
- In women with pre-existing AITP, thrombocytopenia is usually severe. Splenectomy may be necessary to improve the platelet count and function in extreme conditions.
- The baby will be affected and delivery must be atraumatic.

Other causes of thrombocytopenia in pregnancy are

- Pre-eclampsia/HELLP.
- Thrombotic thrombocytopenic purpura (TTP) (see Chapter 22, p 665–666).
- DIC.
- Drug induced.
- The differential diagnosis is important to consider because the management of each is different.
- Close liaison with a haematologist is important for all cases of significant thrombocytopenia of $<80\text{x}10^9$/L.

Congenital coagulopathies

The common congenital coagulopathies are:

- von Willebrand's disease.
- Haemophilia A and B.
- Other single factor deficiences.

> All women with a significant congenital clotting disorder should be delivered in a maternity centre associated with a comprehensive care haemophilia centre, as the management of the mother and baby is likely to be complicated.

von Willebrand's disease (see Chapter 22, p 671)

von Willebrand's disease is the most frequent of all inherited haemostatic abnormalities and is therefore the most likely coagulopathy to affect women in pregnancy. In normal pregnancy, a rise in both factor VIIIC and von Willebrand factor (vWF) is observed.

Pathophysiology

vWF plays two primary roles in coagulation:

- It facilitates platelet adhesion by binding to platelets and collagen.
- It forms a complex with factor VIII, which decreases the excretion of factor VIII.

vWF helps platelet binding to sites of vascular damage. The symptoms of deficiency therefore mimic disorders of platelet function (bleeding from skin and mucosa). A deficiency can also result in decreased factor VIII levels, and patients with severe disease can present with haemorrhage into muscles and joints, similar to that seen in classical haemophilia. However, the bleeding time is prolonged in von Willebrand's disease and normal in haemophiliacs.

Classification

- Type 1—partial deficiency of vWF, mild to moderate bleeding disorder.
- Type 2a—qualitative defect in vWF.
- Type 2b—qualitative defect in vWF with increased binding to platelets causing mild thrombocytopenia.
- Type 3—complete absence of vWF and reduced levels of factor VIII, severe bleeding disorder.

Interaction with pregnancy

- Pregnancy causes a 3- to 4-fold rise in vWF. As a result, patients suffering from type 1 disorder improve during pregnancy as the vWF increases to normal levels.
- Levels at 32 weeks are usually adequate to confirm this.
- Women suffering with types 2 and 3 disorders do not improve during pregnancy and their care should be at a specialist centre.

Anaesthetic implications

- DDAVP (desmopressin) and vWF concentrates are used to increase the levels of vWF.
- Vaginal delivery is considered safe if vWF is >40IU/dL.
- If operative delivery is necessary, the level has to be increased to >50IU/dL.
- PPH is not more common than normal but if it occurs it is likely to be severe as vWF falls to prepregnancy levels.
- Regional anaesthesia is generally safe in patients with type 1 disease after levels in pregnancy have been checked.
- An epidural is not recommended for women with types 2 and 3 disease; however, a spinal anaesthetic could be sited for operative delivery if there is an interval of up to 20min between the administration of vWF concentrates and DDAVP.
- The haematologist's input in the care of this patient is an absolute necessity.

Ref: OHC

Please affix
stamp
outside UK

FREEPOST RRCA-ZSES-GXEY
Medicine Department (OSH)
Oxford University Press
Great Clarendon Street
Oxford OX2 6DP
UK

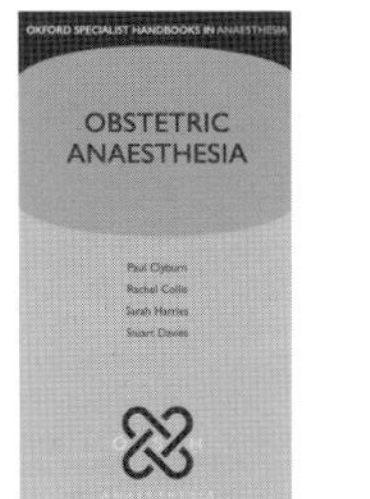

Reader's comments card

Help us to make *Obstetric Anaesthesia* even better!

Send this card, or a letter with your comments, to the address overleaf.

Alternatively you can email helen.liepman@oup.com

or submit your comments online at **www.oup.com/uk/medicine/handbooks**

Where relevant, please give references to back up points.

We may wish to contact you to ask for your views on this and other OUP books. Please tick here if you would prefer not to be contacted regarding future development of our books. ☐

OUP may wish to send you information in the future, by post or email, on OUP products and services. Please tick here if you do not wish to receive such information:

By email: ☐

By post: ☐

1: Are you currently a medical student/junior doctor/specialist trainee/nurse/other (please specify)?

2: What do you like about *Obstetric Anaesthesia*?

3: What do you dislike about *Obstetric Anaesthesia*?

4: Are there any topics not included that you feel should be?

5: Would you like to add any further comments, or suggestions for the next edition?

Personal details (optional):

Name: .... Position: ....

Institution/Address: ....

....

.... Post/Zip Code: .... Country: ....

Email: ....

Medical specialties/subjects of interest: ....

Haemophilia (see Chapter 22, p 620–621)
Haemophilia A and B are X-linked disorders due to a deficiency of factor VIII and IX, respectively. Females are usually carriers of this disease as they have only one affected chromosome. The clotting factor level is expected to be ~50% of normal.

The risks in pregnancy for the female carrier of haemophilia are 2-fold:
- She may have very low factor VIII or IX levels and be at risk of excessive bleeding due to lyonization (random deletion of the X chromosome), especially following a surgical or traumatic delivery. These women with low factor VIII/IX levels have the same risk of bleeding as affected males.
- Half her male offspring will inherit haemophilia. This has important implications now that prenatal diagnosis of these conditions is possible.

Clinical classification of either haemophilia A or B
- Mild— ~5% factor level.
- Moderate— 1–5% factor level.
- Severe— <1% factor level.
- It is important to identify carriers prior to pregnancy, not only to provide appropriate management for the rare mother with pathologically low coagulation activity but also to provide genetic counselling.
- Changes in factor VIII complex may make the identification of carriers more difficult during pregnancy.
- Clinical problems occur more often in carriers of Christmas disease, since factor IX does not rise in response to healthy pregnancy in the same way that factor VIII does.
- There must be a clear atraumatic delivery plan for male babies.

Anaesthetic implications

- During labour, factor VIII levels should be maintained at 50% of normal.
- If CS is required, treatment should be instituted to increase the factor VIII level to 80% of normal.
- The factor VIII level should be checked daily during pregnancy, and levels <25% or any signs of bleeding should be treated actively.
- Delayed PPH is the most common bleeding complication in obstetric patients as factor levels fall quickly in the postpartum period.
- Treatment for haemophilia A is factor VIII concentrate, cryoprecipitate and DDAVP.
- Treatment for haemophilia B is factor IX concentrate and fresh frozen plasma (FFP).

Other single factor deficiencies
- Factor XI deficiency (plasma thromboplastin antecedent deficiency) is the most common and can cause PPH (see Chapter 22, p 614–615).

Acquired coagulopathy

Obstetric causes of acquired coagulopathy include:
- Pregnancy-induced hypertension.
- Placental abruption.

- Retained dead fetus.
- Amniotic fluid embolus.
- Liver disease.
- DIC.
- Therapeutic anticoagulation.

Pre-eclampsia/pregnancy-induced hypertension

There is increased destruction of platelets due to an immunological mechanism. Coagulation screening shows prolonged bleeding time and partial thromboplastin time with increased levels of fibrin degradation products. For further details, see chapter 17.

Liver disease

Liver impairment in pregnancy can be due to:
- Hepatitis.
- Acute fatty liver of pregnancy.
- Cholestasis.
- Hepatic rupture secondary to cholestasis.
- HELLP syndrome.

There is decreased synthesis of coagulation factors due to the damaged liver.

Disseminated intravascular coagulation (DIC)

DIC results from an abnormal activation of the coagulation system, which results in:
- Formation of large amounts of thrombin.
- Depletion of coagulation factors.
- Activation of fibrinolytic system.
- Haemorrhage.

In the obstetric population, the most frequent causes of DIC are pre-eclampsia, placental abruption, sepsis, retained dead fetus syndrome and amniotic fluid embolism. DIC in pregnancy is always a secondary process. Severe DIC is frequently difficult to manage without early delivery of the baby. Uterotonics play a major role in preventing severe PPH.

The laboratory findings include:
- Decreased platelet count, fibrinogen and antithrombin III concentrations.
- Variable increase in prothrombin, partial thromboplastin and thrombin time.
- Increased concentrations of D-dimer, fibrin monomer and fibrin degradation products. Extremely low levels <0.5g/L of fibrinogen are characteristic of pregnancy-associated DIC, and early replacement is paramount.
- Early liaison with a haematologist is important.

Anaesthetic implications

- Some mothers with DIC, i.e. abruption, will labour rapidly. Any form of regional anaesthesia is contraindicated.
- These patients often have multiorgan system failure and require mechanical ventilatory support. DIC always mandates the administration of GA for those patients requiring CS.

Therapeutic anticoagulation

Patients requiring chronic anticoagulation receive heparin throughout pregnancy. There are well recognized guidelines as to the timing of regional anaesthesia. See Chapter 7 for further details.

Hypercoagulable disease

Effective coagulation is maintained by a balance of procoagulant and anticoagulant activity. Pregnancy is a hypercoagulable state and certain diseases increase the risk of thrombosis. Venous thromboses are more common than arterial thromboses and their incidence increases with surgery, pregnancy, use of oral contraceptives and immobilization.
Diseases that increase risks are:
- Protein C deficiency.
- Protein S deficiency.
- Antithrombin III deficiency.
- Factor V Leiden mutation.
- Hyperhomocysteinaemia.
- Prothrombin G20210A variation.

Protein C deficiency (see Chapter 22, p 650)

Protein C is a vitamin K-dependent protein with a short half-life (8h) produced in the liver. It acts by inhibiting activated factors V and VIII. Protein C levels increase by 35% during normal pregnancy. Thrombosis occurs in 25% of pregnant patients with the deficiency, unless anticoagulation therapy is administered.

Heparin should be administered during the first and third trimester, and either heparin or warfarin can be given during the second trimester. If warfarin is administered without prior heparin anticoagulation, protein C levels fall before the levels of factors II, VII, IX and X fall. This results in thrombosis with skin necrosis.

Protein S deficiency (see Chapter 22, p 650)

Protein S is also a vitamin K-dependent protein synthesized in the liver. It acts as a cofactor for protein C. Levels of protein S decrease in normal pregnancy. The treatment of protein S deficiency is identical to that of protein C deficiency.

Antithrombin III deficiency (see Chapter 22, p 590)

Antithrombin III is synthesized in the liver and endothelial cells. It inactivates thrombin and factors IXa, Xa, XIa and XIIa. Its activity is potentiated by heparin. Anticoagulation or antithrombin III replacement is indicated during pregnancy. Since heparin acts by potentiation of antithrombin III, more heparin may be required for the desired effect if levels of antithrombin III are low.

Factor V Leiden mutation (see Chapter 22, p 614)
This is the most common hypercoaguable disorder, affecting 5% of the white population. This mutation leads to a form of factor V, which when activated is resistant to degradation by activated protein C, thereby increasing procoagulant activity.

Anaesthetic implications

- Depending on the mother's personal thrombosis history, she will be on prophylactic or therapeutic low molecular weight heparin during pregnancy.
- Guidelines for the management of mothers with a risk of thrombosis can be found on the Royal College of Obstetrics and Gynaecologists website.
- Many women want the opportunity to receive regional analgesia or anaesthesia, and the timing of anticoagulation is important.
- Information on anticoagulants and regional anaesthesia can be found in Chapter 7.

Further reading

Sharma SK. Haematological and coagulation disorders. In: Chestnut DH. *Obstetric Anaesthesia, Principles and Practice*. 3rd edn. Mosby, 2006, 842–859.

Chapter 5

Antenatal issues including pain management

Rachel Collis, Leanne Rees

David Hill

Aims of antenatal anaesthetic assessment in high risk pregnancies

Advances in medical care have resulted in an increasing number of women with concomitant diseases becoming pregnant. Antenatal anaesthetic assessment plays a vital role in the successful management of such patients. This has been highlighted by successive reports of the Confidential Enquiries into Maternal Deaths (CEMD), and its successor—the Confidential Enquiry into Child and Maternal Health (CEMACH). A National Audit Commission report in 1997 found that anaesthetists were involved in 38% of deliveries, and in some units up to 60% of women received care from an anaesthetist in the peripartum period. The role of anaesthetists has continued to increase. Although it is often not possible to predict in the antenatal period which mothers will eventually have an anaesthetic, those at high risk and with other medical problems should be assessed. The benefits include:

- It avoids short-notice and suboptimal anaesthetic plans being put into place for delivery.
- It enables a detailed history and appropriate physical examination of the patient, which is often difficult or impossible in labour or in an emergency situation.
- It allows review of appropriate information or to prearrange special investigations, e.g. magnetic resonance imaging (MRI) of the lumbar spine.
- The effects of physiological changes in pregnancy on the disease can be given due consideration in patient evaluation and management.
- It enables multidisciplinary input and meetings—anaesthetists, obstetricians, haematologists, cardiologists, allergists, etc.
- It enables the formulation of a management plan tailored to the individual's needs. This plan must be possible on any day at any time because of the unpredictable nature of labour and delivery (even if an elective CS is planned).
- Explanation of issues to the patient, increasing her ability to make informed choices and decreasing anxiety when labour pain or emergency anaesthesia makes it difficult to put complex issues across.
- It avoids disappointment, especially if the patient's expectations are very different from those of her physicians.
- It highlights special requirements, especially if additional monitoring or senior help is required.

Clinic set-up

- Can vary from *ad hoc* calls to the antenatal clinic, to regular formal clinics which are more popular in larger units and tertiary referral centres because of the volume of work and complexity of the cases.
- Senior anaesthetic input and continuity is vital to ensure optimal outcome. Many units will now have a regular consultant anaesthetic session dedicated to a clinic.
- Attention is generally targeted at high risk pregnancies due to limitation of resources.

- A formal clinic environment with clerical support is important. A room in an antenatal clinic is appropriate, and most women feel comfortable with this arrangement.
- It is usual that obstetric and medical notes are separated. It is important that every effort is made to have the medical notes available.
- Regular communication of appropriate referrals to obstetricians and midwives is important.
- Good communication and clear lines of referral should exist between professionals. It is important that referrals can be made from midwifery and consultant obstetric clinics, and that everybody is aware of the mechanism of referral.

Timing

Most patients benefit from review at ~32–34 weeks. An appointment >8 weeks from delivery, where details of likely anaesthetic input are discussed, will have been forgotten or will often not seem relevant to the patient. An appointment after 34 weeks will miss some mothers because of premature delivery, and will not allow enough time to communicate with other professionals and organize special investigations. Any patient with significant medical conditions, especially cardiac disease, should be referred at 24–26 weeks gestation and are likely to need regular review every 4–6 weeks after this because of the changing physiological demands of the pregnancy on the disease.

Documentation

- Date of assessment.
- Patient details.
- Expected date of delivery and current gestation.
- Previous obstetric history and anaesthetic involvement.
- Current delivery plan.
- History of medical problem requiring referral.
- Findings of examination and appropriate investigations.
- Management plans to include suitable anaesthetic techniques and seniority of anaesthetist required.

- Communication of the management plan is important. The attending anaesthetist should have immediate access to such information when the mother is in labour.
- A designated page in the maternity notes or a specific coloured clinic sheet in the main notes will make it immediately clear to midwives, obstetricians and anaesthetists that the patient had been designated high risk in some way and that there is an anaesthetic plan.
- Notes are not always immediately available and it is useful if a copy of the plan is also stored in a folder or filing cabinet on the delivery suite, of which all anaesthetists and labour ward staff must be aware.
- A delivery suite ward folder is also useful to warn anaesthetic staff of potential problems. There should be a flagging process for alerting staff that the patient has been seen antenatally and that the anaesthetist should be informed on admission.

Suggested referrals to the high risk obstetric anaesthetic clinic

The following are the conditions for which patients are likely to need referral to the obstetric anaesthetic clinic:

Cardiac

- Congenital or acquired heart disease even if the patient is asymptomatic.
- Significant history of dysrhythmias.

Haematological

- All patients on heparin, low molecular weight heparin or warfarin in pregnancy.
- Any patient under regular review in a haematology clinic, e.g. idiopathic thrombocytopenic purpura (ITP), thrombotic thrombocytopenic purpura (TTP), antithrombin III deficiency, von Willebrand's disease.
- Sickle cell disease.

Respiratory

- Severe asthma, especially requiring hospital or ICU admission.
- Other significant history of respiratory disease, e.g. sarcoidosis, fibrosing alveolitis, pneumothorax, cystic fibrosis, restrictive chest wall deformities.

Neurological

- History of, or current intracranial pathology.
- History of neuroinflammatory disease, e.g. multiple sclerosis.
- Poorly controlled epilepsy.

Spinal

- All patients with any degree of spina bifida.
- Any patient with a history of back surgery.
- Patients with back problems with specific concerns.
- Patients with neck problems or possibility of difficult intubation.
- Severe kyphoscoliosis especially if causing restrictive lung disease.

Endocrine

- Significant endocrine disease, with the exception of diabetes mellitus or treated thyroid disease.

GIT/liver

- Any patient with a history of major abdominal surgery.
- Chronic liver disease of any cause.

Renal

- Any patient with chronic renal failure.
- All renal transplant recipients.

Anaesthetic

- Previous history or family history of anaesthetic-related problems, e.g. suxamethonium apnoea, malignant hyperthermia.
- Previous history of airway or intubation difficulties.

Drug reactions

- Severe reactions on previous exposure especially to LA and GA drugs.

Obstetric

- Risk of major PPH, e.g. major placenta praevia with a previous CS scar.

Miscellaneous

- Morbid obesity, i.e. BMI >45kg/m^2.
- Substance abusers.
- Patients who refuse blood transfusion, e.g. Jehovah's Witnesses.
- Patients with severe anxiety or phobias.
- Patients with a previous history of inadequate epidural or spinal anaesthesia who are concerned about their experience.
- Pregnant patients with chronic pain. e.g. symphysis pubis dysfunction.

Specific problems in the antenatal period

Cardiac

All mothers with a history of cardiac disease should be assessed, even if they are asymptomatic. They can be roughly divided into three categories of risk: low, medium and high risk. The assessment and allocation of mothers into these groups is important because this will determine where the mother should be looked after, both during her pregnancy and for delivery, and how often key members of a multidisciplinary team should see her.

A multidisciplinary team comprising an obstetrician, obstetric anaesthetist and a cardiologist with an interest in pregnancy must assess these mothers early in pregnancy, especially if there are significant problems. A pulmonary physician may need to be included if the mother has pulmonary hypertension. Flexible and ongoing assessment will be required throughout her pregnancy as plans may rapidly change even if initially she is very well.

Assessment

- Functional New York Heart Association (NYHA) class.
    - NYHC 1: no limit during ordinary activity.
    - NYHC 2: slight limitation during ordinary activity.
    - NYHC 3: marked limitation of ordinary activity.
    - NYHC 4: no physical activity without symptoms.
- An accurate assessment of the level of physical activity prepregnancy and how this has changed. Some deny symptoms of breathlessness but are very limited, whilst other women feel anxious about the breathlessness normally seen in pregnancy. Ask about ordinary daily activities.
- An accurate assessment of the underlying lesion. Most patients require at least one echocardiogram during pregnancy to confirm history unless previously well documented.
- Important to determine results of most recent investigations and cardiology opinion.

Plan should indicate

- Appropriate anaesthesia for both labour and operative procedures.
- Seniority of grade of anaesthetist who should be directly involved in labour.
- The grade of anaesthetist may vary with the procedure and situation. This should be outlined.
- Appropriate monitoring (invasive/non-invasive).
- Requirement for endocarditis prophylaxis.
- Plan for oxytocin bolus/infusion.
- Level of care postdelivery: routine/high dependency/intensive care setting.

Low risk cardiac disease

These mothers should have a normal pregnancy and are frequently perplexed as to why they have been asked to attend an anaesthetic clinic. All mothers with cardiac disease should be seen antenatally so that analgesia and anaesthesia can be planned and then given without delay once in labour, if required.

- The obstetric anaesthetist assessment can occur at any gestation but in a well mother the ideal time is 32–34 weeks gestation.
- A home delivery or delivery in a midwifery-led unit may be possible for some women.
- Some women with asymptomatic lesions require antibiotic cover during labour and many midwifery units cannot provide this treatment.
- In extreme situations, for example major obstetric haemorrhage, she may not tolerate the physiological insult as well as a mother with an entirely normal heart, and this should be discussed with the mother prior to delivery.
- Routine epidural analgesia or anaesthesia for CS can usually be planned.
- Routine monitoring of mother and fetus.

Categorization of low risk women

- NYHA 1.
- Mothers with well controlled and stable ischaemic heart disease.
- Good biventricular function.
- No history of heart failure or pulmonary oedema.
- No history of major dysrhythmias.
- Congenital heart disease which has been surgically completely corrected.
- Complete closure of PDA.
- Complete closure of atrial or ventricular septal defect without residual pulmonary hypertension.
- Correction of coarctation of aorta.
- Small atrial or ventricular defects without a major shunt.
- Minor and asymptomatic pulmonary, aortic (valve area >2cm^2) and mitral stenosis.
- Minor and asymptomatic mitral or aortic incompetence.

Medium risk cardiac disease

Patients can present with deteriorating parameters during pregnancy or delivery, but usually tolerate the physiological demands of pregnancy without major problems.

- These mothers can usually tolerate labour, but the anaesthetic care may need to be modified.
- They are best looked after in a hospital that can offer 24h specialist care in case of sudden cardiac problems and obstetric emergencies.
- In most situations, a caesarean delivery is required only for obstetric indications.

- An exception to this is the mother with a dilated aortic root >4cm, especially associated with Marfan's syndrome, who is usually recommended to have an elective CS.
- All mothers in the medium risk group should be seen from the mid second trimester by a multidisciplinary team, including an obstetric anaesthetist.
- The obstetric anaesthetist should then see the mother again at 32–34 weeks where plans can be modified depending on how the mother is coping with pregnancy, and a more detailed description of anaesthetic plans given to her.

Categorization of medium risk women

- NYHA 2 or greater at the start of pregnancy: any cardiac lesion.
- Deteriorating NYHA: any cardiac lesion.
- Continuing episodes of symptomatic cardiac ischaemia.
- Moderately impaired left ventricular function: ejection fraction (EF) <40%.
- Treated heart failure or pulmonary oedema.
- Episodes of symptomatic dysrhythmias.
- Palliative or partial correction of congenital heart disease.
- Partial correction of tetralogy of Fallot without cyanosis.
- Mustard's or Senning's procedure for transposition of the great vessels.
- Cardiomyopathy with mild to moderate ventricular impairment.
- Congenital, e.g. hypertrophic cardiomyopathy.
- Acquired, e.g. peripartum cardiomyopathy or secondary to viral infection or multisystem disease.
- Moderately stenotic lesions of the aortic (valve area 1–2cm^2), pulmonary or mitral valves.

- In many situations, a routine low dose epidural for labour analgesia is a safe and appropriate choice, with pulse oximetry and non-invasive BP for monitoring.
- If a mother needs an emergency CS, the different physiological demands resulting from an extensive and dense regional block, a GA or blood loss more commonly associated with emergency caesarean delivery often requires a greater level of experience and monitoring than can routinely be provided in many smaller hospitals.
- The major demands on this level of service provision are problems that arise outside office hours, even if an elective CS/delivery is planned.

High risk cardiac disease

These mothers usually deteriorate during pregnancy. The mother may present in the first or the early part of the second trimester with heart failure, where termination of pregnancy may be necessary, or she may need delivery, usually by CS, early in the third trimester when the baby is viable.

- These mothers have many complex problems.
- They will need to be seen every 2 weeks in the second trimester and weekly in the third trimester.

- They may need to be admitted to a high dependency area in hospital (Coronary Care Unit) for monitoring and bed rest at any time during their pregnancy.

Categorization of high risk women

- NYHC 3 or 4.
- Primary pulmonary hypertension.
- Secondary pulmonary hypertension.
  - Eisenmenger syndrome (cyanotic congenial heart disease with increasing pulmonary hypertension eventually causing reversal of the shunt).
  - Chronic veno-occlusive disease associated with antiphospholipid syndrome and other connective tissue diseases.
- Cyanotic congenital heart disease not associated with pulmonary hypertension.
- Palliative shunts from vena cava to pulmonary artery.
- Severely impaired ventricular function, EF <30%.
- Severe mitral or aortic stenosis (valvular area <1cm^2) especially if associated with pulmonary oedema, angina, dysrhythmias and collapse.

Haematological

Referrals should include those on anticoagulant medication for previous thromboembolism or thrombophilia, and patients with an abnormality of coagulation, e.g. idiopathic thrombocytopenia, von Willebrand's disease, factor deficiencies, etc.

- A history of the condition needs to be taken together with current haematological input.
- The appropriateness of regional anaesthesia needs to be determined. If contraindicated, alternative methods of pain relief should be discussed, particularly patient-controlled IV opioid analgesia.
- An assessment of the patient's airway is important in case GA is required for operative delivery.
- Close liaison with a haematologists is generally required.

Plan to include

- If regional anaesthesia is considered.
  - Absolute contraindications in bleeding disorders.
  - Timing of regional techniques relating to anticoagulation administration.
  - Timing of epidural catheter removal.
- Requirement for investigations on admission in labour/for CS.
- Documentation of the level of hematological support required on admission.
- Requirement for IV access.
- Assessment of the increased risk of PPH.
- Plan for postpartum oxytocin infusion.
- Whether NSAIDs are contraindicated.

Respiratory

The most common respiratory problem is severe asthma, but with advances in treatment more women with cystic fibrosis are becoming pregnant. It is important to obtain:

- A detailed medication history.
- The level of activity prior to pregnancy.
- Admissions to hospital/ICU.
- Pulmonary function tests may be useful and should be arranged in good time.

Patients should be encouraged to take maintenance medications as some will avoid taking drugs whilst pregnant.

Plan to include

- Continuation of regular medications. May need extra steroid cover for labour where appropriate.
- Benefits of regional analgesia and anaesthesia. Epidurals to be encouraged, particularly in severe asthmatics. GA for operative delivery may be poorly tolerated.
- Explain the relative problems of Entonox use—it has a drying effect on bronchial secretions if taken over a prolonged period.

Neurological

Women with ongoing or quiescent neurological disease should be assessed, so that a detailed description of the problem can be obtained and full documentation of any neurological deficit made.

- Many women and anaesthetists are fearful that regional anaesthesia is contraindicated or may make the condition worse. A detailed discussion with documentation is required.
- Where there is evidence of current or previous space-occupying lesions, intracranial haemorrhage or infarction, an assessment for evidence of raised intracranial pressure (ICP) must be undertaken.
- Results of recent investigations, e.g. computed tomography (CT) or MRI brain are essential with a history of recent intracranial pathology.
- Input from a neurologist or neurosurgeon may be required before a decision regarding anaesthetic management is made.

Multiple sclerosis

- Patients with a history of multiple sclerosis frequently present to the obstetric anaesthetist.
- The history should elicit medication, respiratory compromise and details of any episodes of relapse.
- A detailed neurological examination is required.
- The patient should be counselled regarding the risks and benefits of regional anaesthesia, together with the chance of relapse with or without an anaesthetic procedure.
- There is no convincing evidence that either general or regional anaesthesia has any influence on the incidence of relapse.
- An informed choice with full documentation of what is discussed is important.

Spinal disease

Spina bifida

- History, neurological examination and documentation are required.
- The level of the defect can be assessed by examination, but the level of the termination of the spinal cord cannot be known without an MRI scan; it may be low due to tethering even in occulta.
- An MRI scan is the gold standard investigation and can be performed in pregnancy. It should be carried out in the second trimester, if possible, because the mother may not be able to lie comfortably and safely on her back in the scanner as pregnancy progresses.
- An MRI scan may be appropriate if the mother is very anxious about pain relief in labour or if she is at high risk of GA.
- A decision regarding appropriateness of regional anaesthesia is dependent on the above. The airway should be assessed in case GA is required.
- Patient-controlled analgesia (PCA) should be discussed with her if regional techniques are contraindicated.

Lumbar disc surgery

- At what spinal level was surgery carried out?
- Was any metal work inserted?
- Previous investigations such as X-rays or MRI.
- Examination to reveal level of scar and neurological deficit.
- Are there any ongoing pain problems?

Plan to include

- Is regional anaesthesia contraindicated?
  - Spinal anaesthesia can usually be performed through a scar if necessary.
  - Epidurals should be inserted away from a visible scar, i.e. one or preferably two interspaces above the site of surgery. This avoids dural puncture as there is a risk of tethering of the dura to the ligamentum flavum due to scar formation.
- Patients should be warned of the increased difficulty of insertion and potential failure due to inadequate spread of LA in the epidural space.
- There is an increased risk of dural puncture with epidural insertion.
- Spinal anaesthesia is generally easier and usually works well, and the patient should be reassured.

Scoliosis

- Assess degree of thoracic and lumbar curvature.
- Determine position of the midline and the presence of palpable spaces.
- Check for neurological dysfunction.
- Is there any respiratory compromise?
- What is the extent of surgery (thoracic/lumbar) and are there anterior or posterior fixation devices?
- Old scans/X-rays are useful.

Plan to include

- Whether regional anaesthesia is contraindicated.
- May require a senior experienced anaesthetist.
- Documentation of any increased risk of inadequate block/failure.
- **Controversial**: epidural may be contraindicated with metal work because of the theoretical risk of introducing infection.

Obesity

The prevalence of obesity is increasing in developed countries, and many patients do not understand the reasons for their attendance at an anaesthetic clinic. This needs to be discussed with care.

- The history should determine any associated antepartum medical disease, e.g. diabetes, hypertension, pre-eclampsia, and whether there has been a history of previous regional anaesthesia.
- Examination should focus on:
  - Venous access.
  - Airway assessment.
  - Anatomy of the back with attention to fat distribution.

It should be explained to the mother:

- Why regional techniques can be difficult and may take time to establish.
- Why GA should ideally be avoided. (The mother should not be frightened into thinking that GA is absolutely contraindicated, as technical failure of regional anaesthesia is common and GA is then the only option.)

Plan to include

- Epidural analgesia is strongly encouraged.
- Epidural may be more difficult to insert with an increased failure rate.
- A written reminder to the on-call anaesthetist that the epidural block should be regularly assessed, re-sited early if inadequate and kept topped up to reduce the risk of GA.
- Early call for senior help if GA is anticipated.
- Non-invasive BP measurement may be unreliable, and an arterial line may be required.
- Risk of PPH is increased.
- Thromboprophylaxis postdelivery is important, and an increased dose may be needed.

Principles of pain management during pregnancy

Poorly controlled pain during pregnancy is associated with self-medication behaviour and, untreated, may induce preterm labour.

Ways of minimizing fetal risk

- Use non-pharmacological options if possible.
- Consider LA infiltration or nerve blocks.
- Avoid drugs during gestation weeks 4–10 (organogenesis) and just before delivery.
- Multimodal and multidisciplinary approach.
- Expect pains to vary in their responsiveness to opioids.
- Combine drugs that act on different receptors.
- Concomitant use of physiotherapy, psychology and complementary medicine.
- Prevent progression to chronic pain.
- Control acute pain adequately and escalate doses.
- Treat any neuropathic component to the pain.
- Treat any psychological vulnerability (poor coping strategies).
- Logical use of analgesics.
- Use slow-release analgesics if pain is constant.
- Use quick-release analgesics for activity-related pain prior to aggravating activity.
- Address sleep disturbance.
- Make realistic goals.

Generic pathway for pain management in pregnancy

Step 1: assessment

- Onset: acute or injury related?—Establish specific diagnosis.
- Flare up of chronic condition?—Escalate usual medication.
- Associated focal tenderness?—Suitable for injection.
- Suitable for physiotherapy?—Spinal or pelvic pain.
- Pain activity or incident related—Short-acting analgesia.
- Pain constant—Slow release analgesia.
- Neuropathic component (burning, shooting, stabbing)—Go to step 5.

Step 2: physiotherapy

Step 3: local anaesthetic ± steroid injection

- Focal areas of tenderness, e.g. myofascial pain, trigger points, abdominal nerve entrapment.
- Spinal pain, e.g. facet joints, paravertebral muscles, sacroiliac joints, coccyx.
- Pelvic pain, e.g. pubic symphysis.

Step 4: systemic analgesia

(a) Short acting

First level

- Paracetamol 1g 6hly (max 4g/day).

Second level: (combine with weak opioid)

- Codeine/paracetamol combination (co-codamol 8/500) 6hly.
- Tramadol/paracetamol combination (Tramacet® 32.5/325) 6hly.

Third level: (escalate weak opioid)

- Tramadol 50–100mg 6hly.
- Codeine/paracetamol (co-codamol 30/500) 6hly.

(b) Slow release

First level: (weak opioid)

- Buprenorphine 5–10 micrograms/h 7-day patch.
- Tramadol MR 50mg BD.

Second level: (moderate opioid)

- Buprenorphine 20 micrograms/h 7-day patch.
- Buprenorphine 35 micrograms/h every 3 days.
- Fentanyl patch 12 micrograms/h every 3 days.

Third level: (strong opioid)

- Fentanyl 25–50 micrograms/h 3-day patch.
- Oxycodene MR 10–20mg BD.

Step 5: neuropathic medication

First level

- Gabapentin 100mg TID escalate up to 600mg TID.
- Combine with paracetamol and weak opioid.
- Consider topical capsaicin 0.025 or 0.075%.
- Consider lidocaine patch 5%.

Second level

- Add in amitriptyline (second and third trimesters only).

Third level

- Add in strong opioid (slow release).
- Consider methadone (long half-life).

Pain therapies

Non-pharmacological techniques

Heat and cold

Local application of heat or cold can be effective in muscular and myofascial pain. Cool gel pads have been found effective in perineal pain after delivery.

Transcutaneous electrical nerve stimulation (TENS)

There is little evidence to support the use of TENS in pregnancy. It has been shown to reduce analgesic consumption in chronic pain patients, and retrospective studies have reported benefit in 70% of patients who purchased TENS units.

Pregnant women as a group are very motivated and may be satisfied with its moderate effect.

TENS may be useful in:
- Spinal pain.
- Myofascial pain.
- Nerve entrapments.
- Pelvic arthropathy.

Most pain management services offer Clinical Nurse Specialist TENS clinics who will advise on the appropriate settings for the TENS unit.

Acupuncture

It is prudent to avoid acupuncture in the first trimester when pregnancy loss is high. Acupuncturists are cautious in pregnancy, although the procedure is widely used in China. There are studies and case reports to support the use of acupuncture for low back and pelvic pain in pregnancy; six or more treatments are required. There is no consensus about the exact 'forbidden points' in pregnancy as different schools and authors vary.

- Avoid direct trauma over the gravid uterus.
- Needling depth and orientation are critical.
- Avoid increasing sympathetic tone by excess stimulation.

Acupuncture during pregnancy is a specialist area and should only be carried out by a qualified and experienced acupuncturist.

Physiotherapy in pregnancy

Physiotherapy has been reported mainly for low back and pelvic pain. Effective reported therapies include:

- Exercise programmes—land and water based.
- Back care classes.
- Postural feedback.
- Massage and relaxation.
- Sacroiliac belts.
- Uterine support pillows.

Physical therapy is effective for pain-associated muscle spasm and maintaining core stability.

Psychology in chronic pain management

Psychology plays a key role in improving coping strategies and maintaining function. Effective techniques include:

- Coping strategies.
- Goal setting and pacing.
- Relaxation.
- Cognitive therapy (negative thoughts).
- EMDR (eye movement de-sensitization and reprocessing).

Patients suitable for referral have poor coping skills, pain behaviour and disproportionate suffering.

Safety of pain drugs used in pregnancy

Categorizing fetal risk

The following categorization of drugs according to fetal risk is adapted from the Australian Drug Evaluation Committee (ADEC) recommendations.

Category	Classification of fetal risk
A	Drugs that have been taken by a large number of pregnant women without proven fetal harm
B	Drugs taken by limited number of pregnant women without proven fetal harm:
	B1 Animal studies have not proven fetal harm
	B2 Animal studies lacking, but available data do not suggest fetal harm
	B3 Animal studies have proven fetal harm, but significance in humans uncertain
C	Have caused harmful fetal effects (pharmacological) but not malformations
D	High risk of fetal damage, only use in exceptional circumstances
X	Very high risk of fetal harm. Don't use in pregnancy

Local anaesthetics and depo-steroids

Bupivacaine/lidocaine (Category A)

Usual dose range for injection in pain management is 2–5mL of 0.25% levobupivacaine or 1% lidiocaine.

Depo-steroid (Category A) (methylprednisolone)

Usual dose for injection is 5–10mg per injection combined with LA. Usual total dose of methylprednisiolone per treatment is 40mg. Treatment intervals usually 4–6 months.

The analgesic effect can outlast the duration of the LA.

Analgesics in pregnancy

Paracetamol (Category A)

Paracetamol has been used since 1893. It is routinely used throughout pregnancy. At therapeutic doses there have been no known teratogenic effects and it is considered safe. When maternal toxic levels are reached, facial cleft, spina bifida and pyloric stenosis have been reported. The fetus is also at risk of toxicity as paracetamol crosses the placenta, as does the antidote, *N*-acetylcysteine.

Aspirin (Category C)

Aspirin has found to be problematic in pregnancy. Commonly self-administered. Consumption during pregnancy may produce anaemia, haemorrhage, prolonged gestation and labour, stillbirth and pre-eclampsia. There is conflicting evidence of the safety of fetal exposure.

Low dose aspirin (40–150mg/day) is used to treat thrombophilia syndromes to reduce the incidence of fetal loss. No fetal abnormalities have been reported after chronic low dose exposure.

The use of high dose aspirin (rheumatological conditions) in the second half of pregnancy is more controversial.

The main concerns are:

- Bleeding during delivery (maternal and fetal).
- Premature closure of the ductus arteriosis.
- Oligohydramnios.

NSAIDs (Category C)

NSAIDs such as indometacin, ibuprofen, naproxen, diclofenac or ketoprofen are not considered teratogenic in humans.

These drugs are used for their antiprostaglandin effects in both rheumatological and myofascial pain syndromes. Ibuprofen has been studied the most in pregnancy; its use has been reported in >100 pregnancies without congenital abnormalities. In usual doses (300–600mg/day), ibuprofen is considered safe in pregnancy. However, persistent pulmonary hypertension has been reported in neonates following fetal exposure.

Higher does (ankylosing spondylitis, rheumatoid arthritis) during the third trimester may cause premature closure of the ductus arteriosis particularly in preterm labour. It is recommended that they are discontinued in the 32nd gestational week.

Opioids (Category C)

These include tramadol, oxycodone, fentanyl and buprenorphine.

Experience of opioids in pregnancy comes from opioid abuse patients who become pregnant. Animal teratogenicity and fetal loss have been reported.

Overall, opioids are considered safe in pregnancy. Opioid use has been linked with low birth weight and strabismus in babies, and possibly associated with schizophrenia in adult life.

Prolonged antenatal exposure risks neonatal withdrawal syndrome; there is some evidence that neonatal withdrawal may not occur with buprenorphine.

Codeine (Category A) is commonly self-administered. Prolonged use of codeine has caused codeine withdrawal in neonates. Up to 9% of adults and 40% of children cannot metabolize codeine to morphine and it is therefore an ineffective analgesic in these patients.

Tramadol (Category C) has been shown to be embryotoxic and fetotoxic in mice, rats and rabbits at maternally toxic doses 3–15 times the maximum human dose or higher. No harm to the fetus due to tramadol was seen at doses that were not maternally toxic.

General advice on opioid use

Pregnant women on long-term opioids should not have them abruptly stopped. During labour and delivery, opioids should be maintained. If operative delivery arises, postoperative doses should be increased. In opioid-maintained mothers, neonatal abstinence syndrome is reported in 30–90% of neonates. Treatment with neonatal morphine (mean 10 days) is preferred to phenobarbital (mean 17 days). Infants born to opioid-maintained/tolerant mothers shouldn't be given naloxone at birth.

Neuropathic drugs

Anticonvulsants

Women who have to remain on these should be counselled on fetal risk. Monotherapy reduces fetal risk. Folic acid supplements (5mg) should be taken 4 weeks prior to and 12 weeks after conception. Regular abnormality scans should be undertaken if therapy is continued through pregnancy.

Gabapentin (Category B1). Limited human data, but no reports of teratogenicity. Usually dosing is 3 times a day. Start at 100mg TID and escalate over several weeks to reach 600mg TID. Somnolence, nausea and weight gain can occur. Normalizes sleep patterns.

Carbamazepine (Category D). 0.5–1% incidence of neural tube defects. Also associated with craniofacial and coagulation defects in the fetus. Often used as the main therapy in trigeminal neuralgia or postherpetic neuralgia at high doses of 1200–1600mg/day. Should be stopped in the first trimester and replaced with opioids (often high dose required), gabapentin or lamotrigine could be introduced from the second trimester.

Lamotrigine (Category B3). Animal teratogenicity has been reported. Lamotrigine in the first trimester has been implicated in cleft lip and palate. Not a first line drug for neuropathic pain.

Other therapies

Amitriptyline (Category C)

Use in the first trimester is associated with limb reduction abnormalities. When used in the second and third trimesters, there have been no reports of excess abnormalities. Prolonged use has led to neonatal withdrawal symptoms. Overdose is harmful to both mother and fetus. Dry mouth and somnolence can be a problem. Usual dose is 10mg at 8pm, but may be escalated up to 70mg, which is an optimum dose. Good at addressing sleep disturbance associated with pain.

Baclofen (Category B3)

Teratogenicity in animals has been reported. It is useful as a second line in trigeminal neuralgia and as a muscle relaxant in myofascial pain/fibromyalgia. Usual dose is 10mg TID. Avoid abrupt withdrawal.

Methadone (Category C)

Has a long half life and should be initiated as an inpatient. It is used off licence for resistant neuropathic pain. Usual dosing starts at 5mg once a day and escalated to TID.

Capsaicin ointment

Fetal risk has not been categorized, but no human teratogenicity has been reported. Available in 0.025 and 0.075% for topical use in diabetic neuropathy and postherpetic neuralgia. May also be useful in myofascial pain.

Common pain problems

Low back pain

Low back pain (LBP) is common throughout pregnancy (50%); ligamentous laxity (relaxin) is the main precipitating factor. Other risk factors are smoking, obesity and previous back pain.

Non-specific LBP

The majority of acute LBP has no cause and improves within 6–8 weeks.

Non-specific LBP is associated with radiation to the buttocks and/or knees.

Degenerative disc disease

This manifests as LBP with radiation below the knee, neurogenic claudication, intermittent numbness and/or weakness of the legs. The severity varies from 'leaking disc', to annular tear, to frank prolapse.

Red flags suggesting serious spinal pathology indicate referral for investigation; yellow flags identify barriers to early recovery suitable for psychology referral.

Red and yellow flags

Red flags: investigation required	Yellow flags: psychosocial factors indicative of long-term chronicity
Features of cauda equina syndrome	A negative attitude that back pain is harmful
Significant trauma	Fear avoidance behaviour
Weight loss	An expectation that passive treatment is necessary
History of cancer	A tendency to depression, low morale and social withdrawal
Fever	Social or financial problems
Possibility of HIV	
Steroid use	
Under 20yrs of age	
Severe night pain	
Pain worse when lying down	

Management

- Maintain mobility (no more than 2 days bed rest).
- Maintain normal activity and remain at work.
- Physiotherapy: manipulation ± therapeutic exercise (limited during first week).

- Injections: trigger points, ligaments and facet joints, epidural steroid injection if nerve root pain (Pain Clinic referral).
- TENS may be useful.

Systemic analgesia: use slow release if pain constant; if activity related use short-acting analgesia. Escalate as per generic pathway.

Diazepam 2mg TID (Category C) for short periods only—for pain-associated muscle spasm.

Acupuncture is not effective in acute LBP. Traction and lumbar corsets are not effective.

Acute prolapsed disc

In pregnancy this is rare (1:10 000). Most patients can be treated conservatively, but those with incapacitating pain, progressive neurological deficits, or bowel or bladder dysfunction may require an MRI and surgical treatment.

Chronic back pain ± leg pain

This is managed with a combination of opioids, LA/steroid injections, physiotherapy and psychological support. Postpartum assessment for invasive pain interventions should be considered.

Headache (migraine)

- Worst in the first trimester, but often improves in the second and third trimesters.
- Prevention with acupuncture and biofeedback are useful.
- Metoprolol and propranolol only in exceptional circumstances.

Acute attacks can be managed using a combination of

- Acupuncture.
- Relaxation and sleep.
- Massage.
- Ice packs/gel pads.
- Biofeedback.

Analgesia is limited to paracetamol ± codeine and ibuprofen for short periods (avoid third trimester). If severe, consider moderate opioid.

Nausea can be managed with ondansetron (Category B1) or prochlorperazine (Category C).

Triptans *and ergot* derivatives are contraindicated.

Abdominal nerve entrapment

A rapidly enlarging uterus can lead to pain and paraesthesia from cutaneous nerves that traverse the rectus muscles or inguinal ligaments. Skin sensitivity and irritating sensations occur.

Common problem sites are

- Abdominal wall (tender points along costal margins).
- Ilioinguinal nerve.
- Genitofemoral nerve.
- Lateral cutaneous nerve of thigh (meralgia paraesthetica).

Symptomatic relief may be achieved with

- LA injections. Tender points around the course of nerves should be sought and injected. The addition of steroids may benefit, but sometimes can make matters worse.
- TENS.
- Ice packs/gel pads.
- Gabapentin ± amitriptyline (not first trimester).

Carpel tunnel syndrome

Compression of either median or ulnar nerves can occur. Paraesthesia is common and pain is experienced in 50% of patients. Exclude pre-eclampsia and heart failure as a cause. Cases presenting postpartum are more likely to need surgery.

- Remove rings and bracelets.
- Elevate hand at night.
- Night-time splint.
- Paracetamol (NSAIDs worsen fluid retention).
- Rarely, surgical release (under regional block).

Pelvic arthropathy

With an incidence of 1:600, this can present during or after pregnancy. Ligament relaxation allows widening of pubic symphysis gap and lumbosacral joints. Ultrasound can be used to measure symphyseal gap.

- Bed rest.
- Acupuncture.
- Physiotherapy.
- Pelvic binders.
- Short-acting analgesia prior to walking (reduces muscle spasm).
- Treat associated neuropathic pain (common).
- Rarely, surgery is required postpartum.

Ureteric obstruction

This often manifests in the second and third trimesters as the enlarging uterus compresses the ureters as they cross the pelvic brim.
Helped by:

- Adopting hand–knee position.
- Paracetamol/Ibuprofen/weak opioid.

Neuropathic pain (NeP)

There are >100 causes of NeP, with varying degrees of neuropathic and nociceptive components:

Purely neuropathic pain	Partially neuropathic pain	Neuropathic component to pain
Postherpectic neuralgia	Atypical facial pain	Fibromyalgia
Diabetic neuropathy	Post-laminectomy pain	Chronic fatigue syndrome
Trigeminal neuralgia	Complex regional pain syndrome	Chronic daily headache
Phantom limb	Postoperative neuralgia	Whiplash injury

Patients with NeP complain of burning or shooting pain, usually unresponsive to the usual pain killers. Skin sensitivity may be present or there are areas of numbness that are painful. Sleep disturbance is common, as are depressive thoughts.

Management is usually a combination of

- *Opioids*: high doses are usually required.
- *Amitriptyline*: 10mg at night escalated to 70mg over 6 weeks.
- *Anticonvulsants*: try and avoid in the first trimester. Monotherapy only—gabapentin or lamotrigine considered safest. Folic acid, and abnormality scans recommended if used.
- *Topical agents*: can be used in postherpetic neuralgia and painful diabetic neuropathy.
  - Lidocaine 5% patch.
  - Capsaicin ointment.

Common pain problems in the puerperium

Perineal pain

This is common after childbirth and persists for a few weeks.

- Cold gel pads or cold/warm baths.
- Paracetamol.
- NSAIDs topical, oral or suppository.
- No proven benefit with LA/steroid injections or ultrasound therapy.

Uterine pain (after pains)

These are a consequence of oxytocin release and common in parous women.

- Paracetamol.
- NSAIDs.

Breast pain

This is common and a frequent reason for stopping breastfeeding. Midwives should assess for infant and lactation problems and advise on preventing breast engorgement.

- Infective mastitis is treated with flucloxacillin and NSAIDs.
- Non-infective mastitis is treated with NSAIDs alone.
- Cabbage leaves and ultrasound are no better than placebo.

Caesarean wound pain (postoperative neuralgia)

Can be problematic and is often associated with areas of sensitivity on the skin of the lower abdomen and areas of numbness around the surgical wound. The pain can be disabling during the first few weeks after delivery. Most cases resolve within a few months. The aetiology is thought to be due to irritation of nerves that pass through the rectus sheath.

- LA injections to tender points in the abdominal wall (steroid can worsen).
- Therapy for 6 weeks with pregabalin or gabapentin.
- Slow release moderate opioid.

Analgesics during lactation

Non-opioids

Paracetamol

Neonatal exposure to paracetamol is estimated to be 2% of the maternal dose. This is considered safe as it is would be below the infant dose of 10mg/kg.

NSAIDs

NSAIDs are considered safe. Ibuprofen has the least neonatal transfer. Diclofenac is also considered safe, with slightly more neonatal transfer.

Indometacin

This has been associated with maternal postpartum psychosis and is not advised.

Aspirin

Aspirin should not be used during breastfeeding because of the risk of Reyes syndrome.

Local anaesthetics

These have acceptably low transfer into breast milk.

Opioids

Opioids are considered safe, most being transferred into breast milk in low doses. Only pethidine has been implicated in neonatal effects; repeated dosing can cause accumulation of the metabolite, norpethidine, in the infant.

Opioids should be avoided in the first week of life in mothers whose babies exhibit episodes of apnoea.

Neonatal exposure to opioids used after CS is ~6%; however, the bioavailability is only 25% in the infant after oral intake.

Further reading

Australian Drug Evaluation Committee. *Prescribing Medicines in Pregnancy*, 4th edn. Canberra: Australian Drug Evaluation Committee, 1999. Copyright Commonwealth of Australia.

Ilett KF, Kristensen JH. Drug use and breastfeeding (Review). *Expert Opinion on Drug Safety* 2005; **4**: 745–768.

Rathmell JP *et al.* Management of nonobstetric pain during pregnancy and lactation (Review). *Anesthia and Analgesia* 1997; **85**: 1074–1087.

Wunsch MJ *et al.* Treatment of pain in pregnancy (Review). *Clinical Journal of Pain* 2003; **19**: 148–155.

Chapter 6

Non-regional labour analgesia

Sarah Harries and Matthew Turner

Pain in labour

Labour presents a physiological and psychological challenge for women. The latter stages of pregnancy can be a difficult time emotionally. Fear and apprehension are experienced alongside excitement. These emotions, both positive and negative, will affect the woman's birth experience.

Pain associated with labour has been described by Melzack as one of the most intense forms of pain that can be experienced. However, removing pain completely from labour does not necessarily mean a better birth experience for the mother. Women need to be included in the decisions regarding their individualized pain management plan. Providing clear information about the types of pain relief available has been found to increase feelings of control.

Women may now choose to deliver their baby in different places, e.g consultant-led units, midwife-led units or at home, depending on their risk assessment and the mother's own wishes. This ultimately means that not all options will be immediately available for all women. Information regarding the options for pain relief offered at each site should be made readily available to all expectant mothers during pregnancy and discussed in detail during the third trimester.

Pain pathways

- Pain during the first stage of labour is initially due to contraction of the body of the uterus, leading to dilatation of the cervix and lower uterine segment, and their subsequent distension and tearing during uterine contractions.
- The pain is visceral in nature and is therefore diffuse or poorly localized, often referred to another area, e.g. the back, and can be associated with profound nausea or vomiting.
- The intensity of pain is related to the speed of cervical dilatation and the strength of uterine contractions.
- Pain impulses during the first stage of labour are transmitted via afferent A and small C fibres from the uterus and cervix to the thoracolumbar sympathetic chain through T10, T11, T12 and L1 spinal nerves, and through their posterior roots enter the dorsal horn neurons of the spinal cord.
- Pain during the latter part of the first stage and the second stage of labour results from continuing uterine contractions and, in addition, pain and pressure related to stretching of the vagina and pelvic floor to accommodate the presenting part.
- This pain is more somatic in nature and is therefore well localized, often sharp, definite, not referred, constant and not usually associated with nausea.
- Pain impulses during the second stage are transmitted via the pudendal nerve and into the spinal cord via S2, S3 and S4 spinal nerve roots.

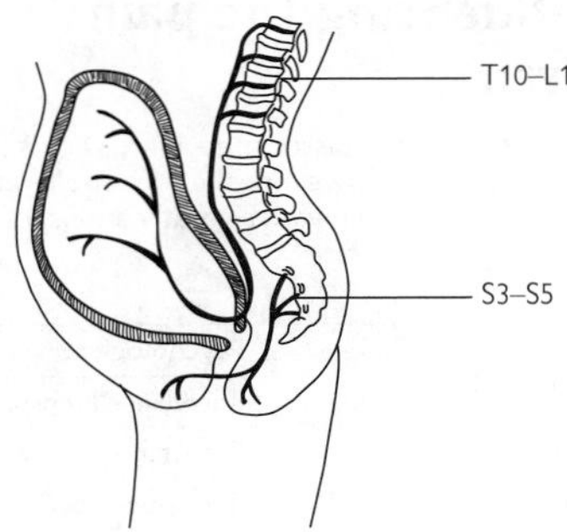

Fig. 6.1 Pain pathways of labour.

Effect of pain on maternal physiology

Labour places massive physical demands upon both mother and fetus. Some of those demands are directly related to pain and can therefore be lessened by effective analgesia.

The CO increases by 25–50% in labour, as a result of tachycardia secondary to pain and increased circulating catecholamines.

- Epidural analgesia has been shown to reduce cardiac index by 3–6%, and mean arterial pressure (MAP) by 1–9% (not influenced by fluid preload).
- This is of particular importance to the parturient with cardiac disease.

The increased minute ventilation associated with labour pain results in a decrease in maternal $PaCO_2$, i.e. <3kPa, which is below the already physiologically low levels of late pregnancy. Hypocapnoea leads to maternal alkalosis with a shift in the haemoglobin A (HbA) oxyhaemaglobin curve to the *left*, i.e. less O_2 is released to fetal haemoglobin (HbF) and less CO_2 taken up by HbA. The fetus is at risk of becoming hypercapnoeic and hypoxic in this environment.

- Effective analgesia aims to return the maternofetal acid–base balance to the term status quo.

Factors influencing the pain of childbirth

For most women, childbirth is associated with very severe pain, often exceeding all expectations. However, the threshold at which women perceive differing intensity of pain varies greatly and is influenced by many physical and psychological factors:

Physical	Psychological
Age	Knowledge/preparation for childbirth
Parity	Expectation of pain
Size of infant/birth canal	Prior pain experiences
Abnormal fetal presentation	Fear and anxiety
Speed of cervical dilatation	Confidence to cope
Frequency of contractions	Supportive birthing partner
Stage of labour	Education and social class
Maternal position in labour	Culture and beliefs

Pain during dysfunctional labour

- Increased intensity of pain may indicate that the labour is not progressing as expected.
- Dysfunctional labour or dystocia in labour is associated with increased pain and therefore the woman should be reassessed for evidence of cephalopelvic disproportion, a macrosomic baby or an abnormal presenting part, e.g. brow or face presentation.
- Women with dysfunctional labour are more likely to request an early epidural.
- Uterine rupture should be excluded if a woman suffers continuous abdominal pain or breakthrough pain despite an adequate epidural analgesic block.

Information

- Women need comprehensive information about the various analgesic choices that are available in their place of delivery.
- Not having their choice of analgesia available to them causes maternal dissatisfaction.
- Many women will attend local midwifery-run classes, and analgesic options will be discussed.
- The midwives running these classes need up to date information on locally available epidural services and protocols.
- Alternatively, locally produced leaflets can be made available in the antenatal clinic which describe in detail the pros and cons of the different analgesic techniques and their local availability. These are particularly useful for those mothers not attending antenatal classes.
- Many women will now use the Internet to supplement information from midwives.
- Reliable and accurate information on all forms of pain relief can be found at:
  - www.oaa-anaes.ac.uk
  - www.midirs.org

Non-pharmacological options

The Complementary Medicine Field of The Cochrane Collaboration defines complementary medicine as 'practices and ideas which are outside the domain of conventional medicine in several countries', and is defined by its users as 'preventing or treating illness, or promoting health and well being' (Cochrane Collaboration, 2003).

- The use of complementary and alternative medicine has become popular with consumers worldwide, often with little or no evidence to support their use.
- Complementary therapies are more commonly used by women of reproductive age, with almost half reporting use. It is possible that a significant proportion of women are using these therapies during pregnancy.
- Many women would like to avoid pharmacological or invasive methods of pain relief in labour. This may contribute towards the popularity of complementary methods of pain management.
- It is important for the obstetric anaesthetist to be familiar with complementary techniques and therapies in order that the efficacy and limitations of therapies might be discussed.

Categories of therapies

- Psychological support
  e.g. partner/midwife continuous support, doula.
- Mind–body interventions
  e.g. breathing, hypnosis, yoga, relaxation therapies.
- Alternative medical practice
  e.g. homeopathy, traditional Chinese medicine.
- Manual handling methods
  e.g. massage, reflexology.
- Physiological and biological treatments
  e.g. TENS, waterblocks.
- Bioelectromagnetic applications
  e.g. magnets.
- Water immersion.

Mind–body interventions

- Was popularized by Grantly Dick-Read after publication of his book 'Natural childbirth' in 1933 and 'Childbirth without fear' in 1944.
- He postulated that the pain of childbirth was largely a product of modern living, leading to a cycle of fear, tension and pain.
- Relaxation, meditation, visualization and breathing are commonly used for labour and are widely accessible through teaching during antenatal classes.
- Yoga, meditation and hypnosis may have a calming effect and provide a distraction from pain and tension.

Aromatherapy

- Essential oils are used, drawing on the healing power of plants. The oils may be massaged into the skin, or inhaled using a steam infusion or burner.
- The mechanism of action of aromatherapy is unclear. Studies have demonstrated psychological improvement in mood and anxiety levels.

Acupuncture

- Fine needles are inserted into different parts of the body. The points used to reduce labour pain are located on the hands, feet and ears.
- Acupressure involves applying pressure on the acupuncture point. The aim is to treat illness and soothe pain by stimulating the specific points.

Homeopathy

- Works on the principle that 'like cures like'. Remedies are prescribed as potencies as a result of tiny and highly diluted amounts of the substances from which they are derived. The more times the substance is diluted, the greater the potency. Remedies are derived from herbs, minerals and other natural substances.
- The principle of treatment is that the substance will stimulate the body and healing functions, so achieving a state of balance with relief of symptoms. It is proposed that homeopathy enables the woman in labour to cope, to soothe and relax her, which may reduce her pain.

Massage

- Massage is commonly used to help relax tense muscles and soothe and calm the individual.
- Massage may help to relieve pain in labour by inhibiting pain signals or by improving blood flow and oxygenation of tissues. Different massage techniques may help different women.

Reflexology

- Reflexologists propose that there are reflex points on the feet corresponding to organs and structures of the body.
- Pain may be reduced by gentle manipulation on certain parts of the foot.
- Pressure applied to the feet has been shown to result in an anaesthetizing effect on other parts of the body.

Cochrane 2003, Authors Conclusions

'The data available suggest hypnosis and acupuncture may be helpful therapies for pain management in labour. The efficacy of aromatherapy, audio-analgesia, bio-feedback and music have not been established'.

Transcutaneous electrical nerve stimulation (TENS)

- Widely accepted by mothers and midwives for pain relief during labour, because of its lack of side effects for mother and fetus.
- Often used in late third trimester to treat LBP or in early labour.
- Four pads are positioned over the lower back and a low voltage electrical current is transmitted constantly to the underlying skin with a 'boost' during uterine contractions.

- Mechanism of action is based on the 'gate theory of pain'.
- Probably most effective in the latent or early phase of labour.
- Allows the mother to mobilize, which may be beneficial and increase its acceptability.
- Meta-analysis failed to demonstrate its efficacy as an analgesic.

Water blocks

- Popular in Scandinavian countries.
- 0.1mL of sterile water is injected intradermally in four spots over the sacrum.
- Intense burning seems to induce pain relief.
- The mechanism is probably similar to TENS.

Water immersion

- The sensation of warm water may soothe the pain of labour.
- The water supports the weight of the gravid uterus.
- The upright posture naturally adopted by the mother may be beneficial to the progress of labour.
- There is some evidence that pain is less and the use of epidurals is reduced in those women who choose water immersion.

Non-pharmacological—summary

Table 6.1 Non-pharmacological options—advantages and disadvantages

Therapy	Advantages	Disadvantages
TENS	Non-invasive, easy to use. Good for back pain	Useful only in early labour. Availability
Immersion	Popular. Backed by Government initiative	Availability. Cannot be used with many other methods
Massage	Perceived as highly effective	Labour intensive
Acupuncture	Drug free	Invasive. Needs trained therapist
Water blocks	Easy to perform. Good for back pain	Temporary relief only (<90min). Initial burning
Continuous support	Almost universal use. Useful at any stage	None
Hypnosis	Non-invasive	Not all susceptible. Time consuming
Aromatherapy	Non-invasive	Oils need to be tested
Homeopathy	Few	Needs individual 'prescription'

TENS = Transcutaneous electrical nerve stimulation.

Table 6.2 Mechanism of action and evidence

Therapy	Mechanism of action	Evidence
TENS	Based on gate theory	Systematic review of 8 RCTs failed to demonstrate analgesic effect
Immersion	Sensation of warm water inhibits pain transmission. Supports gravid uterus	Cochrane review of 3 trials found no difference in pain relief between immersion and non-immersion groups
Massage	Inhibits pain transmission. Provides support and distraction	One RCT with 28 women found physical and emoti-otional benefits
Acupuncture	May inhibit pain transmission by neural method (gate theory) or by release of endorphins or endogenous opioids	One RCT in Sweden comparing acupuncture with no acupuncture found former needed less anal-gesia including epidurals

Table 6.2 (*Contd.*)

Water blocks	Injection of 0.1mL sterile water in 4 spots over sacrum. Action similar to TENS	Two double-blind RCTs showed reduction in labour pain, but other work showed they were not rated by women as effective as other methods
Continuous support	Presence of a trained support person can improve the physiological and psychological aspects of labour, e.g. partner, friend or doula (a doula is a professional non-medical support and advocate)	Cochrane review of 15 RCTs involving 12 791 women. Those with continuous support, as opposed to conventional care, were less likely to have interpartum analgesia, operative birth or be dissatisfied with their experiences
Hypnosis	Hypnotic state has better control over pain	Cochrane review of 3 RCTs. One: less anaesthesia; one: less narcotics; overall: no difference in need for pain releif
Aromatherapy	Essential oils for therapeutic effect	One small RCT (ginger vs lemongrass) found no difference in pain scores
Homeopathy	Minute amount of substance to relieve symptoms	No research

TENS = Transcutaneous electrical nerve stimulation; RCT = Randomized controlled trial.

Further reading

Smith CA, Collins CT, Cyna AM, Crowther CA. Complementary and alternative therapies for pain management in labour. *Cochrane Database of Systematic Reviews*. 2006 Issue 2. John Wiley and Sons, Ltd.

Fortescue C, Wee MYK. Analgesia in labour: non regional techniques. *Continuing Education in Anaesthesia, Critical Care and Pain* 2005; **5**: 9–13.

Carroll D, Tramer M, McQuay H, Nye B, Moore A. TENS in labour pain: a systematic review. *British Journal of Obstetrics and Gynaecology* 1997; **104**: 169–175.

Cluett ER, Nikodem VC, McCandlish RE, Burns EE. Immersion in water in pregnancy, labour and birth. *Cochrane Database of Systematic Reviews* 2002.

Systemic opioids

The use of IM or IV opioids to reduce the pain of labour is common and widely accepted by mothers. When regional analgesia is contra-indicated, it is important that alternative pain relief methods, e.g. systemic opioids, are offered to women who request them. The choice of IM opioid used in delivery units is largely historical. Pethidine and diamorphine are the most widely used in the UK.

In recent years, administration of IV opioids via a patient-controlled analgesia (PCA) device has gained increasing popularity. It has the benefit of giving the mother a degree of control over her pain relief, which may improve satisfaction.

Remifentanil is the opioid that comes closest to the ideal drug profile when used via IV PCA to manage the pain of labour, without neonatal respiratory depression being a major problem.

All opioids share the same side effect profile to differing extents:

- Dose-dependent respiratory depression of mother and neonate.
- Delayed gastric emptying, increased gastric volumes, nausea and vomiting.
- Sedation, dysphoria, euphoria and amnesia.
- Hypotension.

Pethidine

- Pethidine (meperidine) is a synthetic, weakly basic phenylpiperidine derivative, related to fentanyl and sufentanil. It is 28 times more lipid soluble than morphine. It is metabolized to the active metabolite norpethidine, which has convulsant properties and is contra-indicated in those with severe pre-eclampsia and other causes of renal impairment.
- Pethidine is bound to A_1-acid glycoprotein but readily crosses the placenta by passive diffusion and reaches equilibrium within 6min. Peak plasma concentrations in the fetus occurs 2–3h following IM injection in the mother. In the acid environment of the fetal circulation, the weak base is more ionized and thus accumulates (ion trapping).
- Pethidine was made legally available in the UK to midwives for independent use in 1950 and remains the most widely used IM opioid in labour.
- It is usually administered in two divided doses of 75–100mg, up to a maximum dose of 200mg.
- Despite widespread use, its efficacy as an analgesic has been questioned. Many obstetric anaesthetists believe its use as a labour analgesic should be abandoned.
- It does seem, however, to help the parturient cope better by other means, e.g. dysphoria, sedation, amnesia, etc.
- Several studies have found it inferior to other IM opiates (e.g. diamorphine) in terms of analgesia and its adverse effects on mother and baby.
- Respiratory depression is more common in the neonate than the mother. The babies of mothers who received pethidine have been shown to be sleepier and slower to establish feeding.

- About 10% of neonates will have a 1min Apgar score of <6 if pethidine is given 2–3h before delivery as this coincides with peak fetal concentrations. The incidence is very much reduced if given before or after this.
- The practice of not giving the mother pethidine in the second stage of labour for fear of neonatal sedation is illogical.
- Norpethidine is also found in the neonate and may contribute to sedation for several days.

Diamorphine

- Diamorphine is more soluble and has a more rapid onset of action than morphine or pethidine.
- After administration it is rapidly hydrolysed to 6-monoacetylmorphine and then later metabolized to morphine. It is eliminated rapidly by the placenta.
- When diamorphine and pethidine were compared, patients who received pethidine were more likely to report no pain relief and the incidence of vomiting was lower in the diamorphine group. Pethidine was also associated with lower Apgar scores at 1min.
- It has been rated by both mothers and midwives as being subjectively superior to pethidine and Entonox.

Morphine

- This naturally occurring opioid is bound to albumin in the circulation and rapidly crosses the placenta.
- It is not trapped in the fetal circulation and diffuses quickly back into the maternal circulation due to rapid elimination and subsequent diffusion gradient.
- It is metabolized to an opioid agonist (morphine-6-glucoronide) and an antagonist (morphine-3-glucoronide) in varying quantities.
- It was popular in the 1920s and 1930s, and used with hyoscine to induce 'twilight sleep' for labour and delivery.
- Women frequently had little memory of labour or of being in pain.

Fentanyl

- Fentanyl is a synthetic phenylpiperidine derivative, without active metabolites. It is very lipid soluble and highly bound to albumin. It has analgesic potencies 100 × greater than morphine and 800 x greater than pethidine.
- Its high lipid solubility results in a rapid onset.
- A long (~8h) terminal half-life (longer than morphine and pethidine) will result in accumulation, in the mother and fetus, after repeated IM doses.
- IV PCA fentanyl has been investigated in two RCTs:
  - When compared with epidural anaesthesia, satisfaction was similar in the two groups (although 3/10 changed from PCA to epidural). There were no differences in Apgar scores or cord gases, but SpO_2 <90% was more common in babies of PCA mothers. The authors recommend monitoring of the fetus postnatally.
  - When compared with alfentanil, analgesia was described as inadequate in 42% of the alfentanil group and 9% of the fentanyl group.

Remifentanil

- Remifentanil is a new μ-receptor agonist that has been used in anaesthesia for less than a decade. It is a derivative of fentanyl and is described as ultra short-acting.
- It is rapidly hydrolysed by the non-saturatable red cell and tissue esterases. It has a terminal half-life of <10min and a context-sensitive half-life of ~3min.
- It was introduced into obstetric analgesia in the late 1990s, which was reflected by a number of case reports of effective analgesia in the literature.
- Various IV PCA remifentanil dosing regimes exist, e.g.
    - 0.25–0.5 micrograms/kg bolus, no background infusion, 2min lockout.
    - 20–40 micrograms bolus over 20s, no background infusion, 3min lockout.
- The optimal delivery regime has yet to be determined, but the above regimes seem the most successful.
- IV PCA remifentanil may be still considered as experimental, and careful monitoring of the mother and fetus is mandatory.
- Continuous maternal oxygen saturation of the mother is recommended.
- Remifentanil should have a dedicated IV line to avoid accidental bolus administration.
- Supplemental oxygen should be available and may be required.
- The mother requires one-to-one care with a midwife trained in the assessment of the mother using remifentanil.

Opioid analgesia—a summary of dosing regimes

Opioid	IM	IV via PCA device
Pethidine	100mg 2 doses may be administered by qualified midwife	10mg bolus Lockout time 5min Optional loading dose of 25–50mg
Morphine	5–10mg	1mg bolus Lockout time 5min Optional loading dose of 5mg
Diamorphine	2.5–5mg	0.5mg bolus Lockout time 5min Optional loading dose of 2.5mg
Fentanyl	Rarely used	20 micrograms bolus Lockout time 5min Optional loading dose of 50 micrograms
Remifentanil	Not used	40 micrograms bolus Lockout time 2min

Further reading

Obstetric Anaesthetists Association, Controversies meeting: 'The use of pethidine for labour pain should be abandoned'. March 2006.

Fairlie FM *et al.* Intramuscular opioids for maternal pain relief in labour: a randomized controlled trial comparing pethidine with diamorphine. *British Journal of Obstetrics and Gynaecology* 1999; **106**: 1181–1187.

Blair JM *et al.* Patient-controlled analgesia for labour using remifentanil: a feasibility study. *British Journal of Anaesthesia* 2001; **87**: 415–420.

Thurlow JA *et al.* Remifentanil by patient-controlled analgesia compared with intramuscular meperidine for pain relief in labour. *British Journal of Anaesthesia* 2002; **88**: 374–378.

Inhalational analgesia

Inhalational analgesia for childbirth was popularized by the administration of chloroform to Queen Victoria by Dr John Snow for the birth of her 8th child, Prince Leopold in 1853.

Entonox

- Nitrous oxide in air was first described for labour analgesia in 1880.
- Its use was popular for 80 years, with up to 80% N_2O and <10% oxygen!
- Many portable devices such as the Queen Charlotte's apparatus were widely used by obstetricians and midwives for home deliveries.
- Invented by Dr Mike Tunstall in 1961, Entonox (50% N_2O in O_2) was approved for unsupervised use by midwives in 1965.
- A survey in 1990 found Entonox available in 99% of obstetric units in the UK and used by 60% of mothers in labour.
- Although it is very popular in Europe, it is not used in North America.
- Distraction, relaxation and sense of control all increase the subjective benefit of Entonox.
- Although popular and subjectively approved by mothers, the analgesic effect is probably limited.
- Mothers in a survey (National Birthday Trust 1990) thought that Entonox was generally superior to pethidine.
- Adverse effects include drowsiness, disorientation and nausea.
- N_2O has a low blood gas solubility coefficient of 0.47, therefore it equilibrates with blood and is washed out of the lungs quickly. There is minimal accumulation with intermittent use in labour.
- There is the theoretical risk of bone marrow suppression with prolonged use.
- There may be an occupational risk to midwives especially if administered in poorly ventilated rooms.

Halogenated agents

- Chloroform was commonly administered via an open face mask or gauze for much of the first half of the 20th century.
- In the 1940s, chloroform-containing glass capsules were introduced so a measured safer quantity could be administered.
- The halogenated agents superseded chloroform after deaths from ventricular fibrillation and oversedation occurred.
- Trichloroethylene (Trilene), then methoxyflurane were routinely used by midwives through fixed low dose draw-over inhalers until the 1970s.
- Midwives are no longer allowed to administer halogenated agents, and an anaesthetist must now be present.
- Can still be administered via a draw-over inhaler mixed with air or Entonox.
- Active scavenging in delivery suites is required to comply with Health and Safety occupational exposure standards.

Isoflurane

- First reported for labour analgesia in 1975.
- 0.75% in air produced better analgesia than Entonox, but caused increased maternal sedation.
- 0.2–0.25% in Entonox produced superior analgesia to Entonox alone but did not increase maternal satisfaction.

Desflurane

- Low blood gas partition coefficient (0.42) allows rapid onset and offset.
- 0.1–4.5% desflurane has been used for the second stage of labour and compared with 30–60% N_2O alone.
- Both desflurane and N_2O were found to be effective analgesics. Increased concentrations of desflurane caused a higher incidence of amnesia (0 vs 23%).

Sevoflurane

- A study investigated 2–3% sevoflurane in air and O_2, administered intermittently aiming for an end-tidal sevoflurane of 1–1.4%.
- Analgesic properties increased to 0.8%, but increased sedation only occurred at higher doses.
- If given 1min prior to contraction, it significantly reduced pain.
- Apgar scores were unaffected.
- 0.8% sevoflurane is more effective than Entonox.

Further reading

Fortescue C, Wee M. Analgesia in labour: non regional techniques. *Continuing Education in Anaesthesia, Critical Care and Pain* 2005; **5**: 9–13.

Yeo ST, Holdcroft A, Yentis SM, Stewart A. Analgesia with sevoflurane during labour: I. Determination of the optimum concentration. *British Journal of Anaesthesia* 2007; **981**: 105–109.

Yeo ST, Holdcroft A, Yentis SM, Stewart A, Bassett P. Analgesia with sevoflurane during labour: II. Sevoflurane compared with Entonox for labour analgesia. *British Journal of Anaesthesia* 2007; **98**: 110–115.

Chapter 7

Regional techniques in pregnancy

Rachel Collis, Sarah Harries,
Saira Hussain, Martin Garry
and Vinay Ratnalikar

Introduction/benefits

Regional analgesia has provided mothers with enormous benefit since its introduction in the UK in the early 1970s. Since then, the number of procedures has continued to increase, and now the majority of mothers who request regional analgesia can have an epidural for labour analgesia on request. In addition, the number of operative deliveries and other surgical procedures has continued to rise, and now the majority of CSs are performed with the mother awake.

The provision of these services has had enormous benefits for mother, baby and partner, on both safety and humanitarian grounds. The avoidance of GA, where possible, has probably contributed to a fall in maternal deaths related to anaesthesia. Allowing the mother to be awake during the birth of her baby by CS has sound medical benefits, but also improves satisfaction for both her and her partner.

Despite the popularity and overall safety of regional techniques, epidurals and spinals that are performed badly, cause injury and don't work properly have led to a large increase in complaints and legal claims against obstetric anaesthetists. The appropriate consent, documentation and conduct of procedures is therefore of paramount importance when performing any regional technique in pregnancy.

Absolute contraindications

Maternal refusal

- The woman's wishes should be respected at all times. However, the woman has the right to change her mind at any time later.
- All decisions and discussions should be accurately recorded in the case notes.

Allergy

- True allergy to amide local anaesthetic is rare.
- Ascertain the history of the reaction, check the case notes and enquire about formal allergy testing.
- Is there a Medic-alert bracelet?
- The majority of epidural packs and kits are latex free.

Sepsis

- Localized infection at the insertion site.
- Exaggerated or uncontrollable hypotension may occur in the overtly septic patient who is already vasodilated, intravascular volume depleted and has myocardial depression.
- There is the risk of introducing infected blood into a sterile epidural or subarachnoid space.
- Coagulation/platelet abnormalities may be present or developing.

Raised intercranial pressure

- Diagnostic imaging may be required.

Clotting abnormalities

- Platelet count $<70\times10^9$/L.
- Evidence of clotting dysfunction.
- Strong history of bleeding tendency, even if tests are normal.

Lack of appropriately trained staff and/or equipment

- Full resuscitation facilities must be available.
- There should be an appropriately trained person to instigate and interpret monitoring for both the woman and fetus for the duration of the epidural.
- Large bore patent IV access must be *in situ* to allow prompt treatment in the event of maternal hypotension/collapse.

Bleeding disorders

- ***Congenital clotting abnormalities***—usually single factor deficiencies. Personal history of bleeding and family history.
- ***Reduced/absent synthesis*** of clotting factors and fibrinogen 2° to pre-existing liver disease, liver involvement in pre-eclampsia, intrahepatic cholestasis of pregnancy, vitamin K deficiency and drugs.

- ***Increased consumption***, i.e. disseminated intravascular coagulation (DIC) 2° to sepsis, intrauterine death, severe pre-eclampsia, placental abruption and amniotic fluid embolism.
- ***Acute loss ± dilution***, i.e. haemorrhage and massive blood transfusion. Packed red cells lack factors V, VIII, XI, platelets and fibrinogen.
- ***Thrombocytopenia***. Gestational thrombocytopenia of pregnancy (GTP) is clinically indistinguishable from mild immune thrombocytopenic purpura (ITP), both of which are relatively common during pregnancy. GTP resolves postpartum.
- ***Hypertensive disorders of pregnancy*** are the second most common cause of thrombocytopenia, with excessive platelet consumption and altered function. HELLP syndrome represents the most extreme end of the spectrum.
- ***Drug-induced thrombocytopenia*** 2° to heparin therapy (HIT), penicillins, H_2-antagonists, thiazide diuretics, hydralazine and cocaine.
- ***Uraemia*** alters platelet function detrimentally.
- ***Severe von Willibrand's disease*** with persistently low levels despite pregnancy.

Relative contraindications

- Platelets $>70\times10^9$/L but $<100\times10^9$/L.
- Hypovolaemia.
- Ongoing haemorrhage.
- Rapidly falling platelet count, e.g. in severe pre-eclampsia or HELLP. Repeat the platelet count if >2h old and check clotting.
- Raised white cell count (WCC), e.g. $>20\times10^9$/L. The level of WCC or C-reactive protein at which it is unsafe to site an epidural in labour has not been determined. If the WCC is raised, the source of any infection should be sought and treated with appropriate antibiotics. The potential risks of introducing infection into the epidural space should be explained to the patient.
- Anatomical anomalies, e.g. spina bifida cystica or previous spinal surgery. Check notes for neurosurgical comment regarding regional techniques. Has she had an epidural or spinal previously? Were there any difficulties during the procedure, with the block or after delivery?
- Cardiovascular disease, in particular stenotic valvular lesions and cardiomyopathies, where the patient cannot cope with a sudden reduction in SVR. This is seldom a problem when fractionated low dose bupivacaine/opioid mixture is used. A high level of vigilance and invasive BP monitoring may be required.
- Active neurological disease. There should be consultation with a neurologist and documentation of current neurological status along with chronological details of relapses and remission periods.
- If a relative contraindication exists, the medical and obstetric history should be reviewed together with any related laboratory investigations.
- The case notes should be checked for any antenatal anaesthetic clinic alerts and/or input from other specialties sought. For example, neurosurgical referral may prompt an MRI scan to determine the anatomy of the spinal column and epidural space if a spinal anomaly exists.
- Senior anaesthetic input should be sought in these cases and there should be detailed documentation of the delivery plan in the case notes.

The management of the mother on anticoagulants

- ***Low molecular weight heparins (LMWHs)*** are used during pregnancy for treatment or prophylaxis of thromboembolic disease, pro-thrombotic disease such as factor V Leiden mutation, protein S and protein C deficiency and antiphospholipid syndrome. LMWHs have a good safety profile with reduced risk of osteoporosis and heparin induced thrombocytopaenia (HIT) compared with unfractionated heparin.
- ***Unfractionated heparin (UF)*** given continuously is the anticoagulant agent of choice during the first trimester for patients with valvular cardiac lesions and high risk, mechanical valves. The use of LMWHs is associated with an unacceptably high risk of valve thrombosis. UF does not cross the placenta, therefore it is safe during organogenesis in the first trimester compared with warfarin. It is the preferred agent in late pregnancy near delivery as its effects can be rapidly reversed.
- ***Warfarin*** can be used from the second trimester to near term. It is avoided in the first trimester as it is associated with dose-related developmental abnormalities during organogenesis; these are associated with a larger dose >5mg rather than the INR (international normalized ratio).
- ***IV heparin infusion*** may also be used in patients at high risk of venous thromboembolism.
- ***Low dose aspirin*** may be used as prophylaxis in women at high risk of developing pre-eclampsia or recurrent miscarriage. Aspirin use is not a contraindication to siting an epidural catheter.
- There is little evidence to support an increased risk of vertebral canal haematoma if aspirin or an NSAID is used as a sole agent. If used together or in conjunction with LMWH, interaction may occur and senior haematological advice should be sought.

Safe timing for insertion of an epidural catheter with heparins

Drug	Time to epidural insertion after last dose	Time to next dose with catheter *in situ*	Cautions/other Remember to consider the overall picture
LMWH			
Prophylactic dose (20–40mg enoxaparin)	12h	4h	Consider waiting longer (up to 24h) if procedure technically difficult or if there is ongoing bleeding
Therapeutic dose (>40mg enoxaparin)	24h		APPT is normal, and monitoring of anti-Xa levels may be required if regional anaesthesia is considered within these time frames or if the mother has renal impairment
UH			
Heparin SC (Minihep 5000IU)	4h	1h	*As above*
IV infusion	Stop infusion, check clotting after 1h. APTT should be normal and platelet count $>100\times10^9$/L. Inform senior anaesthetist	Infusion should not be started until 12h after siting an epidural and extended to 24h if there was bloody tap Catheter can be removed 4h after stopping infusion if APTT is normal and platelet count $>100\times10^9$/L.	Ideally, heparin should be stopped 4–6h prior to surgery. If delivery imminent, spontaneous or otherwise, discuss with senior anaesthetist and obstetrician Protamine 1mg per 100IU heparin by *slow IV injection* will reverse the effect. Beware severe hypotension, bronchospasm and flushing. Caution if fish/shellfish allergy

Safe timing for insertion of an epidural catheter

Drug	Time to epidural insertion *after* last dose	Time to next dose *with catheter in situ*	Cautions/other *Remember to consider the overall picture*
Other drugs which may affect clotting/platelet function			
Aspirin NSAIDs	No wait necessary	No wait necessary	May be synergy with concomitant administration or other antiplatelet agent. Interaction with LMWH may occur. Beware in disease states causing alteration of platelet number/function
Warfarin	INR <1.5	Use heparin regimen until INR re-established	After stopping warfarin, INR takes 3–5 days to fall to <1.5 If delivery imminent, discuss with haematologist In an emergency, warfarin can be reversed with vitamin K and prothrombin complex Remember the baby is anticoagulated which may not be reversed with these measures Takes 3–4 days for the INR to rise to >2.0 after warfarin recommenced

The same time frames relate to removal of the epidural catheter.

Further reading

Horlocker TT, Heit JA. Low molecular weight heparin: biochemistry, pharmacology, perioperative prophylaxis regimes, guidelines for regional anesthetic management. *Anesthesia and Analgesia* 1997; **85**: 874–885.

Norris LA *et al.* Low molecular weight heparin (tinzaparin) therapy for moderate risk thromboprophylaxis during pregnancy. A pharmacokinetic study. *Thrombosis and Haemostasis* 2004; **92**: 791–796.

Tryba M, Wedel DJ. Central neuraxial block and low molecular weight heparin (enoxaparine): lessons learned from different dosage regimens in two continents. *Acta Anaesthesiologica Scandinavica, Supplement* 1997; **111**: 100–104.

Consent

There is a legal, ethical and professional requirement to obtain informed consent prior to performing a procedure on any patient.

For consent to treatment to be valid:

- Adequate information must be supplied including the benefits, risks and complications of the procedure.
- A person should be considered to have the capacity to give consent and to make a balanced decision free from coercion. A person is deemed to have capacity if they are able to understand and retain the relevant treatment information. They must understand the procedure or treatment, and be able to balance the risks and benefits to arrive at a decision before issuing consent.
- Capacity may be compromised by drugs, fatigue, pain or anxiety, but these would need to be extreme to incapacitate her.
- A woman deemed competent to give consent is free to change her decision at any time.

Special considerations

Birth plans

- If epidural analgesia is requested during labour but refused in the birth plan, the woman's most recent wishes are to be respected and the usual consent procedure followed.
- The change of decision from the original birth plan should be documented in the notes and the woman should be asked to countersign the record if possible.
- If during labour the woman loses capacity, the decision in the birth plan should be adhered to and treated as an Advance Decision ('advance directive'), and considered legally binding.

Non-English-speaking women

- Information leaflets in a variety of languages regarding analgesia in labour are available from the OAA(www.oaa-anaes.ac.uk).
- An interpreter should be made available, ideally from outside the family group, and every attempt should be made to discuss analgesia in the antenatal period.

Parturients under the age of 18

- 16- and 17-year-old women are considered to be adults with regards to making decisions regarding medical intervention.
- Younger teenagers may be considered competent to give consent; however, the physical and psychological demands of labour may compromise capacity.
- Excessive control by a parent that appears to be against the wishes of the young parturient should be strongly discouraged as a child is generally thought to be able to give consent from age of 12 years.

Lack of capacity

- If a patient lacks capacity, whether permanent or temporary, and in the absence of an 'Advance Decision' ('advance directive'), treatment can be carried out without consent, directed in the patient's best interests.

- The treatment should be discussed with family or carers, but this is not a legal requirement.

Obtaining informed consent for epidural analgesia during labour

- Women want information and to be brought into the consent process, even if they are distressed or apparently incapable of retaining information.
- Roughly a third of information will be retained accurately.
- Signed consent is not necessary. However, a record of the discussion, including the risks and complications, should be documented in full in the medical case notes with the date and time of the assessment.
- The discussion should ideally be witnessed by the birthing partner or midwife, and the notes countersigned by the attending midwife.
- Talk between contractions—if contractions are fast and furious or the woman is using Entonox continuously, try to involve the birth partner in the process and keep explanations short and simple.
- Try to confirm their understanding of epidural analgesia initially. Has she received any antenatal education or advice regarding epidural analgesia either from antenatal groups or via other media, e.g. magazines or websites?
- Answers to specific questions should be full, frank and honest, and recorded in the notes.

What information should you give?

Essential information

- The procedure—the correct position, local anaesthetic infiltration, the need to keep as still as possible, etc.
- The risk of a severe headache following accidental dural puncture, e.g. 1 in 100.
- Inadequate or incomplete analgesia and how this can be remedied.
- The increased risk of instrumental delivery associated with epidural analgesia.

Consider telling her

- The need for intermittent monitoring of BP and continuous CTG.
- Nausea and vomiting.
- Itching associated with opioids.
- Tenderness or bruising at insertion site for 24–48h but no increased risk of long-term backache.
- The risk of neurological complications in 1: 10 000.
- The risk of epidural-related infections—very rare.

Further reading

Bethune L *et al.* Complications of obstetric regional analgesia: how much information is enough? *International Journal of Obstetrics and Anesthesia* 2004; **13**: 30–34.

Kelly GD *et al.* Consent for regional anaesthesia in the United Kingdom: what is material risk? *International Journal of Obstetrics and Anesthesia* 2004; **13**: 71–74.

Association of Anaesthetists of Great Britain and Ireland. *Consent for Anaesthesia.* Association of Anaesthetists of Great Britain and Ireland, 2006.

Monitoring

- A midwife fully trained in the management of epidurals and their complications should remain with the woman once an epidural is sited.
- The anaesthetist should stay in the room after the first test dose and ideally until an adequate analgesic block is established.
- There must be adequate facility for BP, heart rate and pulse oximeter monitoring in the delivery room.
- Lack of monitoring equipment or appropriately trained personnel is a contraindication to siting an epidural.

Before siting the epidural

- Request a maternal BP prior to commencing the epidural, ideally taken when the woman is not having a contraction, and compare this with antenatal BP recordings. An unexpected elevated BP may indicate pre-eclampsia, warranting further obstetric and anaesthetic investigation.
- Look at a recent CTG tracing to determine the baseline FHR and features indicative of fetal distress. A 10–15min CTG trace is ideal and can be commenced whilst consent is taken and IV access is established.
- Establish patent IV access. There is a lack of evidence that fluid preload is beneficial, but rapid access to IV fluids may be required in an emergency.

After the first test dose

- Maternal BP should be checked and recorded every 5min for 20min.
- After 5min, check for evidence of accidental intrathecal injection. Presence of a motor block should quickly differentiate between an intrathecal and epidural injection of local anaesthetic.
- FHR should be monitored continuously for 20min. Maternal hypotension will reduce uteroplacental perfusion and may lead to sudden fetal distress.
- Reduce aorto-caval compression with careful positioning of the mother.
- Consider more frequent BP monitoring if BP labile or evidence of fetal distress.
- Check maternal heart rate if BP low; the block may be unusually high, causing a bradycardia.

Once the epidural is established

- For continuous epidural infusion and patient-controlled epidural analgesia (PCEA), the BP should be checked and recorded every 30min.
- For an intermittent 'top-up' regime or any additional 'top-ups', the BP and FHR should be checked every 5min for 10min after each 'top-up'.
- Any change in the mother's condition, e.g. nausea, dizziness, breathing difficulties, warrants a full set of observations immediately and continue until the problem is rectified.
- Remind the midwife of the importance of ongoing maternal observations as the epidural can migrate intrathecally, subdurally or intravascularly at any time.
- National Institute for Health and Clinical Excellence (NICE) recommends continuous fetal monitoring if the mother has an epidural.

Ambulatory analgesia—'mobile epidural'

- Monitor BP and FHR as previously.

In addition

- Measure BP whilst recumbent and again whilst upright to ensure adequate sympathetic response.
- Tests of adequate motor function using the Bromage scale, straight leg raises and deep knee bends whilst standing should be performed prior to ambulation.
- 'Top-ups' can be given with the woman sitting or reclining. Monitor BP and FHR every five 5min for 20min.
- Motor function should be assessed fully after each 'top-up'.
- Reclining/upright BP should be checked to ensure the absence of postural hypotension after 'top-ups'.

Further reading

Association of Anaesthetists of Great Britain and Ireland and Obstetric Anaesthetists' Association. *OAA/AAGBI Guidelines for Obstetric Anaesthetic Services*. 2005.

Documentation

- Documentation of the epidural procedure should be contemporaneous, legible and complete.
- Most obstetric units have a dedicated regional analgesia/anaesthesia chart with space for initial anaesthetic assessment, discussion and consent, subsequent recording of top-ups, vital signs and information relating to complications and/or adverse events.
- If such a chart is not available, the relevant information should be recorded in the patient case notes with date and times documented appropriately.
- It is a legal requirement to keep an anaesthetic record. In addition, this information is invaluable to other members of the team, e.g. at handover, for ongoing audit, research and training.

Documentation should include

- Name and grade of anaesthetist.
- Date and time of procedure.
- Verbal request for epidural or indication for therapeutic epidural with evidence of verbal consent.
- Risks and side effects discussed and incidences quoted, e.g. PDPH 1%.
- IV access site and gauge of cannula.
- Patient position.
- Full aseptic technique (gloves, gown, hat, mask, drape).
- Level of intervertebral space and approach (midline/paramedian).
- Volume and percentage of local anaesthetic infiltration.
- Tuohy needle gauge.
- Loss of resistance technique (saline/air).
- Presence/absence of paraesthesia.
- Depth of needle to epidural space.
- Presence/absence CSF or blood.
- Length of catheter left in space.
- CSF/blood in catheter.
- Initial bolus dose.
- Subsequent doses including pain scores, block height and deficits, and any remedial action.
- Vital signs.
- Any complications at time of insertion or thereafter.
- In addition there should be written evidence of a full anaesthetic assessment, including airway assessment and inspection of the spine.

Positioning the mother

- The techniques of epidural, spinal and combined spinal–epidural (CSE) analgesia and anaesthesia can be used in labour and for caesarean delivery.
- The problems encountered by the obstetric anaesthetist are unique when compared with other patient groups.
- The mother may find it very difficult to remain still during the procedure because of frequent contractions.
- She may find it difficult to maintain an ideal position during insertion because of her pregnancy.
- A labour room bed is not ideal for optimizing the position of either the mother or the anaesthetist.
- Because of these recognized difficulties, meticulous care and explanation is required in positioning the mother before commencing any procedure.
- Poor positioning may result in multiple, unnecessary attempts and is responsible for the majority of failures to site an epidural or spinal.
- Ensure the woman is in the correct position and identify the relevant interspace *prior* to scrubbing up and draping.

Sitting position (Fig 7.1)

- Ensure the woman is sitting on a flat, level mattress (avoiding dips or grooves in the delivery bed).
- Place her feet flat on a high stool with calves close to the side of the bed. Try to prevent her knees falling laterally.
- Always ensure the knees are higher than the hips to reduce the lumbar lordosis.
- Ask her to hold a pillow in front of her chest, place her chin on her chest and relax her shoulders.
- Her shoulders, hips, knees and ankles should be in line. The mother will frequently feel her spine is twisted, even if it is not obvious to the observer; ask her.
- If sitting on the operating table, tilt the table 5° towards the anaesthetist to reduce lumbar lordosis.
- Ask the mother to relax or slump. When all the other elements are in place, the required movement is small and easily possible for the majority of mothers.

Common errors

Twisting of the spine is caused by

- The mother is sitting on the uneven detachable end of a delivery bed.
- The bed is not level (head end is tilted up), which tends to encourage the mother to lean sideways.
- The mother is encouraged to maintain her position by an assistant (frequently the partner or midwife) placing their hands on her shoulders. This can be a helpful manoeuvre but, if the assistant is not directly in front of the mother, she tends to twist towards them.

Leaning forward rather than flexing the spine is caused by

- Her shoulders are hunched and tense.
- Her feet are not on a high enough support. This commonly occurs when the bed is raised to accommodate the anaesthetist's position.
    - The mother does not feel secure and she tends to lean rather than curl forward.
    - The natural flexion of the lumbar spine when the knees are brought above the hips is lost.
- The mother's feet are high enough but she slides her feet and calves away from the side of the bed.

The anaesthetist is not in an optimal position

- The mother is sitting too far across a wide delivery bed. This can be improved by bringing the mother towards you, but care is required to ensure she is still able to sit with her feet firmly on a stool.
- The anaesthetist has learned the technique whilst sitting. With the limitations a labour room bed usually provides, hand position and needle direction are frequently compromised.

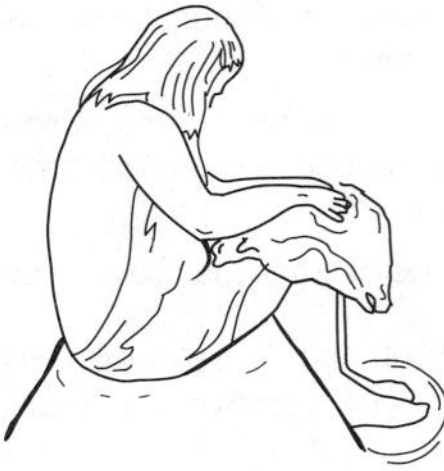

The ideal sitting position

- Knees above hips
- Feet flat and heals close to bed
- Shoulders relaxed
- Pillow close to abdomen
- Back gently curled outwards

Fig. 7.1 The sitting position.

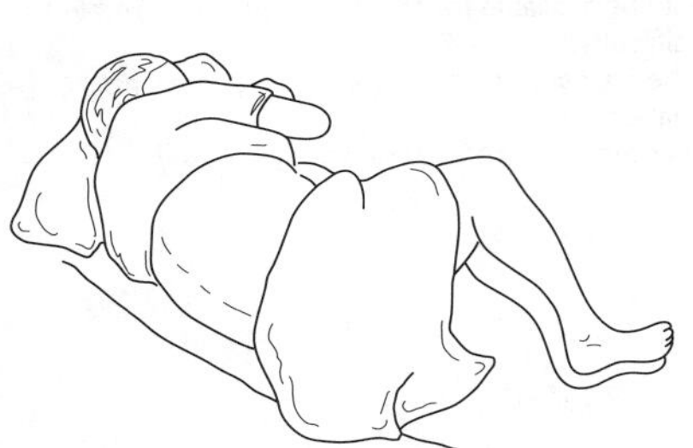

Ideal lateral position

- Head on a pillow and chin brought forward
- Back parallel and close to the edge of bed
- Legs brought up as far as possible and together

Fig. 7.2 The lateral position.

Lateral position (Fig 7.2)

- When the woman is lying on her left side, ensure her back is parallel to and as close to the edge of the bed as possible.
- Her knees should be drawn up in front of her abdomen as far as they will go, and her chin should rest on her chest.
- Place a pillow under her head to level the spine and another between her knees to prevent the pelvis tilting.

Common errors

- The back is not parallel to the edge of the bed, making it difficult to identify the perpendicular approach to the spinous processes.
- The knees are not drawn up adequately to facilitate lumbar flexion.
- The knees are not drawn up evenly, resulting in twisting of the spine.
  - Bring the lower leg to the abdomen first then bring the upper leg to join it. This improves the degree of hip flexion and reduces the risk of twisting the pelvis and lumbar spine.

Problems common to both positions

- The mother changes her position because of painful contractions.
- The mother changes her position because of the pain of local anaesthetic infiltration or needle insertion.

The anaesthetist has to be constantly aware of these problems. Time spent rectifying any movement may reduce the overall time it takes to insert an epidural or spinal anaesthetic.

If the midline is difficult to feel and the mother may have moved, remove the drapes and start again.

- If the epidural is unexpectedly difficult and the spinous process or laminar is encountered more than twice, remove the drapes and start again.
- If difficulties continue, an experienced anaesthetic assistant can be very helpful. They can optimize the mother's position, encourage her to maintain that position and move her back into the correct position if she moves a little. In many units, it is not usual practice for an operating department assistant (ODP) to help the anaesthetist routinely in delivery rooms, but as one should be available for theatre, it may be possible to ask for help in case of difficulty.
- It is unacceptable for the anaesthetist to have multiple attempts.
  - Re-evaluate the situation.
  - Ask for help from someone more experienced.

Skin preparation

Visual inspection and examination of the back should be undertaken at the preprocedural assessment. Localized infection at or near the proposed site of epidural insertion is an absolute contraindication to its placement.

- Position the patient and identify landmarks prior to disinfecting the skin.
- Ensure the CTG straps are well away from the area of insertion, but CTG monitoring should continue during the procedure.
- Maximum aseptic technique is mandatory, with gloves, gown, hat and mask. Scrub up to the elbows with a surgical scrub solution.
- Chlorhexidine is superior to other agents (e.g. povidone iodine) at killing bacteria and reducing the incidence of infection. Alcohol solutions are more effective than aqueous solutions.
- Chlorhexidine (0.5%) in ethanol (80%) is maximally effective within 15s.
- A chlorhexidine and alcohol spray applied directly to the skin should be kept well away from the epidural or spinal tray, reducing the rare complication of chemical meningitis.

Preparation of the skin

- Spraying or painting the skin twice with the chosen disinfectant solution reduces the absolute bacterial count on the skin. The skin must be allowed to dry completely between applications for full effect. It is unclear if double spraying reduces the incidence of rare bacterial infections around epidural sites.
- If the skin is painted, a fresh swab should be used for each application and painted from the insertion site outwards in a circular motion.
- Try to avoid any further rubbing or abrasive pressure to the skin once the skin prep has dried.
- Apply a sterile drape to the back and ensure that it is secure.
- If there is an unsterile area of bed between the anaesthetist and the drape on the back, cover it with another sterile drape.
- If sterility is compromised, you must re-prep the field.

Further reading

Grewal S *et al*. Epidural abscesses. *British Journal of Anaesthesia* 2006; **96**: 292–299.

Reynolds F. Infection as a complication of neuraxial blockade. *International Journal of Obstetric Anesthesia* 2005; **14**: 183–188.

Association of Anaesthetists of Great Britain and Ireland. *Infection Control in Anaesthesia*. 2002.

Techniques of epidural insertion

Most centres have a fully equipped mobile epidural trolley, which can be moved between delivery rooms as required.

Equipment

You will need the following

- Stable work surface.
- Sterile dressing pack with swabs and forceps.
- Range of syringes and needles for local anaesthetic infiltration.
- Filter needle.
- Sterile drapes—ideally with a window and adhesive sides.
- 16G or 18G Tuohy needle.
- Loss of resistance syringe.
- Epidural catheter.
- Luer lock and filter.
- 0.9% saline.
- 1% lidocaine.
- Epidural dressings.
- Epidural drugs.
- Ephedrine 3mg/mL.

Technique

- ***Position***. Both sitting and lateral positions are acceptable.
    - Sitting is easier to identify the midline, but may have a slightly higher incidence of dural puncture and bloody tap.
- ***Interspace***. A mid-lumbar interspace is ideal L2/3 or L3/4. The L4/5 interspace is advocated by some to reduce the risk of accidental spinal cord damage should an accidental dural puncture occur. Even if palpable, this space is frequently difficult to use and may lead to more failures.
- ***Midline vs paramedian***. The midline approach is the most frequently practised technique. A full understanding of the anatomy of both techniques will help if difficulties are encountered.

Midline

- A midline approach is anatomically more straightforward.
- May have an increased risk of false loss of resistance due to small deficits in the interspinous ligaments.
- There may be a midline deficit in the ligamentum flavum with an increased risk of accidental dural puncture.

Paramedian

- Is a successful technique only once the anaesthetist has a strong three-dimensional image of the anatomy of the vertebral column.
- May be more painful as the vertebral lamina is purposely identified.
- As a bony landmark is established, advocates feel there is a reduced chance of a false loss of resistance and dural puncture.

- ***Air vs saline***. The incidence of dural puncture is thought to be lower and there is less risk of a patchy block with saline.
  - Air makes it easier to identify a dural puncture should it occur as any clear fluid emerging from the needle can only be CSF. 30% of dural punctures are not identified during insertion and the discrepancy may be in part caused by earlier recognition when air is used.
  - Both techniques are acceptable, the skill of the operator being the most important factor.
  - A recent survey showed that many anaesthetists use both techniques in different circumstances, and the more experienced the anaesthetist the more likely they are to vary.
- ***Fluid preload***. There is no need to administer a fluid preload unless the woman is hypovolaemic. An IV cannula is mandatory and, in many units, it is still recommended that IV fluids should be connected to ensure IV access.

Procedure

- Ensure no contraindications to insertion and that informed consent has been given.
- Full resuscitation equipment must be available.
- Confirm patent large bore IV access attached to crystalloid infusion.
- Position the patient.
- Identify the relevant interspace (L3/4).
- Put on theatre hat and mask, scrub up and put on gown and gloves.
- Prepare the back using scrupulous aseptic technique.
- Assemble equipment and check patency of epidural catheter by flushing with saline.
- Infiltrate the skin with a 25G needle using 2–5mL of 1% lidocaine at and around the midpoint of the interspace (a common problem is failure to anaesthetize the dermis by infiltrating too deeply).
- Insert the Tuohy needle (obturator *in situ*) through the skin and supraspinous ligament so that the needle is held firm. On average this is 2–3cm but may be less in the very slim or considerably more in the obese. If the tip of the needle is not in the interspinous ligament before pressure is put on the syringe there will be a false loss of resistance.
- Remove obturator and observe hub of needle for clear fluid/blood.
- Attach loss of resistance syringe:
  - If using saline, exert a continuous pressure on the plunger of the syringe as it is advanced until there is sudden loss of resistance.
  - If using air, advance the needle carefully 1mm or less at a time. Each time the needle is stationary, check for loss of resistance by intermittently balloting the plunger of the syringe.
- It is important to keep control of the Tuohy needle so the epidural space is entered slowly. Too fast an approach or lurching into the epidural space from lack of control will increase the risk of dural puncture.
- If air is used, a minimal amount of air (max 1mL) should be injected into the epidural space.

- If saline is used, 2–3mL can be safely used, but more will result in pain and the mother is likely to move, resulting in an increased risk of dural puncture. Saline is more likely to emerge via the Tuohy needle, raising concerns of a dural puncture.
- Remove the syringe from the Tuohy needle and observe for clear fluid or blood. If saline is used for loss of resistance, a few drops of clear fluid may emerge from the hub. CSF flow is continuous and brisk. If in doubt, check for the presence of glucose with a BMstix.
- Note the depth of the space and thread the catheter to around the 15cm mark. Inform the woman that she may feel a slight electric shock down her legs as you pass the catheter but that this is transient.
- Remove the Tuohy needle carefully over the catheter, taking care not to pull the catheter out. Pull back the catheter so that 3–5cm remains in the epidural space. Longer lengths may pass through the intervertebral foramen, while shorter lengths may come out of the epidural space altogether.
- Observe the catheter for blood or flow of clear fluid. Lift the catheter up to determine a drop in the saline meniscus. Hold the open catheter below the patient to see if excessive clear fluid or blood drips out.
- Never withdraw the catheter through the Tuohy needle as there is a risk of shearing the catheter. If unable to insert the catheter freely into the epidural space but the tip has already passed through the Tuohy needle, remove the Tuohy needle and catheter as a unit.
- Fix the Luer lock mechanism to the catheter and perform a tug test to confirm that it is secure. Attach the bacterial filter.
- Secure the catheter to the skin such that the depth markings on the catheter can be clearly seen—dressings should ideally be transparent and semi-permeable. Strap the catheter over the shoulder of the non-dominant hand.

- Although continuous saline and intermittent air are often described as separate techniques, many anaesthetists will use a combination of both techniques and different hand positions (see Figs. 7.3–7.5).
- Multihole epidural catheters are most commonly used because there is a reduced incidence of unsatisfactory or unilateral blocks as the three holes face different directions.
- Single hole catheters may have the advantage of reducing the risk of a multicompartment catheter (proximal hole in the epidural space and the distal hole in the intrathecal space).

The Figs. 7.3–7.5 demonstrates three common methods of holding a Tuohy needle and syringe during insertion. In all techniques continuous pressure is placed on the plunger with one hand, while the needle is controlled by the other.

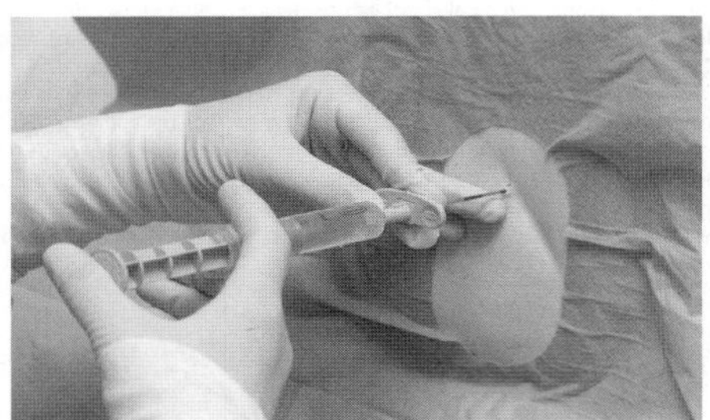

Fig. 7.3

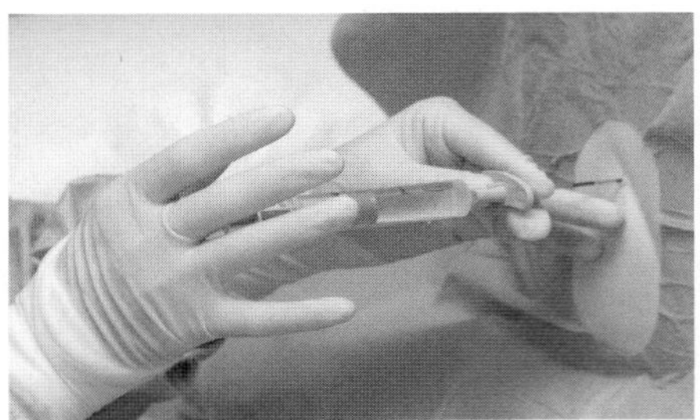

Fig. 7.4

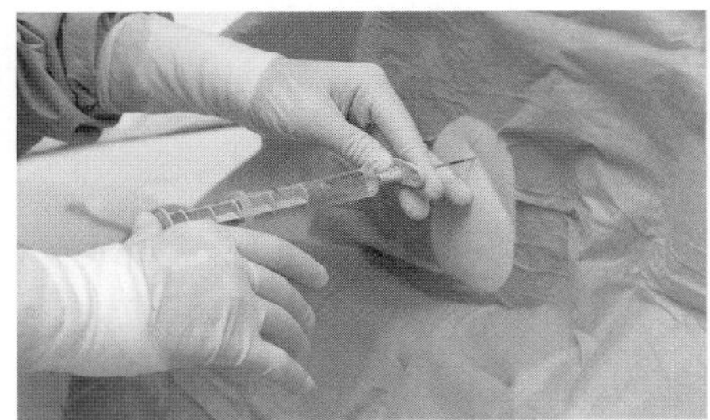

Fig. 7.5

Further reading

Fernando R, Price CM. Regional analgesia for labour. In: Collis R, Platt F, Urquhart J, ed. *Textbook of Obstetric Anaesthesia*. London: Greenwich Medical Media, 2002.

Wantman A *et al.* Techniques for identifying the epidural space: a survey of practice amongst anaesthetists in the UK. *Anaesthesia* 2006; **61**: 370–375.

Yentis SM, Barnes PK. Snippet (epidural anesthesia techniques). *Anaesthesia* 2005; **60**: 406.

Van de Velde M. Identification of the epidural space: stop using the loss of resistance to air technique! (Review). *Acta Anaesthesiolica Belgica* 2006; **57**: 51–54.

Stone PA *et al.* Posture and epidural catheter insertion. The relationship between skill, experience and maternal posture on the outcome of epidural catheter insertion. *Anaesthesia* 1990; **45**: 920–923.

Bahar M *et al.* The lateral recumbent head-down position decreases the incidence of epidural venous puncture during catheter insertion in obese parturients. *Canadian Journal of Anaesthesia* 2004; **51**: 577–580.

D'Angelo R *et al.* A comparison of multiport and uniport epidural catheters in laboring patients. *Anesthesia and Analgesia* 1997; **84**: 1276–1279.

Difficulties with insertion

The most common causes for difficulty in siting an epidural are

- Suboptimal positioning of the woman.
- Failure to insert the needle in the midline.
- Directing the needle too far laterally even if the insertion point is correct.
- Failure to identify the mid-interspinous point correctly.

Top tips

- Establish a rapport with the mother and explain what you are doing—this will help gain her co-operation with positioning. Talk to her face to face initially, explaining what you want her to do.
- Infiltrate the skin and subcutaneous tissues adequately with lidocaine 1%. An 'orange peel' wheel should be seen. Failure to anaesthetize the dermis adequately is a common reason for the mother to move.
- If bone is encountered on the second attempt, either superficially or deep, STOP and re-evaluate your position.
- It may be helpful, especially in the obese, to ask the mother where the midline is. (They always know!)
- If lamina is encountered, ask the mother if she feels the sensation to the RIGHT or LEFT then redirect the needle slightly cephalad and towards the midline.
- She may be unable to tolerate the sitting position due to pain, especially if the baby is in the occipito-posterior (OP) position. Try the left lateral position.
- The sitting position may be the best to identify the midline in the obese woman.
- Delivery mattresses often consist of several detachable parts—make sure that she is not sitting across a join in the mattress as this will destabilize her position.
- The stool she has her feet on is slipping, she feels unstable and therefore leans rather than bends. Her feet can also slip if she is wearing socks and her feet are on a smooth surface.
- If she is unable to keep still, consider performing a low dose spinal to produce rapid analgesia. The epidural is then performed when she is more comfortable and co-operative.
- In the morbidly obese parturient, it may be necessary to use a long (12 or 15cm) Tuohy needle. The principles are the same; however, senior help or supervision should be sought if you are unfamiliar using it.
- If difficulties continue, call for help early. It is unacceptable to submit a woman to multiple, prolonged attempts at insertion.

- Once the Tuohy needle is in the epidural space, there may be difficulties advancing the catheter through the needle.
  - If severe pain is experienced, STOP and remove catheter and needle together.
  - If there is no pain, try gently injecting a few more mLs of saline and rotating the needle through 45°.
  - If the catheter continues not to thread, start again.

Pain on insertion

- Pain may be felt as:
  - The Tuohy needle punctures the skin and subcutaneous tissues.
  - Fluid or air is lost into the interspinous ligaments.
  - The needle hits the periosteum.
  - The needle or catheter hits a nerve root.
  - The spinal cord is damaged.

- If pain is experienced, stop advancing the Tuohy needle and ask if the pain persists. If it does, withdraw the needle until the pain goes.
- Ascertain the location and type of pain.
- Infiltrate more local anaesthetic to the skin and subcutaneous tissues with a 24 or 25G needle. Avoid using a green (19G) needle as there is a risk of accidental dural puncture.
- Try not to 'walk' the needle off the bony vertebrae. The periosteum may feel sore for some days after.
- 'Shooting' or 'electric shock' type pain may be felt down one or other leg if a nerve or nerve root is accidentally brushed (neuropraxia), as well as tingling or numbness. Withdraw the needle slightly and redirect away from the side that the pain is felt. If the sensation recurs, try a different interspace.
- If the needle pierces the spinal cord, there will be sudden severe pain, paraesthesia and possibly paralysis. The spinal cord usually ends at L1/2 in adults; however, anatomical anomalies do exist. If there is a suggestion of conus damage, seek senior neurological advice immediately.

On insertion of the epidural catheter

- The epidural catheter should pass freely through the Tuohy needle.
- On advancing the catheter into the epidural space, the woman may experience a transient shooting sensation down either leg. Warn her about this and, when it occurs, advance the catheter a little further. If it does not very rapidly disappear, withdraw the needle and catheter together.
- Never force the catheter as it may kink or twist, shedding particles into the epidural space. Similarly, never tug or yank the catheter when withdrawing it.
- If the woman experiences pain on injection through the catheter, stop injecting immediately. Confirm that there is no drug error and remove the catheter. Seek senior advice regarding resiting at a different interspace.

Bloody tap

The valveless veins of the epidural venous plexus—Batson's plexus—are engorged and distended during pregnancy and their thin walls make them vulnerable to damage if traumatized by a needle or catheter. There is an increased risk of bloody tap in the obese parturient in the sitting position.

Through the Tuohy needle

If bleeding occurs through the Tuohy needle once the obturator is removed it should be withdrawn and inserted at a different interspace.

Through the epidural catheter

It is essential to ensure that the epidural catheter has not been placed into a vein prior to injecting any drugs through it. If blood is seen in the epidural catheter during insertion:

- Continue to insert the catheter and remove the Tuohy needle.
- Pull the catheter back so that the desired length is in the epidural space, i.e. 3–5cm.
- Flush the catheter with saline.
- Lower the catheter to see if blood flows freely.
- Aspirate gently so as not to collapse the delicate walled vessel.
- If blood is aspirated, flush the catheter with normal saline and re-aspirate. If the catheter is free of blood, give the first dose cautiously.
- If blood is still aspirated or free flowing, pull back the catheter 1cm at a time, flushing and aspirating until blood is no longer seen. Remember to leave a minimum of 3cm within the epidural space.
- If blood is still seen within the catheter, remove it and resite the catheter at a different interspace.
- If there is any doubt as to whether the catheter is sited in a vein, it is safer to remove it and start again.

Remember to document events contemporaneously and clearly. Although epidural haematomas are rare, remain vigilant for neurological signs or symptoms.

Accidental dural puncture

The incidence of accidental dural puncture (ADP) in the pregnant woman is quoted as between 0.5 abd 2.6%, with ~70% of women subsequently developing a PDPH. There is an increased incidence if loss of resistance to air is used. The dura may be punctured by the Tuohy needle or the epidural catheter.

Practical management

Dural puncture with the Tuohy needle

- Clear fluid will be seen to appear and flow continuously from the hub of the Tuohy needle once the obturator or syringe is removed.
- If saline is used for loss of resistance, it is common for a few drops to appear at the needle hub, but that is all.
- If there is any doubt, check the fluid for the presence of glucose using a glucose indicator strip.

If ADP is confirmed, there are two ways to proceed:

Either

- Pass the epidural catheter through the needle, aiming to leave 2–2.5cm in the subarachnoid space. Secure and label the catheter clearly as 'SPINAL'. Establish the block with divided doses of 2mg bupivacaine and 5mcg fentanyl. All subsequent doses should be given ONLY by an anaesthetist. Consideration should be given to leaving the spinal catheter *in situ* in the postdelivery period as this has been shown to reduce the incidence or severity of post-dural puncture headache.

Or

- Remove the needle and repeat the procedure at a different interspace. Proceed carefully as there is always the risk of performing another dural puncture. Once sited, the first dose should also be given cautiously as some of the epidural dose may migrate intrathecally through the meningeal tear. Less local anaesthetic may be needed if the epidural is later used for CS.

Dural puncture with the epidural catheter

- If the epidural catheter has passed into the subarachnoid space, clear CSF will be aspirated easily.
- If saline has been used for loss of resistance, the presence of glucose will confirm the fluid as CSF, and the catheter should be managed as above.

Remember

- Tell the woman what has happened, what to expect and what the treatment options are. Document the complications and ensuing discussion.
- An anaesthetist should perform all epidural or spinal top-ups in the presence of a dural puncture, and the resulting block should be carefully documented.
- Ensure that the midwife understands the nature of the block if a spinal catheter is used and is vigilant for the onset of headache in the postnatal period.
- There is no need to prevent the woman pushing during the second stage.
- Inform a senior anaesthetist and complete relevant paperwork, e.g. follow-up book or audit.

Distinguishing features between CSF and normal saline if suspected accidental dural puncture

	CSF	**Normal saline**
Dural puncture with needle	Gushing and persistent	Few drops then ceases
Dural puncture with catheter	Ongoing aspiration possible. No falling meniscus if catheter raised above head height	Nil aspirated. Falling fluid meniscus if catheter raised above head height
Temperature	Warm	Cold
Protein	Present	Absent
Glucose	Present	Absent
pH	7.5	<7.5

There is a small physiological leak of CSF into the epidural space which may contribute to a false-positive result.

Techniques of spinal insertion

Spinal anaesthesia is commonly performed for CS, but in addition it can be used as the first part of a CSE technique in labour and as a single shot for other obstetric procedures, e.g. forceps delivery, retained placenta and suturing of the perineum.

Relative and absolute contraindications, consent, monitoring, documentation, positioning the mother, skin preparations, pain on insertion and difficulties with insertion are as above.

Equipment

You will need the following:

- Stable work surface.
- Sterile dressing pack with swabs and forceps.
- Range of syringes and needles for local anaesthetic infiltration.
- Filter needle for drawing up intrathecal drugs.
- Sterile drapes—ideally with a window and adhesive sides.
- 24–27G pencil-point spinal needle.
- Spinal drugs.
- 1% lidocaine for skin infiltration.
- Ephedrine 3mg/mL.

Technique

There is a clear end-point (the appearance of CSF at the hub of the spinal needle, which in health has a sparkling quality).

Position

In general terms a spinal anaesthetic is easier to teach and perform than an epidural anaesthetic (Figs. 7.6 and 7.7), but if the mother is not optimally positioned it may be impossible.

Sitting position

- In general, the midline can be more readily identified.
- CSF pressure is higher and it appears more quickly at the hub of the spinal needle, therefore confirming position.
- 'Heavy intrathecal solutions' will produce a low or saddle block if the mother is not laid down quickly, although this may be useful in some situations.

Lateral position (Fig. 7.8)

- May be more comfortable for the mother, especially if she is very distressed.
- The end-point of CSF in the hub of the needle can appear very slowly, which can cause some difficulties and sometimes result in multiple unnecessary attempts.
- 'The Oxford position' (Fig. 7.9) is described for intrathecal injection where the shoulders and head are raised, thus preventing intrathecal solutions from moving too far cephalad. This may cause twisting of the lumbar spine, and extra care during positioning and identification of landmarks is needed.

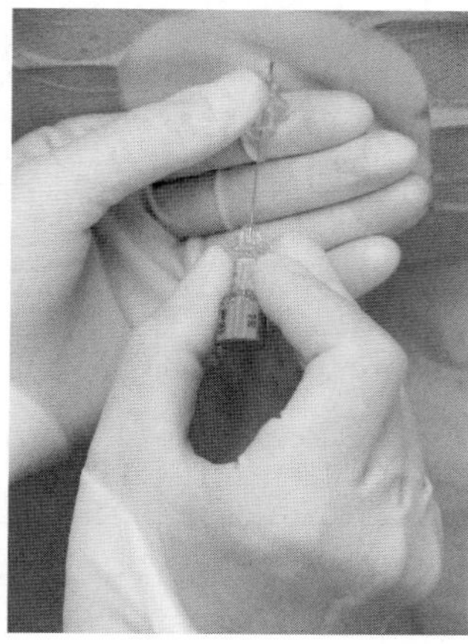

Fig. 7.6 Spinal needle grip. The needle is gripped like a pencil. The advantage is that the subtle differences in the feel of the tissue layers are more easily felt, as well as the 'dural click' as the thecal sac is entered.

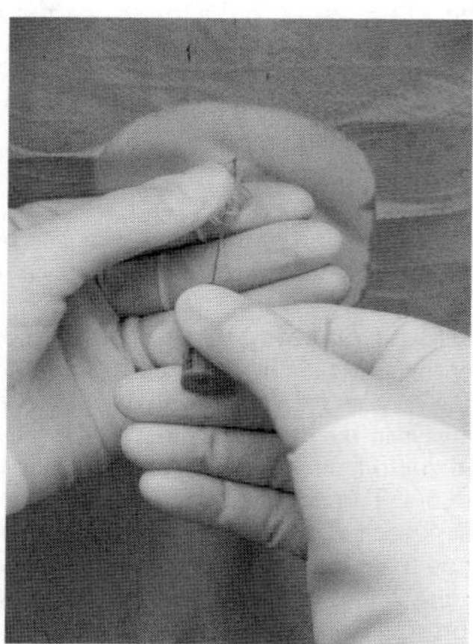

Fig. 7.7 This is a firmer grip—more like a dagger. It is much more difficult to feel subtle changes, but fine needles bend less and can therefore be easier to control.

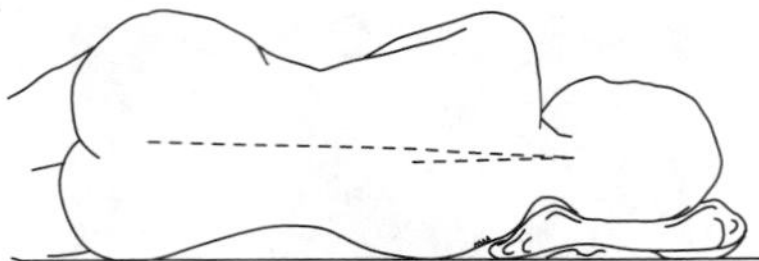

Fig. 7.8 With a pillow under the head and neck only, the spine typically slopes downwards.

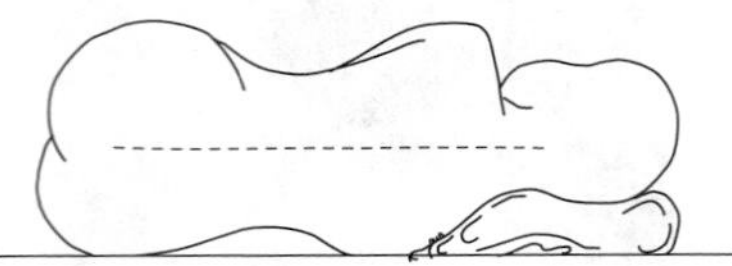

Fig. 7.9 The Oxford position. With the pillow under the lower shoulder, the spine now comes to the vertical.

Interspace

Much has been written about the safe intervertebral space for spinal injection. The L3/4 interspace is ideal, but the L4/5 interspace is advocated by some to reduce the risk of accidental spinal cord damage.

- The spinal cord (conus) ends most commonly between the lower boarder of the T12 vertebra to the lower boarder of L1. In the majority of women, it is safe to perform a spinal anaesthetic in the mid to lower lumbar vertebra, although in ~3%, the conus is as low as L2.
- Tuffier's line is an imaginary line from right to left iliac crest. On plain X-ray, it most commonly bisects the body of L4, thus aiding in the identification of the L3/4 (just above) and L4/5 (just below) this line.
- The accurate identification of the iliac crests can be very difficult, especially if the bony landmarks are difficult to feel because of adipose tissue.
- A landmark MRI study showed that anaesthetists were frequently unable to identify a marked intervertebral space accurately and, more worryingly, were frequently one, two or even three spaces out, nearly always in the cephalad direction. In other words, the space marked could have been L1/2 and the anaesthetist thought they were at L3/4. This could clearly endanger a normal spinal cord.
- Other landmark techniques such as counting down from the 12th rib, counting up from the posterior superior iliac spines and marking an imaginary line 2/3rds of the way down the back from C7 to where the buttocks meet the bed may add additional information.
- Relying on any one technique could lead to inaccuracy, and probably adopting a number together whilst taking an overview of the back is safest.

It is therefore recommended that the back is examined, landmarks identified and the interspace chosen before sterilizing the skin and draping the back.

Choosing the lowest palpable interspace may also help, but this may be as low as L5/S1 where spinal anaesthesia may be impossible, or L4/5, which can be difficult because of the limited flexion of the spine at this level and the shape of the vertebral canal.

Midline vs paramedian

- The midline approach is the most frequently practised technique. A full understanding of the anatomy of both techniques will help if difficulties are encountered.

Midline

- A midline approach is anatomically more straightforward.

Paramedian

- Is a successful technique only once the anaesthetist has a strong 3D image of the anatomy of the vertebral column.
- The approach is different from a paramedian epidural and needs to be taught separately.
- May be more painful as the vertebral lamina is purposely identified.
- The approach can be useful if the interspinous ligaments are unusually calcified or the vertebra are fixed because of unusual anatomy or surgical fixation.

Procedure

- Ensure no contraindications to insertion and that informed consent has been given.
- Full resuscitation equipment must be available.
- Confirm patent, large bore IV access attached to crystalloid infusion.
- Position the patient.
- Identify the relevant interspace.
- Put on theatre hat and mask, scrub up and put on gown and gloves.
- Prepare the back using scrupulous aseptic technique.
- Draw up intrathecal drugs using a filter needle.
- Infiltrate the skin with 25G needle using 2–5mL of 1% lidocaine at and around the midpoint of the interspace. (A common problem is failure to anaesthetize the dermis by infiltrating too deeply).
- Insert the introducer of the spinal needle until it is firmly gripped within the interspinous ligament.
- Hold the spinal needle with the aperture usually directed cephalad.
- Carefully introduce the spinal needle identifying the anatomical layers during insertion.
- Having identified the ligamentum flavum, push the needle forward a couple more millimetres until a gentle pop is felt.
- Remove the stillette of the spinal needle and confirm placement by the appearance of CSF at the hub of the needle.

- Wait for CSF to appear at the hub, BUT before the hub is completely filled with CSF, attach the syringe containing the intrathecal injection. (If the hub is entirely filled by CSF the contents of the syringe tend to leak during injection even if the syringe has been tightly applied.
- Stabilize the needle and syringe during injection.
- It is usual to confirm CSF by gently aspirating on the syringe just before injection. It may be very difficult to aspirate through a 27G or smaller spinal needle.
- Barboutage is controversial. The advocates claim the spinal block works more quickly. The detractors claim it can more readily lead to spinal needle movement and failure.
- Re-confirming needle position by re-aspirating at the end of injection will confirm that the needle has not moved, but the detractors believe it adds nothing as it is in assessment of anaesthesia that will ultimately verify adequate injection.
- Remove syringe, needle and introducer as one at the end of the injection.

Spinal needles

'Pencil-point' spinal needles which divide the vertically arranged dural fibres are now most widely used rather than the Quincke or bevelled needles which tended to cut the fibres, leaving a trap door cut in the dura. This has caused a huge reduction in the incidence of PDPH and was a major factor in the increasing popularity of spinal anaesthesia in obstetric anaesthetic practice from the late 1980s onwards. The most commonly used sizes are 24 and 25G, although some anaesthetists use as small as 27G. The smaller needles offer a marginal advantage in terms of decreased rate of PDPH, but can be more prone to deformity when passing through more solid tissues, and give a slower flashback of CSF. The use of 22G spinal needles is more controversial in the obstetric population because of the increased risk of headache, even with a pencil-point tip.

- This needle can be useful if the interspinous ligaments are unusually tough.
- If the mother is obese. This needle can be used without an introducer, and a standard 90mm needle can be successfully inserted into the CSF ≥9cm from the skin. Although a longer spinal needle can be used in this situation, they are more flexible and difficult to use. Obese mothers have a lower risk of PDPH and a 22G needle is acceptable.

Top tips

- Take as much care with positioning the mother as with an epidural, just because it is fundamentally an easier technique does not mean it will be more successful if the mother is inadequately positioned.
- If probable dural puncture has occurred, take the stillete out quickly. This action draws the CSF down the spinal needle, especially if the needle is of a small diameter, making it easier to confirm correct placement.

- If paraesthesia is more than momentary, do not inject into the CSF and remove the needle.
- If the feeling of dural puncture has occurred but no CSF obtained, rotate the needle through 90°. If CSF is still not seen, withdraw the spinal needle and redirect as it is likely that the ligamentum flavum has been punctured but because of lateral placement the dura has not been punctured.

Continuous spinal anaesthesia

This is not currently popular in obstetric anaesthetic practice, although there are case reports that have described its successful use in parturients with complex cardiac or other problems. This technique allows controlled and gradual development of a dense regional block while maintaining haemodynamic stability.

Various microcatheters have been described. A 22G catheter can be inserted over a 27G spinal needle. The risk of headache is acceptably low when used for specific clinical indications, but probably too high for routine use.

Combined spinal–epidural technique (needle through needle)

CSE is a technique that has increased in popularity for both labour analgesia and CS. It combines the advantages of rapid complete anaesthesia characteristic of spinal anaesthesia with the flexibility to continue anaesthesia for as long as required. It is described either as a separate technique where the spinal and epidural are inserted at different times and sometimes using a different interspace, or as a needle through needle technique.

- The technique of CSE as a separate technique should follow the description of epidural and spinal anaesthesia above.
- The technique of needle through needle CSE is described below.

Relative and absolute contraindications, consent, monitoring, documentation, positioning the mother, skin preparations, pain on insertion and difficulties with insertion are as above.

Equipment

You will need the following:

- Stable work surface.
- Sterile dressing pack with swabs and forceps.
- Range of syringes and needles for local anaesthetic infiltration.
- Filter needle.
- Spinal and epidural needle. Either:
  - Separate 80mm Tuohy needle and 120mm spinal needle.
  - Specially designed CSE kit with a locking device for the spinal needle.
- Loss of resistance syringe.
- Epidural catheter.
- Luer lock and filter.
- 0.9% saline.
- 1% lidocaine.
- Epidural dressings.
- Epidural drugs and/or saline for the epidural space.
- Ephedrine 3mg/mL.

Technique

- The technique for epidural insertion is described above and is not fundamentally different.
- The major difference is that as dural puncture is part of the technique the choice of intervertebral space should follow the spinal technique.

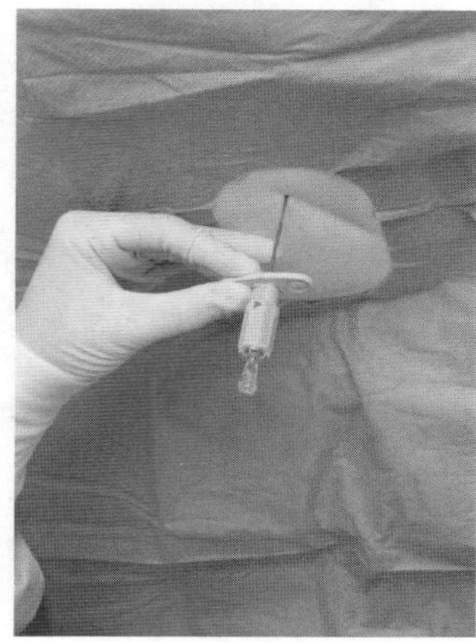

Fig. 7.10 Hand position for a locking CSE: The left hand is stabilized against the patient's back.

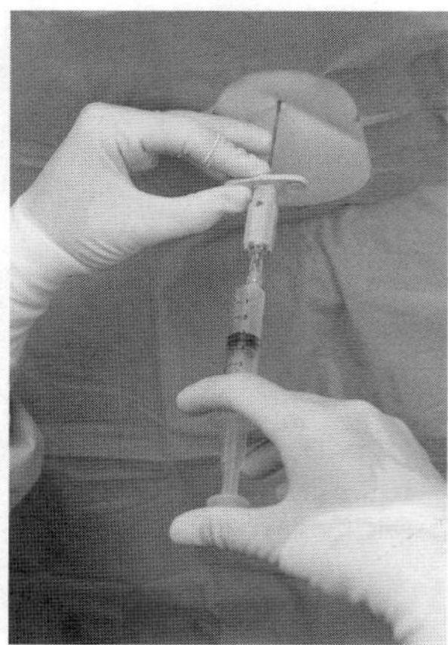

Fig. 7.11 Hand position for a locking CSE: The left hand position does not have to change and the spinal needle is firmly held by the interlocking mechanism during intrathecal injection.

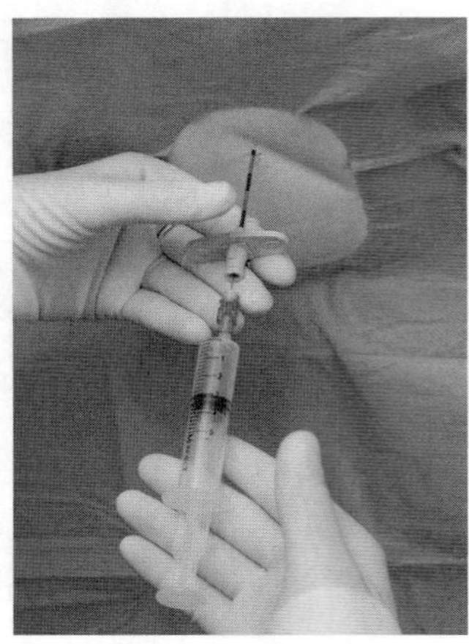

Fig. 7.12 Hand position to stabilize spinal needle for a non-locking CSE: Stabilize spiral needle as it leaving the Tuohy needle with the fingers behind.

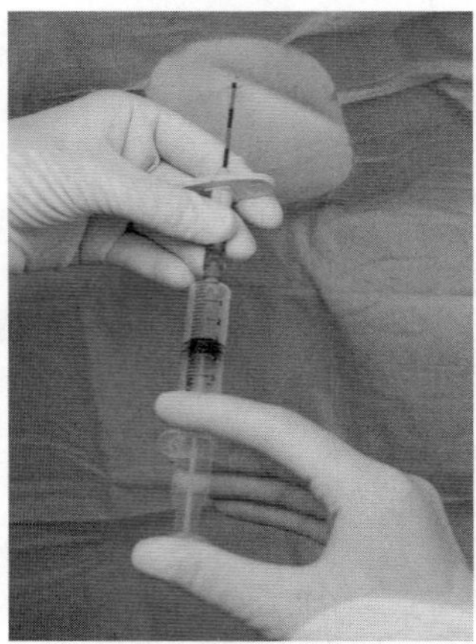

Fig. 7.13 Movement is prevented by gripping the spinal needle with the hub of the Tuohy needle between thumb and fingers.

Procedure

- Initially as for the epidural technique.
- Once the epidural space is identified, control the volume of saline injected (1–2mL).
- Remove the stillette of the spinal needle BEFORE inserting it through the Tuohy needle (hastens CSF backflow).
- Gently insert the spinal needle until the end of the Tuohy needle is identified. From this point, continue to advance with care.
- There is frequently a feel of a 'dural click' on entering the CSF.
- If a dural click is felt OR CSF appears at the hub of the spinal needle, STOP advancing the spinal needle.
- The spinal needle is frequently NOT fully advanced at this point but DO NOT advance further.
  - With a locking CSE kit, lock the spinal needle and inject intrathecal drugs (see Figs. 7.10 and 7.11).
  - If a non-locking spinal needle is used, stabilize spinal and Tuohy needle together (see Figs. 7.12 and 7.13) and inject intrathecal drugs.
- Remove the spinal needle as quickly as possibly and insert the epidural catheter as above.
- If the CSE has been carried out in the sitting position and the block is required to spread upwards, the mother can be placed in the lateral position before the catheter is flushed, aspirated and fixed.
- Injecting saline into the epidural space can increase the spread of the intrathecal drugs. Limit the saline injection during flushing to 2–3mL to minimize this effect.

The major problems encountered during CSE are

- 'Dry tap': the epidural space is identified but the spinal needle does not pass into the CSF.
- This can occur if:
  - The Tuohy needle is too lateral.
  - If too low an interspace is chosen. There is some evidence that the thecal sac becomes move triangular in some patients at L4/5 (see Figs. 7.14 and 7.15). If this is the case, the needle through needle technique may be less successful at this level. If it is likely that the L4/5 interspace has been used, attempt the technique again at the L3/4 interspace.
- Intrathecal injection fails because of movement of the spinal needle. A locking kit reduces this problem but not entirely as needle movement can occur during locking. Practise holding, locking and injecting whatever equipment is available before using it on a patient.

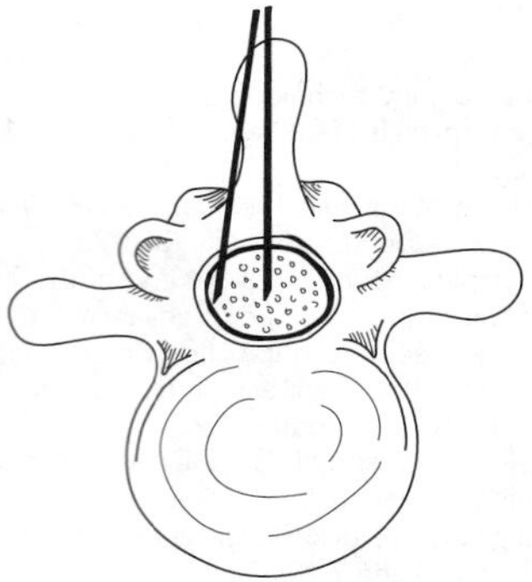

Fig. 7.14 If the thecal sac and bony canal are oval, a slightly lateral approach will be successful.

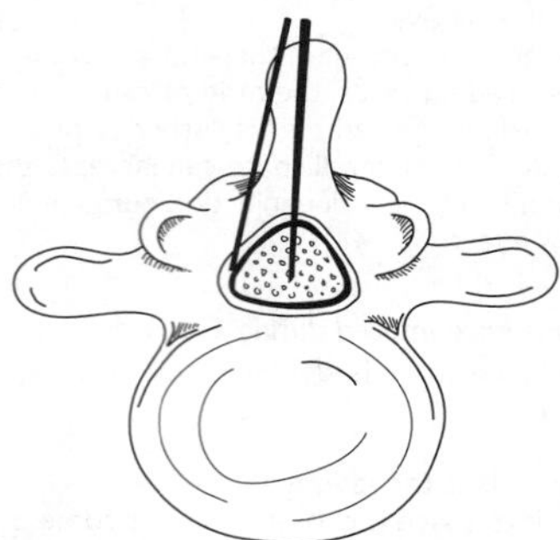

Fig. 7.15 It is common at lower interspaces for the thecal sac and bony canal to become more triangular, with the apex of the triangle posterior. If this is the case, a similar lateral approach with a spinal needle will result in a 'dry trap'.

Removing the epidural catheter

The epidural catheter can be removed as soon as possible after delivery of baby and placenta, unless the following apply:

- Platelet or clotting dysfunction.
  - Await return to normal values.
- Pre-eclampsia.
  - Can be associated with decreased platelet count or coagulopathy.
  - Await return to normal values.
- Accidental dural puncture.
  - If a spinal catheter has been used as first-line management, consider leaving *in situ* for 6–8h post-delivery.
  - Evidence would suggest that the incidence of PDPH is reduced.
- Additional procedures anticipated.
  - E.g. further perineal suturing, return to theatre for examination or ongoing bleeding.
- If difficulties with postdelivery pain management anticipated.
  - E.g. opioid addiction, chronic pain-related problems.
  - Discuss postdelivery analgesia plan with senior anaesthetist.
- Heparins may be required for postpartum thromboembolic prophylaxis or treatment. They may be given safely 4h after an epidural is removed (see page 181).

If the epidural catheter does not come out easily, place the mother in the exact position she was in during insertion. (Don't assume you know if you didn't put it in, ASK HER). It is then very unusual for the catheter not to come out easily. Never pull hard, as there are many reports of broken catheters.

Chapter 8

Regional analgesia for labour

Rachel Collis, Sarah Harries,
Eleanor Lewis, Saira Hussain

Introduction

Epidural analgesia

- Epidural analgesia is the most effective form of analgesia during labour.
- It is the only technique which can potentially provide complete analgesia and has a number of physiological maternal and fetal benefits.
- An effective epidural can also be extended to provide rapid epidural anaesthesia if urgent CS is required.
- Epidural analgesia was first described as caudal analgesia, then continuous lumbar analgesia from the late 1940s.
- Its use was strictly limited because of a lack of expertise in the techniques and the short-acting local anaesthetics available, which over a few hours became ineffective because of tachyphylaxis.
- Interest and development of epidural analgesia for labour began in earnest in the mid 1960s with the introduction of longer lasting local anaesthetics, e.g. bupivacaine.
- Pharmacological and technological advances, as well as a greater understanding of anatomy and physiology, have contributed to its safety and efficacy, with ~25% of women receiving epidural analgesia during labour in the UK today.

Physiological and psychological benefits of epidural analgesia

- As well as minimizing the sensory component of labour, epidural analgesia confers a number of benefits to both mother and fetus.
- Catecholamines and prostaglandins are released in response to the pain of uterine contractions and cervical distension.
- Epidural blockade can limit rises in CO and SVR associated with increased circulating catecholamines.
- Increased oxygen consumption associated with pain and maternal effort can be reduced by effective epidural blockade.
- Maternal and fetal acidosis is minimized and intervillous blood flow is enhanced by arteriolar vasodilatation.
- Uterine contractions may become more coordinated or may be abolished completely.
- These factors are of particular importance in the sick parturient or in those with pre-existing cardiorespiratory disease.

The effect of epidural analgesia on labour and delivery

- Epidural analgesia ***does not*** increase the likelihood of a CS.
- There are associations between epidural analgesia and a prolonged first and second stage of labour, augmentation of labour and need for instrumental delivery. However, there is little evidence to suggest that epidural analgesia is the sole causative factor in these cases.
- Epidural analgesia is not the cause of postpartum backache, nor does it increase the likelihood of developing long-term back problems.
- There is a rise in maternal temperature after epidural analgesia for labour. The exact cause is unknown, although alterations in maternal thermoregulation has been implicated, but it is important to distinguish it from infection to prevent unnecessary use of antibiotics.

Indications for epidural analgesia

- Maternal request.
  - There is no circumstance where it is considered acceptable for a person to experience untreated severe pain, amenable to safe intervention, while under a physician's care.
  - A fully dilated cervix is not a contraindication to site an epidural, unless delivery is imminent.
- Augmentation of labour.
  - Oxytocic drug infusions, e.g. oxytocin, can cause painful, forceful contractions, and epidural analgesia is often encouraged to aid compliance.
- Hypertensive disease.
  - Sympathetic blockade may aid BP control, e.g. in pre-eclampsia.
  - An effective epidural will avoid the hazards of GA if a CS is required.
- Morbid obesity.
  - An epidural should be recommended early in labour, as an effective block may minimize the need for GA in the event of emergency CS.
  - It should be reassessed regularly to ensure that it continues to function optimally.
- Predicated difficult airway or intubation risk.
  - To avoid the need for an emergency GA.
- History/family history of significant GA problems.
  - E.g. malignant hyperpyrexia, suxamethonium apnoea or anaphylaxis.
- Cardiac and respiratory disease.
  - An effective epidural minimizes the increase in CO and minute ventilation associated with labour and delivery.
  - It is essential to ensure that changes to preload and afterload are minimized and aorto-caval compression is avoided at all costs.
  - In severe cardiac disease, invasive BP monitoring may be indicated.
- Cerebrovascular disease.
  - Pushing and straining will cause a rise in the ICP, which may be deleterious in the presence of cerebral aneurysms, arteriovenous malformations or other intracranial disease. Regional analgesia will facilitate an operative delivery in these cases.
- Multiple pregnancy and breech presentation.
  - To facilitate assisted or operative delivery which is often required.

Further reading

Segal S *et al.* The effect of a rapid change in availability of epidural analgesia on the caesarean delivery rate: a meta-analysis. *American Journal of Obstetrics and Gynecology* 2000; **183**: 974–978.

Howell C, Chalmers I. A review of prospectively controlled comparisons of epidural forms of pain relief during labour. *International Journal of Obstetric Anesthesia* 1991; **2**: 1–17.

Anim-Somuah M *et al.* Epidural versus non-epidural or no analgesia in labour. *Cochrane Database Library*, 2005.

Drugs in the epidural space

- The most common class of drugs used to provide epidural analgesia in labour are the amide local anaesthetics (LAs).
- Addition of an opioid results in a synergistic action leading to superior analgesia as well as reduced overall local anaesthetic requirements.
- There is increased maternal satisfaction, less likelihood of motor block and cardiovascular instability with an improved safety profile from low concentration LA mixtures.

Local anaesthetic drugs

- LAs block fast sodium channels, causing a reversible inhibition of neuronal transmission.
- Once injected into the epidural space, the LA diffuses across the dural cuff to gain access to the lumbosacral nerve roots and the dorsal root ganglia.
- It also diffuses directly across the dura into the CSF and thus to the spinal cord and its blood vessels.
- LAs are non-selective in that sensory, motor and autonomic neurons are blocked. C fibres (pain) are blocked first, followed by the larger Aδ (motor, proprioception) and Aβ (pressure, light touch) fibres.

Racemic bupivacaine

- Currently the most widely used LA for labour analgesia in the UK.
  - Pros: highly lipid soluble, potent with long duration of action. Provides effective analgesia at low concentrations in combination with opioids.
  - Cons: dose-dependent motor block, cardiotoxicity due to affinity for cardiac Na^+ channels causing resistant life-threatening arrhythmias.

Levobupivacaine

- S-enantiomer of bupivacaine, which is gaining popularity over the racemic mixture.
  - Pros: clinically equipotent to bupivacaine for labour analgesia but with less arrhythmogenicity, thus better if large dose boluses required, e.g. extension of epidural block for CS.
  - Cons: currently more expensive than racemic bupivacaine.

Ropivacaine

- S-enantiomer of propivacaine.
  - Pros: less cardiotoxic than racemic bupivacaine.
  - Cons: gained popularity due to its apparent differential blockade of sensory fibres but not motor fibres. Studies have shown, however, that this is due to a significantly reduced potency (40% less potent). Common solutions are between 0.1 and 0.2%. The incidence of motor block is the same at equipotent doses of racemic bupivacaine.

Lidocaine

- Short-acting amide LA.
    - Pros: rapid onset of action is useful to extend a pre-existing epidural block for CS.
    - Cons: high degree of motor block and tachyphylaxis precludes its use for labour analgesia in current modern obstetric practice. Lidocaine may be neurotoxic in high doses.

Opioids

- Opioids may act spinally or supraspinally depending on the dose, lipophilicity and frequency of administration, i.e. bolus dosage or continuous infusion.
- Epidural opioids cross the dura and diffuse through the CSF to reach their site of action in the substantia gelatinosa of the dorsal horn of the spinal cord.
- A proportion of the administered epidural/intrathecal dose will be absorbed into the blood to exert a systemic effect.
- There is some evidence to suggest that epidural fentanyl causes segmental analgesia when given as a bolus and non-segmental systemic analgesia when given as a continuous infusion.

Morphine

- Typically used to provide longer lasting analgesia post caesarean section rather than during labour.
    - Pros: long lasting due to poor lipophilicity.
    - Cons: slow onset of action and high incidence of side effects—respiratory depression may appear up to 12h after epidural administration.

Fentanyl

- Most widely used opioid for labour analgesia in the UK.
    - Pros: highly lipophilic with rapid penetration of spinal cord leading to fast onset of analgesia, and reduces LA requirements.
    - Cons: short duration of action. Nausea, vomiting, pruritis (most commonly) and respiratory depression may occur with high doses.

Diamorphine

- Intermediate lipophilicity, mostly used to provide analgesia post caesarean section.
    - Pros: more rapid onset of analgesia than morphine and less risk of late respiratory depression.
    - Cons: shorter duration of analgesic effect than morphine.

Other opioids

- Pethidine is avoided as it has an LA effect causing unpredictable sympathetic and motor block. Nausea is also very common.
- Epidural sufentanil (~5 times as potent as epidural fentanyl) is used widely in the USA but has no product licence in the UK.
- Tramadol is thought to produce less respiratory depression associated with opioids due to its selective μ1-agonism and it prolongs duration of analgesia when used in conjunction with 0.25% bupivacaine.

Other drugs (for doses see Table 10.1, p. 299)

A number of other drugs, typically used in combination with LAs and/or opioids, have been or are being investigated.

Clonidine

- An α_2 agonist which acts at receptors in the dorsal horn of the spinal cord causing analgesia with no motor block.
- Descending noradrenergic pathways are subsequently activated with release of inhibitory neurotransmitters.
- Problems limiting its widespread use include hypotension and sedation.

Adrenaline

- α_1 adrenergic agonism causes vasoconstriction, which decreases systemic absorption of LA and thus prolongs its effects.
- Traditionally used as part of a test dose to determine intravascular injection—manifest as a tachycardia.
- Adrenaline can also provide analgesia via α_2 adrenergic agonism; however, it is associated with a dense motor block.

Neostigmine

- An anticholinesterase, which produces dose-dependent analgesia by inhibiting the breakdown of acetylcholine.
- Acetylcholine is involved in spinal modulation of pain processing predominantly by stimulating cholinergic neurons of the muscarinic type.
- It has been used to counteract the haemodynamic depression produced by epidural clonidine, though nausea and vomiting are common side effects.
- Neostigmine is also poorly lipid soluble, so onset is delayed.

Ketamine

- An NMDA antagonist, which blocks glutamate-mediated excitatory transmission of nociceptive impulses.
- Other effects include opioid agonism and sodium channel interactions.
- The S (+) enantiomer prolongs caudal epidural block in children by up to 4 times, and it has the added benefit of lack of respiratory depression.

Further reading

Murphy JD *et al.* Bupivicaine versus bupivicaine plus fentanyl for epidural analgesia: effect on maternal satisfaction. *British Medical Journal* 1991; **302**: 564–567.

Capogna G *et al.* Determination of the minimum local analgesic concentration (MLAC) of epidural ropivicaine in labour. *British Journal of Anaesthesia* 1998; **80**: 148.

Ginosar Y *et al.* The site of action of epidural fentanyl in humans. The difference between infusion and bolus administration. *Anesthesia and Analgesia* 2003; **97**: 1428–1438.

Roelants F. The use of neuraxial adjuvant drugs (neostigmine, clonidine) in obstetrics (Review). *Current Opinion in Anaesthesiology* 2006; **19**: 233–237.

The test dose

The purpose of the test dose is to exclude or confirm intravascular or intrathecal placement which is most common after initial catheter placement. However, every time a dose is injected into the epidural space it should be considered a test dose as the epidural catheter may migrate intrathecally, subdurally, intravenously or completely out of the epidural space.

The ideal test dose should allow the anaesthetist to detect abnormal placement rapidly before endangering the patient because of drug toxicity.

An ideal drug/mixture of drugs would

- Equally detect intravascular and intrathecal injection.
- Have 100% specificity with 100% positive and negative predictive values.
- Allow detection of abnormal placement immediately (IV) or within 5min (intrathecal).

The fact that there are huge variations in the choices obstetric anaesthetists make confirms there is not an ideal solution.

Detection of accidental intravascular injection

Symptoms of local anaesthetic toxicity

- Circum oral tingling, numbness, tinnitus.
- Lightheadedness, confusion, agitation and tremor.
- Loss of consciousness.
- Convulsions.
- Arrhythmia.
- Cardiovascular collapse.

- After careful aspiration of the epidural catheter, the LA solution should be injected.
- The earliest signs of intravascular injection (circum oral tingling and tinnitus) should warn the anaesthetist to stop injecting.
- The addition of 15 micrograms adrenaline has been popular and is still advocated by some.
  - This small amount of adrenaline will cause a transient increase in maternal heart rate after intravascular injection.
  - It is highly sensitive but only 65% specific (the mother's heart rate commonly varies with the pain of contractions).
  - The increase in heart rate is difficult to detect unless ECG monitoring is used.

Detection of accidental intrathecal placement

5 signs of accidental intrathecal injection

- Very rapid analgesia.
- Excessive sensory block.
- Early motor block (hip flexion).
- Early sacral block (ankle plantaflexion).
- Hypotension.

NB: hypotension may be absent, so the block must be formally tested after the test dose to evaluate the other modalities.

- The ideal test dose would be easily detected within 5min without excessive spread of the block and severe hypotension.
- The general principle is to use a dose of LA that could be used for a CS if given intrathecally.
- There is wide variation in practice.
- 10–15mg bupivacaine can safely be given as a 0.1% solution or 0.5% solution.
- 60mg lidocaine (3mL lidocaine 2%).
- Common practice is 10mL of 0.1% bupivacaine with fentanyl 2 micrograms/mL.
- There is not a test dose that is completely reliable at 5min, and it may be safer to assess the block formally at 10min after injection.

There is an increasing move away from small volume high concentration solutions to large volume low concentration solutions.

The advantage of the latter is that the test dose will:

- Significantly contribute to early analgesia.
- Reduce the overall LA dose required to establish analgesia.
- Reduce the early development of motor block.

Management of a suspected positive test dose

- Stop injecting.
- Re-aspirate.
  - The initial aspiration test may have been negative but is now positive.
  - If aspiration is still negative, the epidural catheter may still be incorrectly positioned.
- If intravascular injection is suspected, pull the catheter back 0.5–1cm and re-aspirate. If uncertainty remains, it is safer to remove the catheter completely and start again.
- If the mother develops signs of intrathecal placement.
  - Place her in the full lateral position to reduce the risk of hypotension.
  - Evaluate the block carefully with particular attention to sacral anaesthesia.
  - Give IV fluids and vasopressors as required.
  - If intrathecal placement is confirmed, label the epidural catheter as SPINAL and use as a spinal catheter (see Management of dural puncture, Chapter 7 p 206).

Further reading

Gardner IC, Kinsella SM. Obstetric epidural test doses: a survey of UK practice. *International Journal of Obstetric Anesthesia* 2005; **14**: 96–103.

Holdcroft A. Use of adrenaline in obstetric analgesia. *Anaesthesia* 1992; **47**: 987–990.

Colonna-Romano P, Nagaraj L. Tests to evaluate intravenous placement of epidural catheters in laboring women: a prospective clinical study. *Anesthesia and Analgesia* 1998; **86**: 985–988.

Norris MC *et al.* Does epinephrine improve the diagnostic accuracy of aspiration during labor epidural analgesia? *Anesthesia and Analgesia* 1999; **88**: 1073–1076.

Yarnell RW *et al.* Sacralization of epidural block with repeated doses of 0.25% bupivacaine during labour. *Regional Anesthesia* 1990; **15**: 275–279.

Daoud Z *et al.* Evaluation of S1 motor block to determine a safe, reliable test dose for epidural analgesia. *British Journal of Anaesthesia* 2002; **89**: 442–445.

Hocking G, Wildsmith JAW. 2004. Intrathecal drug spread (Review). *British Journal of Anaesthesia* 2004 **93**: 568–578.

Pain scoring

A pain score trend can provide valuable information for the clinician regarding:

- Effectiveness of analgesia.
- Escalation of pain due to a new stimulus, e.g. uterine rupture.
- Change in the nature of pain, e.g. sacral pressure with descent of the fetal head.

The most easily applied score is the verbal numerical pain score, where the woman is asked to give a number from 0 to 100 to indicate the severity of the pain—0 being no pain and 100 being the worst pain ever. Aim to reduce the pain score to ≤30 with epidural analgesia.

Practical pain scoring

- Ask the woman to score her pain prior to analgesia.
- Determine the nature and site of the pain—is it.
  - the tightening, crescendo pain of uterine contractions.
  - sacral and rectal pressure from a descending fetal head or malpresentation.
  - or an atypical pain—epigastric or pubic symphysis diastasis?
- Different stimuli may require different management.
- During establishment of the block, score the pain every 10min after top-ups until the pain score is <30.
- Do a pain score 10–15min after each top-up in labour or hourly with an epidural infusion.
- The most obvious sign is a comfortable, smiling woman—observe the woman through contractions (on CTG) and ask her how each one felt.

Pain scores >30

- Establish the epidural in divided doses with up to 30mg bupivacaine with an opioid. If pain scores have never been less than 30 within 40min after initial epidural placement, consider replacing the epidural at this stage.
  THE EPIDURAL WILL NEVER BE SATISFACTORY
- If the epidural has worked well but the mother is now in pain.
  - Check the position of the epidural catheter—it may have come out of the space.
  - Ensure that the woman is getting regular intermittent bolus top-ups—severe pain should not be allowed to return prior to administering further top-ups.
  - If she is using a PCEA, make sure that she is pressing the button as required.
  - If the pain score suddenly increases after being stable with effective established analgesia, determine the nature of the pain. Sacral pain may be managed with a stronger LA top-up (bupivacaine 0.25% with fentanyl) in the sitting position. Sudden onset severe pain may be indicative of another pathology, e.g. liver capsule haematoma [if pre-eclampsia toxaemia (PET)] or uterine rupture, and may warrant further investigations.
- Resite a poorly functioning epidural early.

Assessing the block

The ideal epidural block for labour should cover the T10–S5 nerve roots with minimal motor block of the lower limbs. It can generally be called a 'light' block with evidence of a sensory block to cold sensation and a sympathetic block that usually accompanies this (warm feet). A dense sensory block (unable to feel a pinch or pinprick) is usually associated with quite a dense motor block. This type of block is typical if 0.25% bupivacaine is used, and should be avoided if possible.

Sensory, motor and sympathetic blockade, as well as maternal satisfaction, should be assessed and documented:

- 10min after the first dose.
- 15–20min after the initial incremental doses to establish a block.
- Prior to and 10min after any top-up dose for breakthrough pain, unilateral block or missed segment.
- If there is sudden maternal hypotension, fetal distress or any other abnormal maternal signs or symptoms.
- Prior to top-up for CS.

Sensory block

- It is important to establish that the woman can articulate and appreciate the differences between, touch/pressure, sharp/dull, wetness, cold and ice cold. Show her the 'normal sensation' by applying the stimulus to normal skin.
- Ensure that the block is assessed bilaterally.
- Ice or ethyl chloride are used to determine the level at which temperature sensation is altered, compared with a standard skin dermatome chart.
- A neurological pin test for pinprick sensation with both sharp and dull sensation elicited.
- Light touch can be assessed using cotton wool, touching with a finger or a Von Frey hair.
- Loss of sensation to temperature usually occurs two dermatomes higher than that to pinprick.
- Loss of sensation to pinprick usually occurs two dermatomes higher than that to light touch.
- If S1 (largest sacral nerve root) is blocked, i.e. the soles of the feet, it is unnecessary to test the perineum formally during labour. The S2 dermatome runs up the back of the leg and is also easy to test.
- In labour, it is usual to test and document the block relative to cold sensation.

Sympathetic block

- Epidural blockade can be indicated by vasomotor changes in the lower limbs.
- A sympathetic block of the feet does not develop until there is a well-defined sensory block to T10 (umbilicus).

- The soles of the feet should look pink, well perfused and feel warm and dry. Drying of the feet is an important part of sympathetic block assessment and can only be accurately determined by examining the soles.
- Differences in foot temperature are indicative of an asymmetrical or unilateral block. Regardless of whether testing to ice demonstrates a difference, the quality of the block is still likely to be not as good on the cooler side and the mother is likely to get breakthrough pain on that side.
- Maternal hypotension is rare due to the low dose mixtures commonly used.
- Severe hypotension may occur following accidental intrathecal injection or high/subdural spread.
- Bradycardias may be seen if the cardioaccelerator fibres (T1–T4) are blocked or if there is decreased atrial pressure from reduced VR due to aorto-caval compression.

Motor block

- Motor block is minimal if low dose mixes of LA and opioid are used.
- There is usually some weakness or heaviness of the legs if higher concentrations of bupivacaine are used.
- Motor block can be assessed according to the traditional Bromage Scale (Table 8.1) or the modification of Breen *et al.* (Table 8.2).
- Epidurals act more rapidly on hip flexion and most slowly on ankle dorsiflexion. This differentiation is termed 'sacralization of the epidural block'.

Table 8.1 Bromage Scale

Grade	Criteria	Degree of motor block
I	Free movement of feet and legs	Nil (0%)
II	Just able to flex knees with free movement of feet	Partial (33%)
III	Unable to flex knees but with free movement of feet	Almost complete (66%)
IV	Unable to move legs or feet	Complete (100%)

Table 8.2 Modified Bromage Scale as used by Breen *et al.*

Score	Criteria
1	Complete block (unable to move feet)
2	Almost complete block (able to move feet only)
3	Partial block (just able to move knees)
4	Detectable weakness of hip flexion while supine (full flexion of knees)
5	No detectable weakness of hip flexion while supine
6	Able to perform partial knee bend-whilst standing

Maternal satisfaction

- A comfortable woman who feels in control and can still move freely (either standing or moving herself on the bed) indicates a successful epidural.
- Assess and document pain scores aiming to reduce the score below 30/100 (3/10).
- If she is still requiring Entonox, the epidural block may be inadequate and needs to be reassessed and further top-ups given.
- Remember that the nature and/or intensity of the pain may change as labour advances, especially with the addition of uterine stimulants.

Further reading

Griffin RP, Reynolds F. The association between foot temperature and asymmetrical epidural blockade. *International Journal of Obstetric Anesthesia*; 1994; **3**: 132–136.

Breen TW *et al.* Epidural anesthesia for labour in an ambulatory patient. *Anesthesia and Analgesia* 1993; **77**: 919–924.

Administering analgesia

- Low dose solutions, e.g. 0.0625–0.1% bupivacaine and 2 micrograms/mL fentanyl mixture, have been found to produce effective epidural analgesia during labour.
- Other popular solutions are 0.1–0.2% ropivacaine with fentanyl or sufentanil.
- Following the administration of a titrated bolus dose of LA and opioid solution to establish a sensory block to T10, the method of administering the epidural solution to maintain analgesia throughout labour varies widely between hospitals.

Intermittent top-ups

- Intermittent 'top-ups' can be administered either by the anaesthetist or by a midwife whenever the mother requests further pain relief or as part of a scheduled dosing regime.
- The top-up given varies depending on local protocols and can be 0.25% bupivacaine to <0.1% bupivacaine with an opioid.

Pros

- Analgesia is titrated to the mother's requirements.
- Higher doses reduce the number of administrations.
- Low incidence of motor block with 'low dose regimes', i.e. ≤0.1% bupivacaine.
- Fewer unilateral blocks and missed segments.

Cons

- Considered labour-intensive.
- Essential that an ongoing training programme for midwives is in place.
- Top-ups may be withheld by the midwife in the second stage because of the mistaken view that the mother is more likely to have a normal delivery.

Continuous epidural infusions

- A continuous background infusion of low dose mixture (≤0.1% bupivacaine with an opioid) is administered into the epidural space via an electronic pump.

Pros

- Popular in many hospitals because of their overall efficacy.
- Fewer top-ups required overall, therefore there is a perceived reduction in workload for both midwives and the anaesthetist.
- When working well, will provide analgesia for many hours with stable haemodynamic effects.

Cons

- Purchase and maintenance costs of epidural pumps.
- Ongoing pump training for all staff is required.

- Total amount of drug administered during labour is higher compared with low dose, intermittent top-ups because analgesia is not titrated exactly to requirements and additional top-ups will be required in 70–80% of epidurals.
- If all 'seems' well, there may be a tendency not to check the block and mother's BP.

Patient-controlled epidural analgesia

- Patient controlled 'top-ups' of low dose mixture are administered into the epidural space via an electronic pump.
- Many differing dosing regimes have been reported, both with and without a continuous background infusion.
- Suggested dosing regimes with 0.1–0.125% bupivacaine and 2–3 micrograms fentanyl = 4–6mL bolus, lockout time 10–20min, background infusion 0–6mL/h.

Pros

- Safe, effective method of labour analgesia.
- Offers the mother greater control and autonomy, which is known to improve overall satisfaction.

Cons

- No significant advantage over 'top-up' regimens or infusions alone.
- Purchase and maintenance costs of pumps and ongoing pump training of all staff need to be considered.
- The mother may administer a top-up without supervision and BP monitoring.

Low dose/mobile epidurals

- A so-called 'mobile epidural' can be started in the intrathecal OR epidural space.
- Epidural analgesia does not prevent the mother from getting out of bed, walking around or sitting in a chair.
- Similarly, continuous CTG monitoring is not an indication to remain in bed for the duration of labour (it is a NICE recommendation that there should be continuous CTG monitoring with an epidural).
- If the mother wishes to stand, sit out or ambulate after an epidural has been sited, the following checks should be performed 20min after completion of the epidural:
  - Ensure adequate pain relief.
  - Ensure strong, sustained ability to straight leg raise.
  - Ask mother to place feet on the floor. If her feet feel like 'cotton wool', this usually means it is NOT safe to walk.
  - Standing and first steps should be attempted initially with the anaesthetist and midwife in attendance until the mother is confident that her legs will support her weight.
  - The mother should do a deep knee bend, i.e. femur to ~45° to the vertical, under supervision.
  - Continue to monitor the BP every 30min, unless required more frequently.

- Maintain epidural analgesia with intermittent 'top-ups' of low dose solution with the mother on the bed or sitting in the chair.
- The usual checks should be performed after each 'top-up'.

Further reading

Torvaldsen S *et al.* Discontinuation of epidural analgesia late in labour for reducing the adverse delivery outcomes associated with epidural analgesia (Review). *Cochrane Database of Systematic Reviews* 2004; **18**: CD004457.

Peach MJ. Patient-controlled epidural analgesia in obstetrics. *International Journal of Obstetric Anesthesia* 1996; **5**: 115–125.

Carvalho B *et al.* 'Ultra-light' patient-controlled epidural analgesia during labor: effects of varying regimens on analgesia and physician workload. *International Journal of Obstetric Anesthesia* 2005; **14**: 223–229.

Bernard JM *et al.* Ropivacaine and fentanyl concentrations in patient-controlled epidural analgesia during labor: a volume-range study. *Anesthesia and Analgesia* 2003; **97**: 1800–1807.

Russell R, Reynolds F. Epidural infusion of low-dose bupivacaine and opioid in labour. Does reducing motor block increase the spontaneous delivery rate? *Anaesthesia* 1996; **51**: 266–273.

Collis RE *et al.* Comparison of midwife top-ups, continuous infusion and patient-controlled epidural analgesia for maintaining mobility after a low-dose combined spinal–epidural. *British Journal of Anaesthesia* 1999; **82**: 233–236.

Price C *et al.* Regional analgesia in early active labour: combined spinal epidural vs. epidural. *Anaesthesia* 1998; **53**: 951–955.

Wilson MJ *et al.* Randomized controlled trial comparing traditional with two 'mobile' epidural techniques: anesthetic and analgesic efficacy. *Anesthesiology* 2002; **97**: 1567–1575.

COMET study group UK. Effect of low-dose mobile versus traditional epidural techniques on mode of delivery: a randomised controlled trial. *Lancet* 2001; **358**: 19–23.

Epidurals that don't work

- There is a well-recognized failure rate with epidural blockade, even in experienced hands.
- Failure rates range from 8 to 23%, reducing to 2% at re-siting.
- Failure is much higher amongst obstetric patients than surgical patients.

It is therefore important to understand why epidurals fail and what can be done to remedy the situation. It is also important to inform the mother about the failure rate before she consents to the procedure.

Reasons why the epidural fails

- The catheter is not in the epidural space.
    - The catheter has never been in the epidural space. Possible locations include the subcutaneous tissues, interspinous ligament and paravertebral space.
    - The catheter was once in the epidural space, but has migrated out. This includes 'transforaminal escape'.
    - There are also cases where the catheter has gone beyond the epidural space into the subdural space.
- There is inadequate spread of the drug.
    - Not enough volume of drug.
    - Presence of anatomical barriers within the epidural space.
    - Blocked epidural catheter.
    - Abnormal spinal anatomy, e.g. scoliosis.

Catheter not in the epidural space

False loss of resistance

- If the catheter is not in the epidural space, the initial placement technique was incorrect.
- False loss of resistance is a common problem.
- The operator experiences a loss of resistance dorsal to the ligamentum flavum whilst still in the interspinous ligament.
- There are lacunae or cavities in the interspinous ligament that when entered can give the impression of a loss of resistance.

Indicators of a false loss of resistance

- Loss of resistance is more superficial than expected.
- The catheter is difficult to thread.
- There is no fall in meniscus level down epidural catheter.

How to decide between true and false loss of resistance

- This comes with experience.
- Ultimately, loss of resistance must be considered to be true, as the consequence of ignoring it is an accidental dural tap, which is far worse than re-siting a failed epidural.
- Before starting the procedure, have an idea where you may expect to encounter loss of resistance.
- The average depth to the epidural space at L3/4 level is 5cm via the midline approach, with a range from 2.5 to 10cm.

- If the mother is obese, the epidural space is unlikely to be superficial. False loss of resistance is common as the needle may have to advanced to 6 or 7cm before the interspinous ligament is found.
- If the catheter does not thread easily and then there is no fall of the saline meniscus due to the negative pressure within the epidural space, have a high index of suspicion that the catheter is not in the right place.
- If satisfactory analgesia is not achieved after 3×10mL epidural bolus doses, consider re-siting the epidural early.

Paravertebral block

- The epidural space is continuous with the paravertebral space laterally.
- If the needle placement is too lateral from the midline, the paravertebral space may be entered.
- A loss of resistance will be experienced and the catheter may thread easily.
- The block will be obviously unilateral and inadequate.
- A marked unilateral sympathetic block with little associated analgesia is highly suggestive.
- The only option is re-siting.

Subdural block

- The subdural space occurs between the dura and arachnoid mater.
- It is possible for the catheter to enter the epidural space, then breech the dura but not go as far as the arachnoid and subarachnoid space, which would result in CSF release and a recognized dural tap.
- If this occurs, the catheter would be sitting in the subdural space.
- A subdural block, which is a rare occurrence, characteristically results in a patchy but unexpectedly high sensory block.
- There is usually a fairly weak motor block.
- Perineal analgesia is usually poor.
- Once recognized, the only option is to re-site the catheter.

Transforaminal escape

- Collier demonstrated this phenomenon by performing epidurograms after delivery in women who had had unsatisfactory epidural analgesia (See Figs. 8.1 and 8.2).
- A major cause of inadequate epidural analgesia was found to be escape of the catheter through the intervertebral foramina.
- The block characteristics are of a limited unilateral block, usually L1/3 dermatomes.
- The occurrence rate is ~6% and is due to too much catheter being inserted into the epidural space.
- After 4cm of catheter has been inserted, the catheter tends to curl up. It is therefore recommended that only 2–4cm of catheter is inserted into the epidural space.
- Interestingly, partial withdrawal of a long catheter only improves the block in 50% of women. It is thought that the catheter opens up a path through the intervertebral foramina which all subsequent epidural doses will track.
- Transforaminal escape is more common in obstetric patients, and epidural venous distention is thought to be a possible causative factor.

Catheter migration with maternal repositioning

- The distance to the epidural space is greatest when lateral, and less when sitting.
- When maternal position is changed from sitting to lateral, the catheter may withdraw.
- If the catheter is taped down with the mother flexed, it will move out as she straightens.
- The key point is to allow the mother to reposition before the catheter is fixed to the skin.

Inadequate spread of the drug within the epidural space

This assumes the catheter is in the correct space.

Not enough drug volume

- Characteristically, the block is bilateral but inadequate, because it is usually too low. An upper sensory block to T10 is required.
- It can also be inadequate due to failure to block the perineum sufficiently. A lower sensory block to S3,4,5 is required.
- In both cases, the management is to inject more volume of low dose local anaesthetic/opioid mixture.

Anatomical barriers within the epidural space

- Contrast X-ray studies indicate the existence of an anatomical barrier in some epidural spaces.
- A dorsomedian connective tissue band has been directly visualized with an epiduroscope.
- Midline pedicles and epidural fat pads have also been described.
- The characteristic block is a unilateral block that occurs in ~3% of all epidurals.
- A true missed segment, which is a rare finding, can also be explained by this mechanism.
- The barrier can usually be successfully overcome by increasing the volume in the epidural space.
- Partial catheter withdrawal may also help.

Spinal deformity

- Scoliosis is one example where unusual distribution of the epidural solution results in an inadequate block.
- Similar difficulties may result after spinal surgery, when scar tissue reduces the spread of epidural solution.

Blocked catheter

- A patent catheter at the point of insertion can become blocked with fibrin or blood clots, resulting in poor distribution of the drug.

Further reading

Collier CB. Why obstetric epidurals fail: a study of epidurograms. *International Journal of Obstetric Anesthesia* 1996; **5**: 19–31.

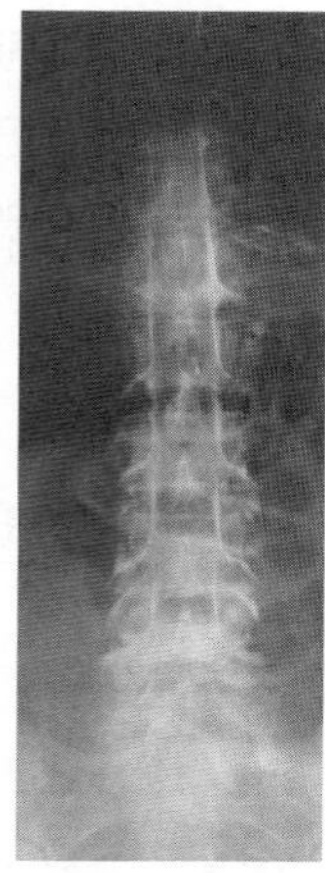

Fig. 8.1 A normal epidurogram. An even spread of contrast in the epidural space with a typical 'Christmas tree' appearance and good root spill of contrast.

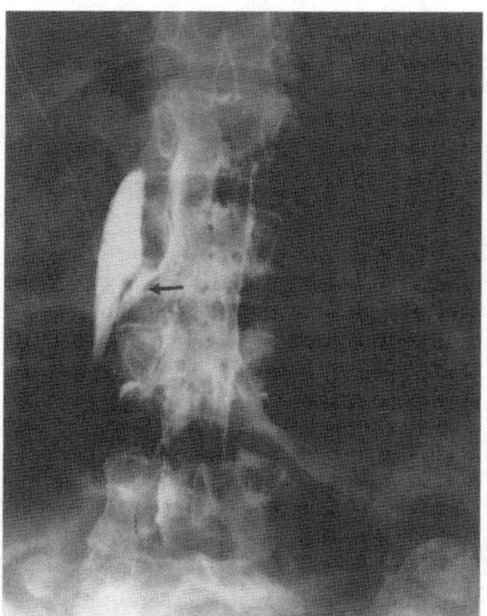

Fig. 8.2 An abnormal epidurogram. The epidural catheter emerges through the L2 intervertebral foramen (arrow). Contrast shows marked psoas and predominantly unilateral epidural spread.

Rescuing the failing epidural

The key to success is to know why the epidural is failing. A decision can then be made either to spend time adjusting the catheter, increase the dose or consider re-siting the epidural immediately. Even after re-siting, 2% of mothers will still not achieve adequate epidural analgesia.

Epidurals can be divided into 3 groups:
- Those that initially worked well.
- Those that have been partially effective.
- Those that have never worked.

Epidurals that have initially worked well

- These are worth spending some time sorting out because, initially, the catheter was in the epidural space.
- The question is 'what has changed?'
  - Has the catheter moved inward or outward? Check the position at the skin.
  - Check the block—is it bilateral or unilateral? Is it too low or not low enough?
  - Have the woman's requirements changed as her labour progresses?
- If the catheter has migrated inward then withdraw it to its original site.
- If it has come out, re-site the epidural, making sure that it is fixed securely after the mother has repositioned herself. Alternatively, consider suturing it in.
- After checking the sensory level of the block, usually to ice-cold, the height and depth of the block on both sides should be recorded and compared with previous sensory levels recorded for that epidural.
- If the block is bilateral but not extensive enough, inject more volume into the epidural space.
  - A low concentration bolus, e.g. 10mL bupivacaine 0.1% + fentanyl 2 micrograms/mL should improve the situation.
  - It is safe to give a second top-up if a recent top-up has been given, provided that the height of the block is known.
  - Re-assess in 10–15min and consider a further 10mL bolus of low concentration mixture to improve the situation further.
  - If the block height is still inadequate, re-position the woman in a lateral position to encourage the spread of the drug in a cephalad direction and inject a similar volume of low concentration mixture.
  - Never lie the mother supine to encourage cephalad spread as this will lead to profound aorto-caval compression.
- If the block is unilateral, check the length of catheter present in the space; 3–4cm is the ideal length.
- After ensuring the appropriate length of catheter is present, more volume should be injected.
  - Most midline anatomical barriers can be overcome, but up to 30mL of low concentration mixture may be required to ensure spread bilaterally.
  - It is logical to assist the spread using gravity; therefore, position the mother lying on the unblocked side.

- Give the low concentration mixture bolus in two divided doses over a period of 30min.
- If some contralateral analgesia has developed, it is worth persisting with this epidural and administering further incremental doses.

- As labour advances, the woman may experience increasing perineal pain due to descent of the presenting part.
- As before, volume is the first step to improve the spread of the block.
  - However, if a satisfactory sensory block can be demonstrated and further analgesia is required, a higher concentration of LA can be advantageous, e.g. 5–10m: 0.125–0.25% bupivacaine with the addition of 50 micrograms fentanyl.

Epidurals that have been partially effective

- There are two common reasons for partially effective epidurals:
  - transforaminal escape of the catheter, or
  - the presence of a midline barrier.

Transforaminal escape

- Transforaminal escape of the catheter is characterized by a unilateral block in the lumbar region, limited to a few segments.
- The catheter needs to be withdrawn to encourage it back into the epidural space. Then, proceed with further bolus doses as above.
- Success is limited to 50%, as further drug tends to escape down the preformed track.
- If no improvement is seen, the epidural catheter should be re-sited.
- The paramedian approach may be considered beneficial as it has been shown to encourage a straight course of the catheter.
- However, the most important factor is to introduce only 3–4cm of catheter into the space in the first instance.

Unilateral block

- Where a true unilateral block persists despite an appropriate length of catheter in the space, a midline barrier is thought to exist.
- Increased volume of solution can improve the spread in ~50% of cases.
- If this is unsuccessful, the epidural catheter should be re-sited.
- Consider using a different approach and intervertebral space.
- If the analgesia has been patchy and unilateral, re-site higher.

A missed segment

- This is a rare phenomenon, and closer examination of the block usually reveals a unilateral block or block that is less dense on one side (a cold or cooler foot is frequently noted on the side of pain).
- For a true missed segment to occur, there must be a demonstrable block above and below the segment with no analgesia.
- The same rules apply for improving the analgesia:
  - Increase the volume of low concentration solution.
  - Adjust the woman's position.
  - Administer additional epidural opioids, e.g. fentanyl 50 micrograms.
  - Try a bolus of higher concentration bupivacaine, e.g. 10mL of 0.125–0.25%.
  - Offer to re-site the epidural catheter.

Epidurals that have never worked

- The aim is to recognize these early and promptly offer to re-site the epidural, rather than persist with many ineffective top-ups.
- The woman should be warned that even after re-siting, 2% of patients still do not achieve effective epidural analgesia.

Checklist for managing the failing epidural

- Check catheter position and length.
- Establish sensory block height and intensity.
- If bilateral block present:
    - Give increased volume 1–2 bolus doses of 10mL 0.1% bupivacaine with fentanyl 2–3mcg/mL.
    - Consider changing woman's position to improve spread.
    - If spread is adequate but breakthrough pain persists, consider 10mL bolus 0.125% or 0.25% bupivacaine.
    - Consider additional epidural fentanyl 50mcg.
- If unilateral block present:
    - Withdraw catheter until 3–4cm remains in the epidural space.
    - Position the woman on her unblocked side.
    - Give up to 30mL bupivacaine 0.1% in divided doses.
    - Reassess early for evidence of improvement.
    - Offer to resite if no improvement.
- No block.
    - Give one bolus dose of 15mL 0.1% bupivacaine.
    - Re-assess after 10min.
    - If no block, re-site the epidural catheter.

A block that has been persistently unilateral and remains only partially effective after a couple of extra top-ups and re-positioning will never be fully effective. If it is not re-sited, many additional top-ups will be required and it will never be suitable to top-up for a caesarean delivery. Explain this to the mother and encourage her to have the epidural re-sited.

Assessing a labour epidural for anaesthesia

- Using an *in situ* epidural for an operative delivery is a useful technique and provides good surgical anaesthesia in many cases.
- However, not all epidurals that provide analgesia for labour will provide adequate anaesthesia for surgery.
- There are several pitfalls involved with augmenting (topping up) epidurals for surgery.
- Careful assessment of the epidural is needed before the decision is made to use it as a method of anaesthesia.
- Changing to either a spinal or a general anaesthetic after a failed epidural top-up can be difficult.
- Therefore, it is important to use the most appropriate method of anaesthesia in the first instance.

Benefits

- No further invasive procedures required.
- Potentially time-saving.
- The block can be extended incrementally if rapid reduction of afterload is undesirable.

Potential pitfalls

- Can take longer to achieve an adequate block for surgical anaesthesia.
- Increased incidence of a patchy or less dense block.
- Later conversion to a spinal anaesthetic may result in a high block.
- Increased requirement for supplementary analgesia intraoperatively:
  - Studies have quoted an 84% success rate for epidural augmentation using 2% lidocaine with adrenaline.
  - 14% supplementation rate with IV analgesia.
  - 2.6% conversion rate to GA.
  - 80% of conversions to GA are due to insufficient cephalic spread of the block.

Questions to be answered when considering an epidural for surgery

- How urgent is the delivery?
  - Most blocks will be adequate in 15min, but some may require 30min.
- How effective has it been for labour analgesia:
  - Very effective: augmentation should be straightforward.
  - Partially effective: may present difficulties.
  - Not effective at all: should not be considered for augmentation of epidural anaesthesia at all.

Signs of an effective epidural

- A comfortable woman, not requiring additional analgesia.
- A recent low dose top-up that has been fully effective.

- A demonstrable sensory block to ice-cold temperature.
- Bilateral warm, dry feet.
- An appropriate administration of LA solution for the duration and progress of labour.
- Epidural that has not moved.

If all of the above are present, it would be appropriate to use the epidural for the operative delivery.

What to do with the partially effective epidural?

- It has been shown that the strongest factor that was associated with a failed top-up for CS was the need for rescue top-ups above the usual protocol, examples would be:
  - Continuous infusion needing any additional top-ups.
  - Intermittent top-ups of 10mL bupivacaine 0.1% with fentanyl more frequent than hourly.
- Other associations were young maternal age, increased BMI and increased gestation.
- A combination of the above factors may put the epidural in a high risk category, and the epidural should be reviewed carefully during labour and before augmentation.
- Partially effective epidurals that could be considered for augmentation:
  - Block too low because of insufficient LA administered.
  - Perineal pain or deep pressure—often a denser block is required.
  - Unilateral block as a result of excessive catheter in the epidural space. Withdraw the catheter to 3–4cm in the space prior to augmentation.
- If the block is only partially effective and the reason is not obvious, it is safer to abandon the epidural and opt for another technique—usually a spinal if time allows.
- The worst scenario, however, is removing the epidural catheter and not being able to establish spinal anaesthesia.
- The decision regarding the dose of spinal to inject after augmentation of the epidural has failed can be difficult.

For suggested doses, volume, timing and location of epidural augmentation and spinal anaesthesia after failed augmentation, see Chapter 10 p 292–294.

Instrumental deliveries

- The same rules apply for instrumental deliveries as for CSs.
- If the epidural is inadequate for an abdominal delivery, do not be tempted to use it for an instrumental delivery.
- A failed instrumental delivery often turns into an urgent and very difficult CS, with minimal time to extend the block.
- Ensure the sensory block is adequate at the beginning of the procedure.

Further reading

Tortosa JC *et al.* Effacy of augmentation of epidural analgaesia for caesarean section. *British Journal of Anaesthesia* 2003; **91**: 532–535.

Orbach-Zinger S *et al.* Risk factors for failure to extend labor epidural analgesia to epidural anesthesia for Cesarean section. *Acta Anaesthesiologica Scandinavica* 2006; **50**: 1014–1018.

Combined spinal–epidural analgesia in labour

- The CSE technique has gained popularity in the obstetric setting as it provides flexible analgesic options for a wide range of labour scenarios.
- A local anaesthetic and opioid mixture or opioid alone can be delivered directly into the CSF, leading to rapid onset of superior quality analgesia with minimal or absent motor blockade.
- No difference has been demonstrated when compared with simple epidural analgesia in duration of labour or mode of delivery.

The technique of CSE is described in Chapter 7 p 214–217. The two separate injection technique is especially useful if the mother is distressed or unco-operative for any reason. Once analgesia has been achieved, the epidural can then be inserted more safely.

Pros

- Rapid onset analgesia.
- Early sacral analgesia.
- High maternal satisfaction.
- Less motor block (with low dose regimes)—some hospitals allow and encourage ambulation.
- Reduced total local anaesthetic dose with intrathecal administration of opioid.
- Supplemental analgesia supplied by epidural catheter.

Cons

- More technically challenging with a higher incidence of failure, in particular the spinal component, probably secondary to tenting of the dura or deviation of the spinal needle in the epidural space.
- Untested epidural catheter *in situ*.
- Possible increased chance of headache from deliberate dural puncture.
- Increased incidence of opioid-mediated pruritis, especially when not given with LA.
- Case reports of meningitis exist, but these are associated with multiple punctures.
- Possible association with fetal bradycardia.
- Increased equipment costs.

Suggested intrathecal doses

- The spread of the intrathecal block and analgesia is better with plain rather than 'heavy' bupivacaine.
- Some authorities add adrenaline 2.5 micrograms to the intrathecal solution to prolong analgesia, although the effect is quite small. In addition, it introduces mixing and dilution errors.

Early labour <4cm

- Sufentanil 5–10 micrograms alone.
- Fentanyl 25 micrograms alone.
- Bupivacaine 1.5mg with 1.5 micrograms sufentanil.
- Bupivacaine 1.5mg with fentanyl 6 micrograms.

Any stage of labour

- Bupivacaine 2.5–5mg with fentanyl 6–25 micrograms.
- Ropivacaine 2.5mg with fentanyl 6–25 micrograms.
- Levobupivacaine 2.5mg with fentanyl 6–25 micrograms.
- The fentanyl can be changed to sufentanil 5–10 micrograms in any of the above.

Late labour

- Bupivacaine 2.5mg bupivacaine with fentanyl 25 micrograms.
- Bupivacaine 5mg alone.

There is no difference between CSE and epidural techniques with respect to

- The incidence of instrumental delivery, maternal mobility, PDPHs, CS rates or admission of babies to the neonatal unit.
- It is not possible to draw any meaningful conclusions regarding rare complications such as nerve injury and meningitis; however, studies are ongoing.

Further reading

Hughes D *et al.* Combined spinal–epidural versus epidural analgesia in labour. *Cochrane Database of Systematic Reviews* 2003; Issue 4.

Cheng CJ *et al.* Either sufentanil or fentanyl, in addition to intrathecal bupivacaine, provide satisfactory early labour analgesia. *Canadian Journal of Anaesthesia* 2001; **48**: 570–574.

Lim EH *et al.* Addition of bupivacaine 1.25mg to fentanyl confers no advantage over fentanyl alone for intrathecal analgesia in early labour. *Canadian Journal of Anaesthesia* 2002; **49**: 57–61.

Wong CA *et al.* The dose–response of intrathecal sufentanil added to bupivacaine for labor analgesia. *Anesthesiology* 2000; **92**: 1553–1558.

Vercauteren MP *et al.* Intrathecal labor analgesia with bupivacaine and sufentanil: the effect of adding 2.25 microg epinephrine. *Regional Anesthesia and Pain Medicine* 2001; **26**: 473–477.

Collis RE *et al.* Combined spinal epidural (CSE) analgesia: technique, management, and outcome of 300 mothers. *International Journal of Obstetric Anesthesia* 1994; **3**: 75–81.

Stacey RG *et al.* Single space combined spinal–extradural technique for analgesia in labour. *British Journal of Anaesthesia* 2003; **71**: 499–502.

Regional analgesia for early labour

- Cervical dilatation of ≤4cm is considered early labour, and pain is mainly visceral as uterine activity increases.
- Traditionally, epidurals were avoided in early labour as it was thought that they prolonged the duration of the first and second stages.
- Blame was partially attributed to dilution of circulating prostaglandins by fluid preloading—nowadays unnecessary due to the low concentrations of epidural drug solutions used.
- Studies have shown that the duration of the first phase of labour appears unchanged with epidural analgesia, but the second stage of labour is likely to be prolonged.
- Requests for an early epidural are associated with
  - Long latent phase.
  - Dysfunctional contractions.
  - Occipito-posterior position of the baby.
  - Large baby.
- Atypical, rapidly escalating pain may be indicative of dysfunctional uterine contractions, abnormal fetal presentation or other intrauterine/intrabdominal problems, and an obstetric opinion should be sought.

Indications

- Maternal request.
  - It is unacceptable not to offer epidural analgesia to a woman because she is <4cm dilated as long as she is considered to be in the active phase of labour or there is an obstetric commitment to deliver.
- Augmentation of labour.
  - Contractions may appear suddenly and with force following the start of an oxytocin infusion to augment labour.
- Pre-eclampsia.
  - To optimize BP control.
- Obstetric request.
  - To facilitate obstetric examination or fetal scalp electrode monitoring.
- Cardiac disease.
  - To minimize the effects of circulating catecholamines and aid in haemodynamic stability.
- Morbid obesity.
  - To pre-empt and avoid significant GA risks.

Techniques

- A standard low dose epidural technique is appropriate for analgesia in early labour.
- If rapid pain control is necessary, a CSE technique can be used.
- Low dose CSE is also beneficial if ambulation is allowed.
- It is essential to check the adequacy of an epidural placed early on in labour as there is a greater risk of it becoming displaced.
- Epidural top-ups may be required more frequently as labour progresses or with increasing oxytocin infusion rates.

Further reading

Ohel G *et al.* Early versus late initiation of epidural analgesia in labor: does it increase the risk of cesarean section? A randomized trial. *American Journal of Obstetrics and Gynecology* 2006; **194**: 600–605.

Wong CA *et al.* The risk of cesarean delivery with neuraxial analgesia given early versus late in labor. *New England Journal of Medicine* 2005; **352**: 655–665.

Panni MK *et al.* Local anesthetic requirements are greater in dystocia than in normal labor. *Anesthesiology* 2003; **98**: 957–963.

Regional analgesia for late labour

- Late labour is considered to be at cervical dilatation of ≥7cm.
- Late labour has been considered by some to be a contraindication to regional analgesia and should be discouraged.
- For some women, careful assessment and midwifery support is all that is required, but each situation must be considered on its own merit.

Indications

- An increasing number of women are labouring in midwifery-led units. Some will be transferred to medical obstetric units in late first stage or second stage labour because of extreme maternal distress or failure to progress in the later part of their labour.
- These women need careful obstetric assessment and many will require regional analgesia for examination and augmentation despite the late stage of the labour. They should never be denied analgesia because the second stage of labour has been reached.
- Some woman in the second stage of labour will not push because of fear and pain; regional analgesia can be beneficial.
- Some women become exhausted, and an instrumental delivery becomes the likely outcome. Regional analgesia can then be used for instrumental delivery.

Techniques

Epidural

- A low dose epidural can be used, but sacral pain can be difficult to treat with the low dose solutions and good analgesia difficult to obtain.
- 10mL bupivacaine 0.25% with fentanyl 50 micrograms can be helpful.
- The benefit of primarily siting an epidural is that the epidural is tested in case of instrumental or caesarean delivery.

Combined spinal–epidural

- Can provide ideal, rapid analgesia in late labour.
    - Bupivacaine 2.5mg with fentanyl 25 micrograms.
    - Bupivacaine 5mg alone.
- Analgesia will be shorter lived than when a CSE is used in early labour, but these doses usually provide 30–40min of complete pain relief.
- Although a proportion of women will deliver on the spinal component alone, a request for late analgesia often indicates a problem with the labour, and a request to convert analgesia to anaesthesia for instrumental or caesarean delivery is likely.
- The epidural component will remain untested for some time and may then not be reliable when required. Early testing of the epidural component of the CSE should be considered in these circumstances.

Chapter 9

Anaesthesia for caesarean section: basic principles

Kath Eggers, Monica Chawathe, Fiona Benjamin, Jon Hughes, Karthikeyan Chelliah, and Rafal Baraz

Urgency, timing and classification

The purpose of classifying the urgency of CSs is to balance the safe management of the mother with the appropriate timing of fetal delivery.

The following 4-point classification of urgency has been adopted in the UK (Table 9.1). Although initially proposed as a postdelivery audit tool, it is widely used to classify the clinical urgency of every CS prior to transfer to theatre.

Whatever system or classification is used in an individual unit, it should be known and understood by all healthcare professionals involved so that there is mutual understanding of the urgency in any particular situation.

Category 1

- The traditionally accepted time of 30min from decision to delivery for category 1 CS and its effect on fetal outcome has shortcomings, which have been highlighted by the NICE guidelines.
- The delivery of the fetus within a 30min interval may not be rapid enough. For a true emergency category 1 CS, e.g. due to maternal haemorrhage or sustained fetal bradycardia, the fetus may require delivery much earlier than this.
- GA will usually be the preferred anaesthetic technique for a true category 1. However, maternal problems such as an anticipated difficult airway or morbid obesity must be taken into consideration when deciding the anaesthetic technique and discussed pre-emptively with the obstetric and midwifery team.
- Inappropriate haste to comply with the 30min rule may unduly compromise the mother's safety.
- Good communication between midwives, obstetricians and anaesthetists is essential.
- Intrauterine fetal resuscitation, if appropriate, needs to be considered during this period, as this may improve the CTG trace such that a category 1 CS may be regraded to a category 2, therefore allowing time for a regional technique.

Table 9.1 Classification of urgency of caesarean section

Grade	Definition (at time of decision to operate)
Category 1	Immediate threat to life of woman or fetus
Category 2	Maternal or fetal compromise, not immediately life threatening
Category 3	Needs early delivery but no maternal or fetal compromise
Category 4	At a time to suit the woman and staff

Intrauterine fetal resuscitation

The anaesthetist should actively take part in both maternal and fetal resuscitation once the decision for CS has been made.

Immediate management should include:

- Turn off oxytocin.
- Position the mother in full left lateral, right lateral or knee–elbow position (if FHR persistently abnormal or cord compression).
- Administer 15L/min oxygen via a Hudson mask with a reservoir bag.
- Give fluid bolus, e.g. 1000mL Hartmann's solution (caution in pre-eclampsia).
- Treat hypotension with an IV vasopressor, e.g. ephedrine or phenylephrine.

Consider tocolysis (especially if fetal distress is associated with prostaglandin or oxytocin administration)—discuss with obstetrician and consider terbutaline 250mcg subcutaneously or GTN sublingual spray.

Further reading

Lucas DN *et al.* Urgency of Caesarean section: a new classification. *Journal of the Royal Society of Medicine* 2000; **93**: 346–350.

Levy DM. Emergency caesarean section: best practice. Review article. *Anaesthesia* 2006; **61**: 786–791.

NHS Caesarean section clinical guideline. National Institute for Health and Clinical Excellence. 2005. http;//www.nice.org.uk

Thurlow JA *et al.* Intrauterine resuscitation: active management of fetal distress. *International Journal of Obstetric Anesthesia* 2002; **11**: 105–116.

Information and consent

Antenatal information

- All pregnant women can expect full involvement in decisions regarding their maternity care, and have an increasing demand and access to information regarding obstetric anaesthesia.
- The antenatal period should be used to provide women with access to written information, such as that provided by the OAA (http://www.oaa-anaes.ac.uk), particularly the OAA leaflets 'Pain relief in labour' and 'Caesarean section: your choice of anaesthesia'. Videotapes are also available for antenatal classes.
- Anaesthetists should be involved in antenatal education on pain relief.
- An antenatal anaesthetic assessment clinic should be available for women who require specific discussions regarding anaesthetic risks, e.g. morbid obesity, cardiac disease, known anaesthetic problems, airway problems and any women with particular concerns who wish to see an anaesthetist.
- A system should be in place for midwives and obstetricians to refer these women for early anaesthetic review.
- Appropriate literature and interpreters should be available for women from ethnic minorities.

Preoperative information

Elective caesarean section

Local guidelines should be followed in the preparation of women for an elective LSCS. The following example reflects typical practice.

- The woman is seen 1–3 days prior to surgery for preoperative clerking, midwifery assessment and confirmation of surgical consent.
- Investigations are sent as appropriate; usually blood tests for a full blood count and group and save, or cross-match as required.
- Antacid prophylaxis is prescribed, i.e. ranitidine 150mg +/– metoclopramide 10mg orally to be taken the night before and on the morning of surgery.
- The patient is informed of the starvation requirements.
- The anaesthetist should complete a thorough preoperative assessment looking for problems related to a regional technique or GA. This includes examining the patient, paying particular attention to the airway, back and auscultation for significant heart murmurs. This is a good time to reinforce the information on timing of antacid prophylaxis and starvation requirements.
- Further information on the planned anaesthetic technique should be discussed.

Regional technique

Information on what to expect when the regional technique is being performed should include:

- Positioning and monitoring, e.g. sitting or lying.
- IV access.
- The aseptic technique, e.g. very cold spray.
- LA to numb the skin of the back.

- Paraesthesia may occur momentarily during insertion of the epidural or spinal.
- Failure of insertion may occur, requiring repeated attempts or a GA.
- When the spinal anaesthetic is inserted, the patient will feel a warm bottom and legs, with tingling, leading to complete motor block of the legs.
- Nausea and vomiting is common in the first 10–15min and will be treated.
- The BP will be closely monitored during this time.
- Numbness will spread up to the chest and will be tested before surgery is allowed to proceed.
- The table is tilted to the left side.
- The drape will obscure any vision of the surgery for mother and partner, and may be lowered at delivery if the parents want to see their baby being born and subject to clinical conditions at the time. (Not all hospitals may allow this).
- The mother will feel pulling and tugging during the procedure and occasionally this may become uncomfortable. We can give extra analgesia through the drip if necessary. Very rarely, it may even be painful and we will administer a GA immediately if this is the case.
- At the end of the operation, we may insert suppositories to aid postoperative analgesia.
- A urinary catheter may be left in until bladder function returns.
- Motor function of the legs will return within 4–6h.
- Postoperative analgesia will include regular paracetamol and NSAIDs (assuming no contraindications).

Side effects explained should include the common and the serious:
- Failure, including conversion to GA.
- Pruritus.
- PDPH (use local audit figures, national figures are ~1%).
- Neurological complications ~1 in 10 000.

- Reassurance that having a spinal or epidural does not give you a 'bad back', although local bruising may occur causing local tenderness for a few days.
- The presence of the partner during the whole procedure if requested should be allowed and encouraged.
- You should enquire whether the mother (and partner) have any questions before concluding the preoperative visit.
- Documentation of this consultation should be written in the case notes, and a preprinted sticky label or preassessment form will aid in mentioning all the relevant risks.

General anaesthesia

- Many of the general points mentioned above also apply to GA, with the exception that the partner will not be present during induction or the operation, but will be allowed to see the baby as soon as is practicable.

- The conduct of the anaesthetic should describe the need for monitoring, IV access, preoxygenation and cricoid pressure.
- Specific informed consent could include mentioning the risks of:
  - Awareness.
  - Regurgitation and aspiration.
  - Sore throat.
  - Muscle aches and pains.
- Specific consent should be sought for the administration of analgesia by suppository during GA.
- It is preferable to use IV opioids, e.g. morphine, via a PCA device for the first 24h following a CS under GA, and balanced analgesia with regular paracetamol and diclofenac.

Emergency caesarean section

- Labour is a difficult time to obtain informed consent. Mothers are often in severe pain, may be exhausted, under the influence of drugs such as opioids or Entonox, or feeling extreme anxiety. However, this does not alter the principles or amount of information necessary to obtain informed consent for obstetric anaesthesia.
- Research has shown that despite the influence of pain or drugs, women like to be informed and are capable of recalling the risks and benefits of regional anaesthesia. Using simple and clear information cards (e.g. giving short notes on the advantages and risks of epidural analgesia) improves recall of information and patient satisfaction.
- If time is of the essence, the consent process should occur at the same time as the woman is prepared for theatre. In an extreme emergency, consent can be verbal and a description in the notes of the conversation made afterwards.
- The volume of information may be less but the principle of informed consent still applies, and the material risks, i.e. common and serious risks, still need to be mentioned.
- Pain under regional anaesthesia is a common cause of litigation, and this needs to be mentioned prior to it occurring, with the reassurance that if it occurs, it will be dealt with swiftly, including a GA if necessary.

Further reading

Seeking patient's consent: the ethical considerations, General Medical Council. November 1998. http://www.gmc-uk.org/guidance/current/library/consent.asp

AAGBI: consent for anaesthesia, Revised edition 2006. Website www.aagbi.org

Chester v Afshar [2004] UKHL 41.

Sullivan WJ *et al.* Maternal autonomy: ethics and the law. *International Journal of Obstetric Anesthesia* 2006; **15**: 95–97.

Antacid prophylaxis

- Regurgitation and inhalation of gastric contents can cause pneumonitis, particularly if the fluid is acidic; this can cause severe morbidity and occasionally death.
- This condition is referred to as chemical pneumonitis or Mendelson's syndrome.
- Although chemical pneumonitis is a serious condition, most deaths in Mendelson's study were associated with aspiration of solid matter.
- Gastro-oesophageal regurgitation can occur during GA if the stomach is not empty, as anaesthetic drugs relax the lower oesophageal sphincter tone.

Pregnant women are thought to be at increased risk of regurgitation because:
- The pregnancy hormones progesterone and relaxin cause relaxation of the smooth muscle of the stomach.
- There is reduced barrier pressure and increased intra-abdominal pressure in pregnancy.
- Pain, anxiety and the use of opioids during labour increase the risk by further delaying gastric emptying.

Incidence

- Since Mendelson first described the acid aspiration syndrome in 1946, the incidence has dramatically reduced.
- The CEMACH report 2000–2002 describes one case compared with 66 cases in 1946.
- The reasons for this dramatic reduction are multifactorial:
  - An increase in the use of regional anaesthesia for CS.
  - Better provision of antacid prophylaxis.
  - Availability of experienced obstetric anaesthetists and their assistants.
  - The identification and treatment of those women at higher risk of aspiration, e.g. women receiving opioids in labour, pre-eclampsia, multiple pregnancies, previous CS, obesity, diabetes.

Methods of reducing the risk of aspiration

Based on animal work, the important factors thought to increase the chance of chemical pneumonitis are:
- Gastric pH <2.5.
- Gastric volume >25mL.

The methods employed to reduce the risk of aspiration include:
- Starvation of mothers for at least 6h before a planned CS to reduce the volume of gastric contents.
- Limits on oral intake during labour (especially solid food).
- Antacid prophylaxis: the administration of the following drugs to reduce the volume and/or acidity of the stomach contents.

Antacids

These are alkaline substances, which reduce or neutralize the acidity of the stomach contents.

Magnesium trisilicate

- First antacid to be widely used in labour but rarely used nowadays.
- It effectively reduces gastric pH.
- Slow to mix with stomach contents.
- Particulate nature is potentially hazardous.

Sodium citrate

- Most widely used antacid.
- Given as 30mL of 0.3M solution.
- Effective quickly (10min from laboratory studies).
- Short acting and effect unpredictable at 60min.
- Does not seem to increase gastric volume.
- Unpalatable.
- Short shelf-life.

H_2 antagonists

- H_2 receptor antagonists, e.g. ranitidine, inhibit the secretion of acid into the stomach, which reduces the volume and acidity of the stomach contents.
- This action is not immediate and so H_2 receptor antagonists are often used in combination with antacids at induction of emergency anaesthesia.
- Oral administration of ranitidine 150mg is effective in 60min.
- IV administration of ranitidine is effective in 30min and should be given at induction of emergency anaesthesia if the mother has not previously received the drug to cover extubation (when the effect of sodium citrate is unreliable).
- Adverse effects of the drugs may include dizziness, fatigue, rashes, headaches, GIT disturbances.

Dopamine antagonists, e.g. metoclopramide

- Has been widely and safely used in pregnancy.
- 10mg metoclopramide orally or slow IV.
- These drugs inhibit vomiting and accelerate gastric emptying.
- May increase lower oesophageal tone.
- Most effective when used in conjunction with ranitidine or omeprazole.
- Adverse effects include drowsiness, restlessness, diarrhoea and arrhythmias.

Proton pump inhibitors, e.g. omeprazole

- These drugs block the production of gastric acid by interfering with the proton pump mechanism in the gastric parietal cells.
- Omeprazole is the only proton pump inhibitor that has been widely investigated in obstetric practice.
- An oral dose of 80mg is effective in 60min.
- An IV dose of 40mg is effective in 30min.
- No clear advantage over ranitidine.
- More expensive.
- Adverse effects include rashes and GIT disturbances.

There is limited evidence to support the routine administration of acid prophylaxis drugs in **normal labour** to prevent gastric aspiration and its consequences.

Aspiration prophylaxis protocol

Varies between individual obstetric units.

Typical aspiration prophylaxis for CS would be:

- Elective caesarean section:
  - 12h preop, ranitidine 150mg orally.
  - 2h preop, ranitidine 150mg orally +/– metaclopramide 10mg orally immediately preop.
  - Some units also add 0.3M sodium citrate 30mL orally. However, as it is only effective for 20min following ingestion, many units will only treat with sodium citrate if a GA is required.
- Emergency CS under GA:
  - Ranitidine 150mg orally if time allows.
  - Immediately preoperatively, 0.3M sodium citrate 30mL.
  - Intraoperatively ranitidine 50mg and metaclopromide 10mg both IV.
  - At the end of CS the stomach may be emptied with an orogastric tube, which should be removed before extubation.
- Typical aspiration prophylaxis for at risk mothers in active labour ranitidine 150mg 6hly orally, e.g. epidural analgesia for labour.

Further reading

Gyte GML *et al.* Routine prophylactic drugs in normal labour for reducing gastric aspiration and its effects. *Cochrane Database of Systematic Reviews*, 2006.

Calthorpe N, Lewis M. Acid aspiration prophylaxis in labour: a survey of UK obstetric units. *International Journal of Obstetric Anesthesia* 2005; **14**: 300–304.

Monitoring mother and fetus

- To ensure patient safety, monitoring for CS should be started prior to induction or insertion of regional technique and continued into recovery for both general and regional anaesthesia.
- Monitoring equipment should be checked before each new patient.
- The 2000–2002 CEMACH report highlights the importance of capnography as deaths occurred following undetected oesophageal intubation.
- Unexpected monitor readings should not be dismissed.

The AAGBI have published guidelines on standards of monitoring that must be used whenever a patient is anaesthetized. These include:

- Presence of an appropriately experienced anaesthetist and a trained anaesthetic assistant during the whole of the procedure.
- Accurate record keeping.
- Monitoring of the anaesthetic equipment, e.g. appropriate alarm settings, oxygen and volatile agent analyser.
- Monitoring the mother and fetus.

Maternal monitoring

Clinical observation

- A drop in BP in a patient under going a CS under regional anaesthesia may be heralded by pallor, yawning, anxiety and a complaint of nausea.
- Frequent verbal interaction with the patient is essential and one of the most reliable methods of monitoring the mother.

Minimal monitoring requires:

- Pulse oximeter.
- Non-invasive blood pressure monitor.
- ECG.
- Capnography.
- Inspired oxygen and volatile agent analyser.
- Neuromuscular monitoring.
- Temperature monitor.

- Blood loss should be measured in every patient and **additional monitoring** applied dependent on patient and obstetric factors:
  - Urinary output measurements—continue monitoring closely in the postoperative period following major haemorrhage (blood loss >1500mL) and PET.
  - Invasive monitoring. e.g. arterial line and CVP.
  - Appropriate blood tests.
  - CO monitor, e.g. suprasternal Doppler ultrasound and oesophageal Doppler.

Fetal monitoring

- Monitoring of the fetal heart should ideally be performed from prior to induction of anaesthesia to the beginning of surgery. In an emergency, induction and placement of fetal monitoring may need to happen at the same time.
- Monitoring can be intermittent, i.e. with a Doppler ultrasound, or continuous monitoring, with a CTG.
- The CTG monitors the fetal heart in conjunction with maternal contractions either transabdominally or via a fetal scalp electrode, which should be removed prior to the start of surgery.
- In an emergency situation, good communication is essential to facilitate adequate fetal monitoring and safe conduct of anaesthesia.
- Intermittent monitoring may be appropriate in the elective setting.
- Continuous monitoring should ideally be applied throughout the conduct of anaesthesia, including any regional techniques in any emergency or labour setting.

Further reading

Association of Anaesthetists of Great Britain and Ireland. *Checking Anaesthetic Equipment 3*. London: Association of Anaesthetists. 2004.

Association of Anaesthetists of Great Britain and Ireland. *Recommendations for Standards of Monitoring During Anaesthesia and Recovery*. London: Association of Anaesthetists, 2000.

Aorto-caval compression

- Gideon Ahltorp in 1931 first noted that signs and symptoms of cardiac insufficiency (nausea, dyspnoea, pallor, unconsciousness and weak pulses) only occurred when the gravid uterus lay on the posterior abdominal wall. These symptoms disappeared when the lateral position was adopted or the uterus lifted upwards.
- In 1953, Howard described the concept of supine hypotensive syndrome in late pregnancy. He found that 11.2% of pregnant women developed hypotension, a decrease in systolic arterial pressure of >30mmHg, when assuming the supine position after some minutes.
- Aorto-caval compression is caused by partial occlusion of the IVC and to a lesser extent the aorta by the gravid uterus.
- Occlusion of the IVC significantly reduces the VR and CO. Despite a reduction in the CO, the BP is often maintained by means of arterial vasoconstriction.
- Occlusion of the aorta increases afterload and consequently reduces CO.
- A baroreceptor-mediated vagal bradycardia secondary to increase in systemic arterial pressure following aortic compression may cause a bradycardia and contribute to hypotension.
- Intense bradycardia <20bpm, often associated with a very low CO and maternal collapse, is thought to be caused by a severe fall in VR to the right atrium (Bezold–Jarisch reflex).
- Supine hypotension can occur as early as 20 weeks, and becomes more severe in the third trimester as the uterus increases in size.
- Hypotension occurs especially in women with poor azygos venous system collaterals.
- Other contributory factors are:
  - Polyhydramnios.
  - Abnormal presentation of the fetus (breech, transverse lie).
  - Multiple pregnancy.
  - Maternal obesity.
  - Uterine myomata.
- Supine hypotension is less severe after membrane rupture, engagement of the fetal head and descent of the head through the pelvis, and is unlikely to take place after delivery. It is most common in a term elective CS.

Lesser degrees of aorto-caval compression, insufficient to cause maternal symptoms, may nevertheless reduce placental perfusion and cause fetal compromise. **There is no place for complacency with regards to aorto-caval compression.**

Physiological considerations

- The degree of hypotension depends on the density and the extent of the preganglionic sympathetic blockade. Sympathetic block up to T5 will result in:
    - Dilatation of the resistance vessels and consequently reduction in systemic vascular resistance.
    - Dilatation of the capacitance vessels leading to venous pooling and reduction in VR.
    - Reduction in endogenous catecholamine secretion from the adrenal medulla due to splanchnic nerve block.
- Sympathetic block above T5, in addition to vasodilatation, causes a fall in BP due to bradycardia and reduction in myocardial contractility.
- The combination of aorto-caval compression, the greater sensitivity to local anaesthetics and the predominance of the sympathetic nervous system during pregnancy contributes significantly to the increased risk of hypotension associated with spinal or epidural anaesthesia.

Definition and incidence

- Hypotension is commonly defined as a drop of systolic BP below 100mmHg or a fall of >20% of baseline.
- The incidence of hypotension following spinal or epidural anaesthesia can be as high as 80% without prophylactic measures, and is more likely if spinal anaesthesia is used.
- If untreated, it can lead to unpleasant maternal symptoms; nausea, vomiting, dizziness and distress, and serious fetal complications; bradycardia and acidosis secondary to placental hypoperfusion.
- The induction of anaesthesia, either general or regional, with the associated arterial vasodilatation will block the main compensatory mechanism and as a result, some hypotension will inevitably occur.
- The aggressive treatment of hypotension to maintain baseline BP has been shown to be beneficial to the fetus.

Further reading

Kinsella SM, Tuckey JP. Perioperative bradycardia and asystole: relationship to vasovagal syncope and the Bezold–Jarisch reflex (Review). *British Journal of Anaesthesia* 2001; **86**: 859–868.

Ngan Kee WD. Comparison of phenylephrine infusion regimens for maintaining maternal blood pressure during spinal anaesthesia for caesarean section. *British Journal of Anaesthesia* 2004; **92**: 469–474.

Ngan Kee WD, Lee A. Multivariate analysis of factors associated with umbilical arterial pH and standard base excess after caesarean section under spinal anaesthesia. *Anaesthesia* 2003; **58**: 125–130.

Reynolds F, Seed PT. Anaesthesia for caesarean section and neonatal acid–base status: a meta-analysis (Review). *Anaesthesia* 2005; **60**: 636–653.

Maternal position

The effects of aorto-caval compression can be minimized or relieved by:

Full lateral position to either side

- Most effective.
- Impractical to perform CS in this position, but keep woman in the full lateral if severe hypotension persists and until BP is restored to normal limits.
- High risk pregnancy (e.g. multiple pregnancy) induce block in lateral position.

Tilt operating 15° to left

A 15° left lateral tilt was proposed by Crawford in the 1970s and has become accepted by many to be the ideal position in which to place a mother prior to and during CS. There are no scientific data to validate this tilt as optimal, but it is a reasonable compromise between lying supine and tilting so far that it is dangerous to the mother. Most obstetric anaesthetists overestimate the tilt unless a tilt-measuring device is used and, if the mother is actually placed in 15° left lateral tilt, most obstetricians complain that the tilt is too severe to operate.

- Partially relieves caval compression.
- May be inadequate in high risk patients.
- Increasing the tilt, i.e. to ≥20° may improve hypotension but make the mother's position unsafe.
- CS possible in this position.

Wedge under right buttock

- Uterine displacement easily achieved.
- Twists the mother's spine, which can cause discomfort.

Manual displacement of uterus to left

- Effective.
- Useful temporary measure.
- Need an additional assistant.

Whichever measure is taken, **visual displacement** of the uterus must occur.

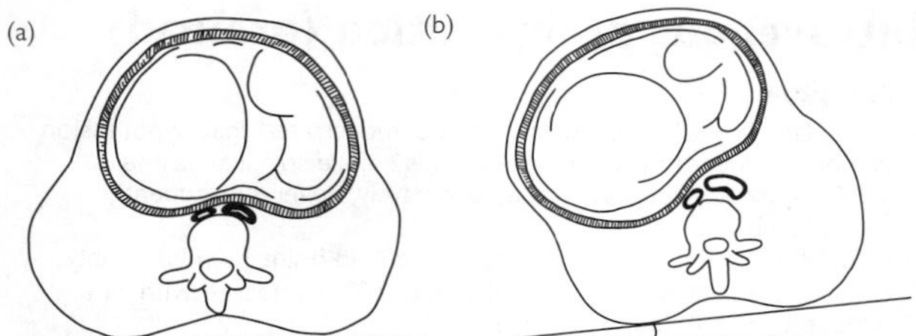

Fig. 9.1 Aorto-caval compression. (a) In the supine position, blood flow through the vena cava and aorta is significantly reduced, causing maternal and fetal compromise. The efficacy of left lateral displacement was demonstrated in 1972. The full left or right lateral position completely relieves aorto-caval compression. (b) Elevating the mother's hip 10–15cm completely relieves aorto-caval compression in 58% of term parturients.

Further reading

Kinsella SM, Lohmann G. Supine hypotensive syndrome. *Obstetrics and Gynecology* 1999; **83**: 774–788.

Rees SG *et al.* Maternal cardiovascular consequences of positioning after spinal anaesthesia for caesarean section: left 15 degree table tilt vs. left lateral. *Anaesthesia* 2002; **57**: 15–20.

Mendonca C *et al.* Hypotension following combined spinal–epidural anaesthesia for caesarean section. Left lateral position vs. tilted supine position. *Anaesthesia* 2003; **58**: 428–431.

Intravenous prehydration (preload)

Crystalloids

- In the late 1960s Wollman and Marx demonstrated that hypotension can be eliminated by a crystalloid bolus before spinal anaesthesia. This remarkable success was, unfortunately, never subsequently reproduced.
- Rout *et al.* found that even a large crystalloid bolus (20mL/kg) only reduces the incidence of hypotension to 55% compared with 71% when no crystalloid bolus was used.
- Many subsequent studies have confirmed the ineffectiveness of this measure, and it is now widely accepted that a formal crystalloid preload is not essential prior to spinal anaesthesia.
- The poor efficacy of crystalloids is mainly due to their very short intravascular half-life. Therefore, if given, this should be whilst spinal anaesthesia is instituted (co-load).
- Large crystalloid preload causes haemodilution and the release of atrial natriuretic peptide, a vasodilator, leading to persistent hypotension.
- In pregnancy, low colloid oncotic pressure can be decreased further by a large preload, potentially leading to pulmonary oedema.

Colloids

- Colloids are more effective in the prevention of hypotension. Preload with 500mL of hydroxylethylstarch 10% reduces the incidence of hypotension to 40% compared with 80% in patients given 1000mL lactated Ringer's solution.
- The greater efficacy of colloids is the result of their slower redistribution out of the intravascular space, leading to a more sustained increase in the CVP.
- This benefit must be weighed against:
  - Increased cost.
  - Allergic reactions.
  - Pruritis.
  - Interference with blood cross-matching.

Lower limb wrapping

- There is evidence to suggest that wrapping of the legs with tight elasticated bandages prior to spinal anaesthesia significantly reduces the incidence of hypotension.
- Raising the legs can be an effective and rapid method of treating hypotension.
- Neither method is commonly employed in the UK.

Further reading

Burns SM *et al.* Prevention and management of hypotension during spinal anaesthesia for elective caesarean section: a survey of practice. *Anaesthesia* 2001; **56**: 794–798.

Siddik SM *et al.* Hydroxyethylstarch 10% is superior to Ringer's solution for preloading before spinal anesthesia for Cesarean section. *Canadian Journal of Anaesthesia* 2000; **47**: 616–621.

Rocke DA, Rout CC. Volume preloading, spinal hypotension and caesarean section. *British Journal of Anaesthesia* 1995; **75**: 257–279.

Jackson R *et al.* Volume preloading is not essential to prevent spinal-induced hypotension at caesarean section. *British Journal of Anaesthesia* 1995; **75**: 262–265.

French GW *et al.* Comparison of pentastarch and Hartmann's solution for volume preloading in spinal anaesthesia for elective caesarean section. *British Journal of Anaesthesia* 1999; **83**: 475–477.

Rout CC *et al.* Leg elevation and wrapping in the prevention of hypotension following spinal anaesthesia for elective caesarean section. *Anaesthesia* 1993; **48**: 304–308.

Vasopressors

Ephedrine

- This non-specific adrenergic agonist mainly increases BP by augmenting CO through its actions on β-receptors.
- A smaller contribution by increasing the SVR via α_1 receptor stimulation also exists.
- Ephedrine, therefore, has minimal or no vasoconstrictive effect on uteroplacental circulation, a feature that has made this drug very popular and used as a first line by most anaesthetists for decades.
- A survey of UK practice in 1999 showed that >95% of obstetric anaesthetists used ephedrine alone to maintain BP during spinal anaesthesia for CS. More than 60% of respondents used it prophylactically and nearly half added it to the bag of IV fluid.
- Commonly and safely given as 6mg IV bolus.

Advantages

- Easy to dilute and use.
- Can be given PO, IM or IV.
- Has a very good safety record.

Disadvantages

- It increases HR and contractility, therefore increasing myocardial oxygen demands. This is of particular importance in women with heart disease.
- Slow onset of action and relatively long duration of action make accurate titration difficult.
- Risk of ectopics and tachyarrhythmias.
- Risk of tachyphylaxis.
- Its use has been linked to a fall in umbilical arterial pH. This is most probably due to its direct effect on fetal metabolism. Ephedrine crosses the placenta, and stimulation of β-receptors in the fetus increases oxygen consumption and lactate production.

Phenylephrine

- Based on animal studies, this pure α agonist was found to cause uteroplacental hypoperfusion because of vasoconstriction, and therefore its use in obstetrics was thought to be contraindicated.
- Clinical trials in humans using smaller doses have failed to show any evidence of adverse fetal or neonatal effects.
- Phenylephrine raises BP by increasing the SVR through its direct effect on the α-1 receptor.
- From its mechanism of action, it seems logical to use phenylephrine, rather than ephedrine, to correct hypotension associated with vasodilatation arising from sympathetic block.

Suggested dose regimens

- IV 100 micrograms/mL (10mg in 100mL normal saline) run at 60mL/h (high dose infusion).
- IV 12.5 micrograms/ml (prepared solution) start infusion at 80–100ml/h (low dose infusion).
- IV bolus 12.5–50 micrograms as required.

Advantages

- Maternal BP is easily maintained, with a positive effect on uteroplacental perfusion.
- Its rapid onset of action and short duration make it easy to titrate when compared with ephedrine.

Disadvantages

- A reflex bradycardia is common and an anticholinergic should always be available.
- Phenylephrine is supplied commercially in different concentrations (10mg/mL, 1mg/10mL, 250 micrograms/mL and 12.5 micrograms/mL), and extreme care is required when using this drug. The fear of a dosing error has probably contributed to the reluctance among some obstetric anaesthetists in the UK to adopt its use.

Combining two vasopressors

- The risk of bradycardia can be reduced when ephedrine is used in addition to phenylephrine.
- To date there is little evidence of benefit when the two drugs are combined.
- Studies that showed an increased incidence of nausea and vomiting with combination therapy did not use an optimal combination ratio and therefore a conclusion cannot be drawn.
- Metaraminol, a mixed α- and β-receptor agonist, has also been used, although there has been little research into its use.

Recent advances

- The combination of a high dose phenylephrine infusion (100 micrograms/min) and rapid crystalloid co-hydration immediately after spinal injection is the first technique to date that was found to be effective in preventing hypotension during spinal anaesthesia for elective caesarean delivery.
- This resulted in a positive outcome for the fetus.
- Studies to date have been conducted in the elective well fetus.
- Some caution must be exercised at present before extrapolation of these results to the emergency distressed fetus.

Summary

- Hypotension associated with neuroaxial blocks for caesarean delivery is common and should be minimized to avoid unpleasant maternal side effects and serious fetal consequences, i.e. fetal acidosis.
- Many methods for its prevention have been investigated and no single technique has proven to eliminate it.
- Crystalloid preload is ineffective.
- Rapid crystalloid administration during spinal anaesthesia (co-load) may be advantageous.
- Colloids are more effective than crystalloids in preventing hypotension at the expense of cost and risk of adverse reactions.
- Phenylephrine has many favourable characteristics over ephedrine and is now considered as the drug of choice when treating hypotension following spinal or epidural anaesthesia in the obstetric patient.

Further reading

Kee WD *et al.* Prevention of hypotension during spinal anesthesia for cesarean delivery: an effective technique using combination phenylephrine infusion and crystalloid cohydration. *Anesthesiology* 2005; **103**: 744–750.

Ngan Kee W *et al.* Comparison of phenylephrine infusion regimens for maintaining maternal blood pressure during spinal anaesthesia for caesarean section. *British Journal of Anaesthesia* 2004; **92**: 469–474.

Lee A *et al.* A dose–response meta-analysis of prophylactic intravenous ephedrine for the prevention of hypotension during spinal anesthesia for elective cesarean delivery. *Anesthesia and Analgesia* 2004; **98**: 483–490.

Lee A *et al.* A quantitative, systematic review of randomized controlled trials of ephedrine versus phenylephrine for the management of hypotension during spinal anesthesia for cesarean delivery. *Anesthesia and Analgesia* 2002; **94**: 920–926.

Cyna AM *et al.* Techniques for preventing hypotension during spinal anaesthesia for caesarean section (Review). *Cochrane Database of Systematic Reviews* 2006; **18**: CD002251.

Drugs for uterine contraction

There are four main pharmacological options to contract the uterus following delivery of the baby:

- Syntocinon®, a synthetic analogue of the posterior pituitary hormone oxytocin.
- Ergometrine, an ergot alkaloid.
- Carboprost, a prostaglandin (PG) $F_{2\alpha}$ analogue.
- Misoprostol, a PGE_2 analogue.

Oxytocin (Syntocinon®)

- Oxytocin injection is indicated to produce or enhance uterine contractions during labour and to control postpartum bleeding or haemorrhage.
- Syntocinon® is a synthetic, (1–6) cyclic nonapeptide.

Doses and time of action

- Following IM injection, the myotonic effect on the uterus appears in 3–7min, and persists for 30–60min.
- With IV injection, the uterine effect appears within 1min and is of more brief duration.
- Dose is 5IU slow IV bolus, and/or 30–50IU in 500mL crystalloid as IV infusion titrated as indicated.

Metabolism and excretion

- Oxytocin is active when administered by any parenteral route but inactivated by chymotrypsin if given orally.
- It is removed rapidly from the plasma by hydrolysis in the liver and kidney by the action of oxytocinase.
- The elimination half-life is 1–7min.

Adverse effects

- Nausea and vomiting.
- Hypotension.
- Uterine hypertonicity.
- Water intoxication and hyponatraemia.

Contraindications

- Cardiac disease.
- Hypotension.

Storage

- Store at 2–8°C (refrigerate, do not freeze).

Ergometrine maleate

- Ergometrine is an amine ergot alkaloid used to prevent PPH by producing intense contractions of the uterus usually followed by periods of relaxation.

Dose and time of action

- Postpartum dose is 200 micrograms administered IM.
- In an emergency, 200 micrograms may be injected IV slowly, over a period of at least 1min.

- Following IV injection, uterine contractions are initiated within 1min and persist for 45min.
- Following IM injection, uterine contractions are initiated within 2–5min and persist for ≥3h.

Metabolism and excretion
- Metabolized in the liver, excreted in the faeces.

Adverse effects
- Highly emetic especially when given IV.
- Vasoconstriction, hypertension and bradycardia.
- Headache.

Contraindications
- Hypersensitivity to ergot alkaloids.
- Eclampsia or pre-eclampsia.
- Severe or persistent sepsis.
- Peripheral vascular disease, heart disease, hypertension.
- Impaired hepatic or renal function.

Storage
- Store at 2–8°C (refrigerate, do not freeze).

Synthetic oxytocin and ergometrine maleate (Syntometrine®)

- Syntometrine® combines the rapid uterine action of oxytocin, a nonapeptide hormone released by the posterior lobe of the pituitary, with the sustained uterotonic effect of ergometrine.
- It is used in the prevention and treatment of PPH associated with uterine atony.

Dose and time of action
- Each 1mL ampoule contains 5IU synthetic oxytocin and 500 micrograms ergometrine maleate.
- 1mL IM is given following expulsion of the placenta, or when bleeding occurs. Another 1mL can be repeated after an interval of 2h.
- The total dose given within 24h should not exceed 3mL.

Metabolism and excretion
- See metabolism of oxytocin and ergometrine.

Contraindications
- Hypersensitivity to any of the components.
- Severe hypertension, pre-eclampsia and eclampsia.
- Cardiac, hepatic or renal dysfunction.

Adverse effects
- Nausea, vomiting.
- Uterine hypertonicity.
- Hypertension, bradycardia, cardiac arrythmias.
- Anaphylactoid reactions.

Storage
- Store at 2–8°C (refrigerate, do not freeze). Protect from light.

Carboprost tromethamine injection (Hemabate®)

- Carboprost, an oxytocic, contains the tromethamine salt of the (15S)-15 methyl analogue of naturally occurring $PGF_{2\alpha}$.
- Carboprost is only used to treat PPH when oxytocin and ergometrine have been ineffective in stopping the bleeding.

Dosage and time of action

- 1 ml of Hemabate® contains 250 micrograms of carboprost and is administered by deep IM injection (dangerous if given IV).
- Subsequent doses of 250 micrograms should be administered at 90min intervals depending on uterine response, although this may be reduced to 15min if bleeding is severe.
- The total dose of carboprost should not exceed 2mg.

Adverse effects

- Nausea, vomiting and diarrhoea.
- Hyperthermia and flushing.
- Bronchospasm.
- Risk of pulmonary oedema with increasing doses.

Contraindications

- Known hypersensitivity.
- Asthma.
- Acute pelvic inflammatory disease.
- Cardiac, renal, hepatic or pulmonary disease.

Misoprostol

- Misoprostol, a PGE_2 analogue, is frequently used for the induction of labour.
- It also has an important role as third or fourth line management of uterine atony, when syntocinon and ergometrine have failed.
- It should be administered rectally in a dosage of 800 micrograms as a stat dose.

Chapter 10

Anaesthesia for caesarean section: regional anaesthesia

Sarah Harries, Martin Garry
and Vinay Ratnalikar

Introduction

Regional anaesthesia is the technique of choice for caesarean delivery in the developed world, provided no contraindications exist. The relationship between the increased use of regional anaesthetic techniques for caesarean delivery and decreased maternal mortality is well recognized, with epidemiological studies indicating regional anaesthesia to be 16 times safer than GA. The three commonly practised techniques—epidural, spinal and combined spinal–epidural (CSE)—all offer significant advantages for both the mother and neonate.

Advantages

- The mother remains awake and is very much part of the delivery of her baby.
- Early maternal–baby contact, e.g. 'skin to skin' contact, encourages bonding and improves success at breastfeeding.
- The baby's father or a birthing partner is permitted into the operating theatre during surgery, providing emotional support for the mother.
- Many birthing partners welcome being part of the delivery.
- Enhanced postoperative analgesia through the use of intrathecal or epidural opioids.
- Reduces incidence of postoperative sedation, which may delay bonding with the newborn baby.
- Reduced incidence of nausea and vomiting.
- Early mobilization.
- Reduced incidence of postoperative deep vein thrombosis (DVT).
- The direct sedative effects of GA drugs on the neonate are avoided, i.e. delayed onset of respiration, thermoregulation and feeding.
- Reduced incidence of regurgitation and pulmonary aspiration.
- Reduced incidence of difficult or failed intubation or failed ventilation.
- Reduced operative bleeding.
- Reduced incidence of awareness.

Disadvantages

- Hypotension is associated with all regional techniques and can confer significant harm to mother and neonate if not promptly treated.
- Intraoperative nausea and vomiting.
- High blocks or total spinal blocks.
- Failed block requiring conversion to GA.
- Intraoperative pain leading to dissatisfaction and complaint.
- PDPH—approximate incidence 1%.
- Neurological complications reported rarely.
- Infection-related complications again reported rarely.
- The time required to perform a regional technique or top-up an existing epidural may prohibit its use in certain situations, e.g. delivery required in <15 min.

Whenever the anaesthetist is faced with a mother reluctant to accept a regional technique for caesarean delivery, the specific risks and benefits of general vs. regional anaesthesia should be clearly emphasized, provided there are no contraindications to the proposed technique. The mother must not be frightened into accepting a regional technique on the grounds that GA is dangerous as there must be a clear back-up to regional anaesthesia, and having to give a GA to a mother who is unduly frightened by the technique is unacceptable.

Preparation for theatre

Whatever regional technique is considered appropriate for surgery, the following should be checked and prepared prior to transfer to theatre:

- A careful history should be taken and a thorough examination performed, including examination of the lower back and an airway assessment.
- A recent full blood count (FBC) should be checked and routine group and blood screen sent to the blood bank to check for the presence of transfusion antibodies. It is acceptable not to wait for an FBC for a category 1 or 2 CS, but a pregnancy FBC should be known.
- Routine cross-matching of blood is not necessary unless significant haemorrhage is anticipated, e.g. grade 4 placenta previa or accreta, in which case blood must be available in theatre or in the delivery suite fridge at the start of surgery. Electronic issue of blood is now available in many large units, reducing the need for unnecessary routine cross-matching of blood, e.g. multiple previous CSs.
- Review the latest ultrasound report to confirm placental position.
- Antacid prophylaxis should be administered preoperatively, either by the oral route or IV according to unit policy.
- A clear explanation of the planned anaesthetic technique should be given, including the associated risks, and verbal consent obtained for the technique and any other procedures, e.g. IV insertion, monitoring, catheterization and rectal medication.
- Document the complications that were discussed, including:
  - Risk of intraoperative discomfort, e.g. pulling, tugging and pressure during surgery.
  - PDPH ~1% for all techniques, dependent on experience of anaesthetist.
  - Failed block, including conversion to GA—between 1 and 5% of regional techniques for CS are inadequate for the duration of surgery.
  - Nausea and vomiting.
  - Shivering.
  - Itching.
  - Neurological complications.
  - Infection-related complications.
- Check the anaesthetic machine and all emergency drugs.
- Prepare all anaesthetic drugs prior to regional technique, e.g. vasopressors, vagolytics, oxytocin, antibiotics.
- Check IV cannula is patent and attach IV infusion.
- Apply minimal monitoring: ECG, pulse oximeter and record the baseline BP.
- Although an elective CS is routine for the attending anaesthetist, it is never routine for the expectant mother and her partner.

See Chapter 7 for further information on the techniques of insertion and contraindications.

Assessment of the block

There has been considerable discussion and debate regarding the most reliable method of assessing both the density and height of the block required to perform a painless CS under regional anaesthesia. At present, there is no single, universally accepted best or most predictable method of testing a block prior to the start of surgery. The fundamental block required for CS is no different if a spinal or epidural is used. The difference is that in most cases the block from a spinal anaesthetic is high, dense and easy to assess. The block from an epidural is frequently more difficult to assess, requiring careful and subtle evaluation.

There are three elements to testing a regional block
- Sensory block.
- Motor block.
- Sympathetic block.

Each should be independently tested and the results documented.

What is an adequate block for surgery?

Traditional teaching was that an unspecified block to T4 was necessary for CS. However, more recent evidence suggests that loss of sensation to light touch up to and including T5 is the best indicator of a pain-free operation.
- Light touch has been shown to be a more sensitive predictor of density of block, with low light touch blocks being associated with the highest proportion of cases of intraoperative pain.
- However, light touch is not very specific in that a large proportion of such cases with too low a block will not feel any pain, but anaesthetists may feel obliged to repeat the regional or convert to a GA unnecessarily.
- Temperature and pain (to T4) are conversely less sensitive and more specific.

It is best practice to measure and document temperature and light touch testing. The method of testing light touch should be recorded, as some methods give lower results than others. The sensory testing should always be done in conjunction with motor and sympathetic block testing.

Sensory block testing

The following modalities of sensation are commonly assessed:
- *Temperature sensation* using:
  - Ice cube, differentiating between wet, cold and ice-cold sensation.
  - Ethyl chloride spray, differentiating between wet and dripping, cold and ice-cold.
- *Pain* with pinprick or a 'pinch' over the site of incision.
- *Light touch* sensation using:
  - Cotton wool.
  - Von Frey hairs.

- Blunt 'pinprick' (Neurotip).
- Patient's own finger.
- Ethyl chloride spray or ice cube, differentiating between the sensation of touch rather than cold.

Practical aspects of testing

- There is considerable scope for interassessor variability when testing a sensory block.
- The extent of the upper limit of the block will be different when tested by the different modalities and possibly different if alternative methods of testing any particular modality are used, e.g. continuous vs intermittent application of ice or cotton wool. Learn to use one method of testing.
- The sensation of ice-cold is normally blocked 1–2 dermatomes higher than pain, which in turn is blocked 1–2 dermatomes higher than light touch.
- The lower limit of the block should be tested for all regional techniques. Many anaesthetists only test the lower limit when using epidural anaesthesia, in the belief that during spinal anaesthesia, LA injected into the CSF at the lumbar level will inevitably block transmission along the sacral nerve roots passing through that area.

Top tips for testing

- Check the block at relatively fixed time intervals, thus gaining experience of what to expect at those intervals.
- Wait for evidence of motor block before testing the sensory block for the first time.
- If the block is denser on one side than the other (noted by more motor block), start the sensory testing on that side. The mother will then appreciate if there are differences and this will help you determine subtle changes.
- Perform the first check early enough to allow positional changes or top-ups prior to fixing of intrathecal LA.
- Be prepared to repeat testing if the picture is initially vague.
- Always check the block bilaterally ~5cm from the midline. If too lateral an approach is taken, the anaesthetized dermatones can be overestimated.
- Compare sensation with adjacent rather than distant areas of skin.
- Continue testing past the initial level of change to seek possible further change at a higher level. This is most commonly noted when testing with an ice cube. The mother will first note cool touching, followed by cold then icy cold as the ice cube is moved cephalad.

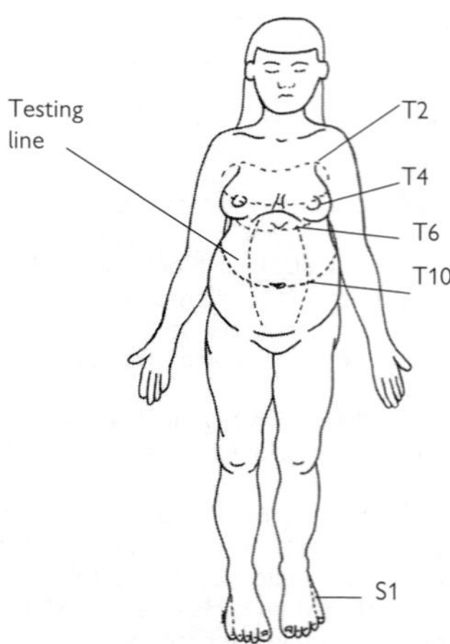

Fig. 10.1 Sensory block for caesarean section. The sensory block should be tested 5cm from the midline. S1 should be blocked to all modalities. No sensation of pinching below T10. No sensation of light touch (rubbing ice cube) below T6. No senstaion of cold below T4. Sensaton of icy cold at T2.

Motor block

- The dense sensory block required for CS is associated with dense motor block of the lumbar–sacral plexus.
- If the mother can straight leg raise, no matter how high the loss of sensation, the block is not suitable for a CS.
- Complete motor block of S1 plantar-flexion is characteristic of spinal anaesthesia but unusual with an epidural. Normal ankle motor function during epidural anaesthesia may indicate absent or inadequate sacral anaesthesia, which will result in pain during surgery.

Sympathetic block

- A sympathetic block of the feet does not develop until there is a well-defined sensory block to T10 (umbilicus).
- The **soles** of the feet should look pink and well perfused, and feel warm and dry. Dryness of the feet is an important part of sympathetic block assessment and can only be accurately determined by examining the soles.
- Differences in foot temperature or dampness of the feet are indicative of an asymmetrical or unilateral block. Even if sensory testing does not demonstrate a difference, the quality of the block will not be as good on the cooler side.
- Observing the sympathetic block can frequently pick up the more subtle differences seen in sensory testing of epidural blocks.

The ideal block for painless caesarean section

- Sensory.
  - Dabbing cotton wool or Von Frey hair—T8.
  - Sensation of ice cube or dripping of ethyl chloride spray—T6.
  - Sensation of cold—T4.
  - Sensation of icy cold—T2.
  - Pinching of skin over abdomen felt as gentle pressure only.
- Motor.
  - Complete lumbar–sacral motor block (spinal).
  - Absent straight leg raise and reduced plantar-flexion (epidural).
- Sympathetic.
  - Hot dry soles of the feet.
  - Equal temperature of both feet.

Documentation

Accurately document:
- The preoperative height of block.
- The precise modalities that were used to test the block.
- The timing of testing.

- Untreated pain during CS under regional anaesthesia is currently the leading cause of complaints and litigation in the UK.
- Due to the variety of body shapes and the difference in our understanding of dermatome positions in the pregnant woman, it has been suggested that the most reproducible way of documenting the height of sensory block is through the use of a dermatome map on the anaesthetic chart.

Further reading

Russell I. Assessing the block for caesarean section. *International Journal of Obstetric Anesthesia* 2001; **10**: 83–85.

Yentis SM. Height of confusion: assessing regional blocks before caesarean section. *International Journal of Obstetric Anesthesia* 2006; **15**: 2–6.

White JL *et al.* Differential sensory block: spinal vs epidural with lidocaine. *Canadian Journal of Anaesthesia* 1998; **45**: 1049–1053.

Epidural anaesthesia

- In the past, epidural anaesthesia was considered to be the technique of choice for CS in mothers with cardiovascular instability, e.g. cardiac disease or severe pre-eclampsia, therefore avoiding the sudden haemodynamic changes associated with spinal anaesthesia. The CSE technique has largely replaced the need for *de novo* epidural anaesthesia in this group.
- The most common indication for epidural anaesthesia for CS is the extension of the sensory block by 'topping-up' an existing epidural that has been sited for labour analgesia. A more concentrated and greater volume of solution is required to produce the dense sensory block necessary for operative delivery.
- An epidural top-up can theoretically be used in any classification of CS (categories 1–4), although it is may be difficult in a category 1 CS where there is immediate threat to the life of the woman or fetus, e.g. massive obstetric haemorrhage or prolonged fetal bradycardia.
- If epidural analgesia has not been effective during labour despite administration of adequate doses of LA, it is unlikely that the 'top-up' will provide adequate anaesthesia for CS. In such a case, re-siting the epidural catheter may be considered, although more commonly a spinal can be inserted instead. If the clinical situation does not permit this, GA should be administered.

Advantages

- No additional procedures required. It is an extension of existing analgesia in terms of its spread and density of neural blockade.
- Greater cardiovascular stability than with spinal anaesthesia is advantageous in situations where regional blockade needs to be established gradually, e.g. parturients with severe cardiac disease.
- It can be topped-up intraoperatively to rescue an inadequate block or if surgery is prolonged.
- An epidural catheter can remain *in situ* postoperatively and be used to provide a longer duration of analgesia than is provided by a single dose of intrathecal opioid or utilized if further examination or surgery under anaesthesia is required.

Disadvantages

- Slower onset of action.
- Larger doses of LA and opioid are required.
- Less dense, patchy block than with spinal anaesthesia with a greater incidence of intraoperative pain.
- Prolonged motor and sensory block postdelivery (sometimes for 8–12h).
- Risk of catheter migration to intrathecal, intravenous or subdural space.

See Chapter 7 for further details on the technique of insertion for epidural anaesthesia and the contraindications.

Checks prior to 'top-up'

The following checks should be performed on the epidural catheter in addition to the checklist already described when preparing the mother for theatre:

- Confirm that the IV line remains patent or re-site prior to top-up.
- From the notes, confirm the depth of the epidural space measured at the time of catheter insertion and examine the back to ensure the depth of catheter is unchanged or that the catheter has not inadvertently fallen out or migrated further inwards.
- Exclude that any fluid or blood has accumulated at the site of insertion.
- Review the effectiveness of the epidural during labour. If recent 'top-ups' have been ineffective, re-assess the level of sensory block. If a block is asymmetrical, poor or absent, it may be best to abandon the epidural and insert a spinal anaesthetic instead (See p 300).

Place of top-up

- An epidural 'top-up' should be administered with full monitoring and preferably in the operating theatre.
- To expedite the onset of the block, an epidural top-up is sometimes administered in the delivery room.
- If this is done:
  - The anaesthetist must confirm that a means of measuring the BP and appropriate IV vasopressors are readily available to treat any hypotension.
  - The anaesthetist must stay with the mother at all times to monitor her vital signs.
  - CTG monitoring of the fetus must continue. Early involvement of the anaesthetist in such situations is always beneficial.
  - Transfer the mother to the operating theatre in the full lateral position, as it is the safest position for her and her baby. Place her on the side of the coolest foot.

Single top-up or divided doses

- Almost all epidurals will require at least 20mL of a high concentration LA solution to produce an adequate block for CS.
- Almost all studies evaluating various solutions for CS have used either a 2mL (test dose) followed by 18mL bolus, or a single 20mL bolus.
- The most reliable and rapid method of topping up an epidural is to give a single large volume.
- A single top-up is not detrimental to the baby.
- If divided doses are given, the time to achieve an adequate block can double but pre-top-up block assessment does not adequately distinguish between epidurals that will top-up easily or not.
- The total LA dose may also increase if the top-up is given in divided doses.

- Occasionally, a single 20mL bolus will produce a sensory block that produces some numbness of the lower cervical dermatones but, apart from reassuring the mother, this should require no further action.
- Some anaesthetists exercise caution, especially if top-ups are started in the delivery room, by dividing the top-ups into 10 or 5mL boluses.
- Divided doses may be safer if haemodynamic stability is important or if there is plenty of time.

Choice of drugs

Local anaesthetics

- An epidural 'top-up' should increase both the extent and density of the block that has provided analgesia for labour to a degree that is adequate for performing CS, without causing any maternal or fetal compromise.
- There are a number of possible LA solutions that may be used to 'top-up' an epidural to provide surgical anaesthesia, provided the epidural has been functioning well in labour.

The following are examples of effective local anaesthetics commonly used:

- 0.5% bupivacaine 20–25mL.
- 0.5% levobupivacaine 20–35mL.
- 2% lidocaine (often with additional 1:200 000 adrenaline) 15–20mL.
- 50/50 mixture of 0.5% bupivacaine and 2% lidocaine 15–25mL.
- 0.5% ropivacaine 15–25mL.
- 0.75% ropivacaine 15–20mL.

- Bupivacaine 0.5% 20mL is generally accepted as an appropriate epidural top-up and has been found to be consistently effective when administered with opioid, e.g. 50–100 micrograms fentanyl.
- Levobupivacaine may be used in the same or an increased dose, up to 35mL of 0.5%, and may add an extra element of safety by virtue of its less cardiotoxic side effect profile.
- Some studies have shown that the onset of anaesthesia is quicker with 2% lidocaine when used as a sole agent or in combination with bupivacaine. Although there is some evidence that lidocaine-containing solutions may be less reliable. If 2% lidocaine is used, adrenaline should be added to reduce the systemic absorption of LA and improve the density of the block.
- If after 20mL of a high concentration solution there is adequate spread but inadequate density of the block, a further 5 or 10mL of the same LA solution can be given.

Opioids

- The addition of lipophilic opioids, e.g. 50–100 micrograms fentanyl or 20–50 micrograms sufentanil to the LA solution has consistently been shown to increase the quality of the sensory block and improve intra-operative analgesia.
- The site of action of all spinal opioids is the dorsal horn of the spinal cord via spinal opioid receptors. Opioids administered via the epidural route undergo systemic absorption and may cause unwanted side effects, i.e. nausea and vomiting, itching, sedation and respiratory depression.
- Longer acting opioids, e.g. diamorphine 2.5–5mg or morphine 3–5mg may be given via the epidural catheter following delivery of the baby for postoperative analgesia. They may cause the same unwanted side effects, including late-onset respiratory depression, and the mother should be monitored postoperatively.

Adjuvant drugs

- *2mL of 8.4% preservative-free sodium bicarbonate* to the epidural top-up solution has been shown to increase the speed of onset of epidural anaesthesia. The non-ionized fraction of the LA drug is increased, which in theory crosses the perineural sheath with greater efficiency. In practice, this advantage is not considered to be of any clinical significance.
- *0.1mL of 1:1000 adrenaline* to a 2% lidocaine mixture reduces the systemic absorption of lidocaine and intensifies and prolongs the neural blockade. It has a direct antinociceptor effect by acting as an α_2 agonist within the spinal cord.
- *Clonidine* is a pure α_2 adrenergic agonist, which is thought to produce analgesia by an action within the dorsal horn of the spinal cord. It is administered as an epidural bolus of 75–100 micrograms. Clonidine has the advantage of causing less nausea and vomiting, pruritus or respiratory depression than opioids, but is associated with hypotension and sedation. It has been evaluated mostly for its postoperative analgesic effect.
- *Neostigmine* has been studied in doses of 30–300 micrograms. It produces dose-related nausea and sedation, and has a modest analgesic value.

Management of the failed block

Prior to surgery

- If the block remains inadequate before the start of surgery, a further incremental dose of LA should be administered, e.g. 5–10mL bupivacaine 0.5% or levobupivacaine 0.5%, if time allows and the patient is positioned appropriately.
- If there is no further extension of the block, most anaesthetists would advocate abandoning any further epidural top-ups and insertion of a reduced dose spinal anaesthetic, e.g. 1–1.5mL hyperbaric bupivacaine 0.5% in the left lateral 'Oxford' position (see Chapter 7, p 210). The mother should then be placed on her back with a left lateral tilt, with two pillows placed well under the thoracic curvature to prevent a high block.
- If there is insufficient time to perform a spinal, a GA is the only option.

During surgery

- An inadequate block may become apparent after surgery has commenced, e.g. during peritoneal incision, exteriorization of the uterus or swabbing of paracolic gutters. At whatever stage pain becomes apparent, reassurance of the mother and partner that it will be dealt with is paramount, and any pain or discomfort should be communicated to the surgeon.
- It is important to differentiate at every stage between pain and the sensation of pressure/tugging, which can cause considerable discomfort. Verbal contact and support from the anaesthetic team are essential during a CS under regional anaesthesia.
- Symptoms of pain during a CS should never be dismissed. Appropriate action should always be taken, and any management offered or refused always documented.
- If pain is apparent during peritoneal incision, i.e. before delivery of the baby, attempts can be made to improve the block with a further top-up of LA +/– opioid. The surgeon should be asked to stop surgery and wait until the patient is comfortable. Entonox and/or a short-acting supplementary opioid, e.g. 0.5–1mg alfentanil, should be offered until the 'top-up' is effective.
- If the supplemental epidural top-up is ineffective or the urgency of delivery is such that surgery cannot stop at this stage, conversion to GA is usually the only option.
- If pain becomes apparent after delivery of the baby, surgery should be stopped and similarly a supplemental epidural 'top-up' given and the administration of Entonox offered, and/or a short-acting supplementary opioid, e.g. 0.5–1mg alfentanil until the 'top-up' is effective. IV ketamine in 10mg increments is an additional option. If this is ineffective, GA should be offered.
- If approaching the end of surgery, local infiltration of LA at the incision site can be offered.
- All patients should be reviewed in the postdelivery period. Specific information about the proposed reasons for the inadequate block should be clearly explained.

Further reading

Goring-Morris J *et al.* A randomized comparison of 0.5% bupivacaine with a lidocaine/epinephrine/fentanyl mixture for epidural top-up for emergency caesarean section after 'low dose' epidural for labour. *International Journal of Obstetric Anesthesia* 2006; **15**: 109–114.

Lucas DN *et al.* Extending low dose epidural analgesia for emergency caesarean section. A comparison of three solutions. *Anaesthesia* 1999; **54**: 1173–1177.

Dickson MA, Jenkins J. Extension of epidural blockade for emergency caesarean section. Assessment of a bolus dose of bupivacaine 0.5% 10 mL following an infusion of 0.1% for analgesia in labour. *Anaesthesia* 1994; **49**: 636–638.

Saunders RD *et al.* Extending low-dose epidural analgesia for emergency caesarean section using ropivacaine 0.75%. *Anaesthesia* 2004; **59**: 988–992.

Lam DT *et al.* Extension of epidural blockade in labour for emergency caesarean section using 2% lidocaine with epinephrine and fentanyl, with or without alkalinisation. *Anaesthesia* 2001; **56**: 790–794.

Karinen J *et al.* Single bolus compared with a fractionated dose injection technique of bupivacaine for extradural caesarean section: effect on uteroplacental and fetal haemodynamic state. *British Journal of Anaesthesia* 1996; **77**: 140–144.

King MJ *et al.* Epidural fentanyl and 0.5% bupivacaine for elective caesarean section. *Anaesthesia* 1990; **45**: 285–288.
Roelants F. The use of neuraxial adjuvant drugs (neostigmine, clonidine) in obstetrics (Review). *Current Opinion in Anesthesiology* 2006; **19**: 233–237.
Tortosa JC *et al.* Efficacy of augmentation of epidural analgesia for caesarean section. *British Journal of Anaesthesia* 2003; **91**: 532–535.

Spinal anaesthesia

Spinal anaesthesia produces a dense block, which has a much faster onset and provides better quality anaesthesia than an epidural technique. In a 1996 survey, it was the first choice technique for the majority of UK anesthetists when performing an elective or urgent CS. The role of spinal anaesthesia in a category 1 CS depends on the experience of the anaesthetist and also the obstetrician making the decision for CS. There are very few situations where the degree of urgency does not allow time for a spinal anaesthetic to be performed. If a working epidural is *in situ*, this should be topped-up for the CS to proceed. However, if the epidural has functioned poorly during labour, it should be removed and a spinal performed if time allows.

Advantages

- Rapid onset of anaesthesia.
- Dense sensory and motor block.
- Predictable extent of sensory block.
- Easy to perform in a pressurized situation, with a clear end-point.
- The addition of long-acting opioids will improve postoperative analgesia and facilitate early mobilization.
- The incidence of thromboembolic disease is reduced.

Disadvantages

- Rapid onset of sympathetic blockade, with associated hypotension and nausea and vomiting.
- Lack of flexibility of duration with single-shot technique.
- An unexpected high block may lead to compromised respiration.
- Untreated hypotension with unrelieved aorto-caval compression can precipitate severe fetal hypoxia and acidosis.
- Maternal bradycardia due to the combination of sympathetic blockade and reduced VR initiates the Bezold–Jarish reflex.

See Chapter 7, p 208 for further details on the technique of insertion, contraindications and management of hypotension.

Choice of drugs

Local anaesthetics

- 0.5% hyperbaric bupivacaine is the only drug licensed for intrathecal use in the UK. A dose of 12.5mg has been shown to produce a reliable sensory block for surgery; however, lower doses (8–10mg) are frequently used and are considered sufficient, especially when combined with an epidural technique, and may be associated with less hypotension.
- The use of 0.5% hyperbaric lidocaine has been abandoned since reports of prolonged neurological deficits associated with intrathecal injection.

- Plain bupivacaine has been extensively investigated and can produce a reliable block which some say is less susceptible to the position of the mother.
- The final block is more dependent on the mass of drug rather than the volume of injectate, i.e.10mg bupivacaine can be given as 2mL of 0.5% solution or 10mL of 0.1% solution with equal effect.
- Levobupivacaine 0.5% and ropivacaine 0.5–0.75% also produce satisfactory blocks but are not at the present time available as hyperbaric solutions.
- The required volume of LA injectate is dependent on a number of additional factors which should be considered:
  - Pregnant term women—need 25% less LA.
  - Height of the mother—although the evidence for this is limited. It may be appropriate to increase or decrease the dose a little at the extremes of height.
  - Gestational age—prematurity is associated with a smaller uterus and therefore less vena cava compression, which reduces cephalad spread of LA. Either increase the dose or use a CSE technique.
  - Increased uterine size—multiple pregnancies and polyhydramnios can cause a more rapid onset and extent of block due to increased cephalad spread.

Opioids

- The addition of lipophilic opiods, e.g. 10 micrograms fentanyl, 2.5–10 micrograms sufentanil or 250 micrograms diamorphine, to the LA has consistently been shown both to increase the quality of the sensory block and to improve intraoperative analgesia. Intrathecal diamorphine will provide postoperative analgesia for up to 12h.
- Morphine is much slower in onset (45–60min) and does not provide good intraoperative analgesia, but is effective for the management of postoperative pain.
- The site of action of all spinal opioids is the dorsal horn of the spinal cord via spinal opioid receptors. Opioids administered via the spinal route undergo a degree of systemic absorption and may cause unwanted side effects, i.e. nausea and vomiting, itching, sedation and respiratory depression.
- Short-acting opioids, e.g. fentanyl or sufentanil, contribute little to postoperative analgesia. Therefore, the addition of a long-acting opioid, e.g. morphine 100 micrograms, is recommended to provide optimal postoperative analgesia, provided appropriate staff and facilities are available for monitoring of vital signs every 2h for the first 24h post-operatively, as there is a small risk of developing late-onset (>12h) respiratory depression following intrathecal morphine.
- Intrathecal diamorphine has been shown to be associated with less nausea, vomiting and itching than intrathecal morphine. However, the duration of action of diamorphine is less, i.e. 12h following surgery, compared with 24h after intrathecal morphine.

Adjuvant drugs

- Intrathecal clonidine is an α_2 adrenergic agonist, which produces analgesia within the dorsal horn of the spinal cord through the release of nitric oxide. Clonidine 75 micrograms added to hyperbaric bupivacaine and fentanyl has been shown to improve intraoperative and postoperative analgesia. Side effects include a prolonged motor block, hypotension, bradycardia and sedation.
- Intrathecal midazolam 1mg has analgesic properties; however, when combined with intrathecal diamorphine, the effect is no different from that of diamorphine alone.
- Intrathecal neostigmine produces analgesia by inhibiting the breakdown of acetylcholine. Doses from 10 to 100 micrograms have been used and have been shown to improve postoperative pain for up to 24h. However, there is a high incidence of dose-related nausea and vomiting, which has limited its clinical use.

Assessment and manipulation of the block

- Perform the first check early enough, i.e. within a few minutes of positioning the mother in left tilt, to allow positional changes prior to fixing of intrathecal LA if block is inadequate.
- The extent of the sensory block should be mapped with great care, including assessment of the lower limit of the block. Bilateral motor block is expected with spinal anaesthesia.
- Although the block is usually bilateral, occasionally it is unequal and postural manipulation, especially if 'heavy' bupivacaine is used, is useful.
- The mother can be tilted or turned on to the inadequate side to improve the block.
- If the upper level of the block is inadequate, tilting the table slightly head down or flexing the hips are both effective measures.
- A sensory block to ice-cold from T4 to S5 and to light touch to T5 should ensure a pain-free CS.
- The mother should be fully prepared for the sensation she may feel during surgery and warned of the possibility of intraoperative discomfort or pain, and how this will be dealt with.

Table 10.1 Comparison of drug doses for epidural vs intrathecal use

Drug	Epidural route	Intrathecal route	Duration of action	Notes
Fentanyl	50–100 micrograms	15–25 micrograms	2–3h	Increased dosage produces increasing side effects, e.g. nausea, vomiting, pruritus
Morphine	3–5mg	100–200 micrograms	19–24h	Increased dosage produces increasing side effects Observe for late-onset (>12h) respiratory depression
Diamorphine	2.5–5mg	250–375 micrograms	12–20h	Associated with less unwanted side effects compared with morphine, but pruritus occurs in >80%
Sufentanil	20–50 micrograms	2.5–10 micrograms	2–4h	Increased dosage produces increasing side effects, e.g. nausea, vomiting, pruritus Not used in the UK
Clonidine	150–600 micrograms, an infusion 40 micrograms/h is required to provide lasting postoperative analgesia	75 micrograms	2–4h following an intrathecal dose with bupivacaine and fentanyl	Prolonged motor block, hypotension, bradycardia and sedation are unwanted side effects
Neostigmine	–	10–50 micrograms	10–24h	High incidence of nausea and vomiting, limiting its use

Management of the failed block

Prior to surgery

- If the block is inadequate for surgery to proceed within the expected time frame, i.e. up to ~15min, there are a number of possible management options:
  - Change to mother's position—positioning head down or in the lateral position, with the unblocked area dependent may improve a sensory block that is not quite at the limits required.
  - Repeat the spinal—if there is no evidence of a sensory or motor block or the upper limit of the block is below T12, repeating the spinal is recommended. If no or minimal block is apparent, the same dose should be repeated. If there is evidence of a degree of sensory block, e.g. up to T12, a reduced dose of LA (1–1.5 of 0.5% heavy bupivacaine) should be considered to avoid a high block. The mother should be carefully repositioned with two pillows under the thoracic curve to avoid a high block (see Figs 10.2 and 10.3).
  - Insertion of an epidural—if the upper limit of the sensory block is between T12 and T4 dermatomes, insertion of an epidural catheter and augmentation of the block with incremental top-ups is recommended if time allows. 5mL of bupivacaine 0.5% or levobupivacaine 0.5% should be given and the block re-assessed every 5min until the required sensory block is reached.
  - GA—if the urgency of surgery does not allow further time to improve the regional anaesthetic, a GA should be performed. The mother and fetus should be risk assessed in consultation with the obstetrician again in theatre, as the decision to convert to a GA in the morbidly obese or severely pre-eclamptic patient carries significant airway risks.

During surgery

- An inadequate block may become apparent after surgery has commenced, e.g. during peritoneal incision, exteriorization of the uterus or swabbing of paracolic gutters. At whatever stage of surgery pain becomes apparent, reassurance of the mother and partner that it will be dealt with is paramount, and any pain or discomfort should be communicated to the surgeon.
- If pain is apparent during peritoneal incision, i.e. before delivery of the baby, conversion to GA is usually the only option. The surgeon should be asked to stop surgery, whilst the GA drugs and equipment are prepared. Entonox and a short-acting supplementary opioid, e.g. 0.5–1mg alfentanil. should be offered.
- If pain becomes apparent after delivery of the baby, surgery should be stopped and similarly Entonox offered, and a short-acting supplementary opioid, e.g. 0.5–1mg alfentanil given. IV ketamine in 10mg increments is an additional option. If this is ineffective, GA should be offered.
- If approaching the end of surgery, local infiltration of LA at the incision site should be performed.

- It is important to differentiate at every stage between pain and the sensation of pressure/tugging, which can cause considerable discomfort. Verbal contact and support from the anaesthetic team are essential during a CS under regional anaesthesia.
- Symptoms of pain during a CS should never be dismissed. Appropriate action should always be taken, and any management offered or refused always documented.
- All patients should be reviewed in the postdelivery period. Specific information about the proposed reasons for the inadequate block should be clearly explained.

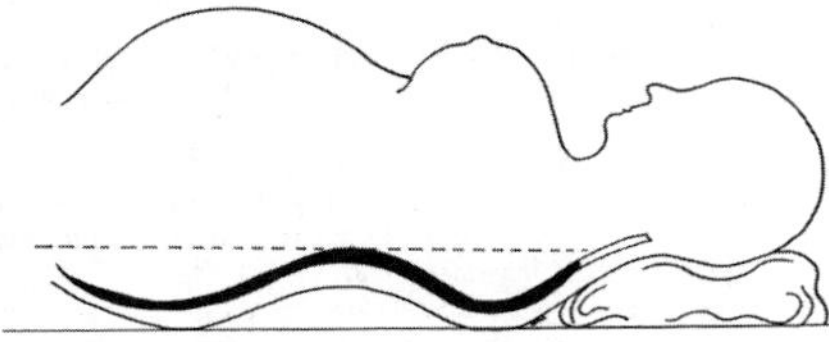

Fig. 10.2 During spinal anaesthesia, a pillow placed under the head and neck will tend to allow the intrathecal solution to travel to T2.

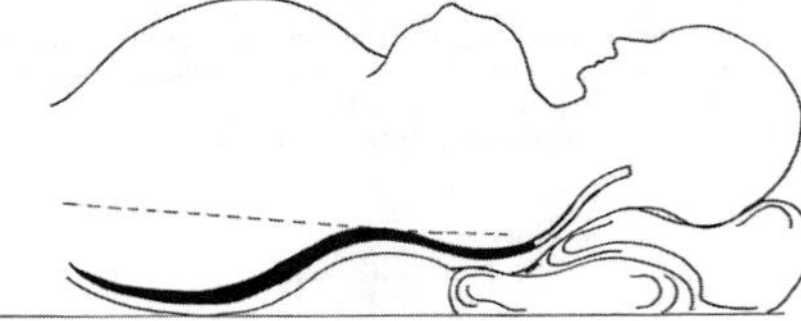

Fig. 10.3 With a second pillow placed under the mid thoracic curve, the spread of intrathecal solutions can be more easily controlled. This will prevent excessive spread of intrathecal injection, especially if performed after a failed epidural top-up.

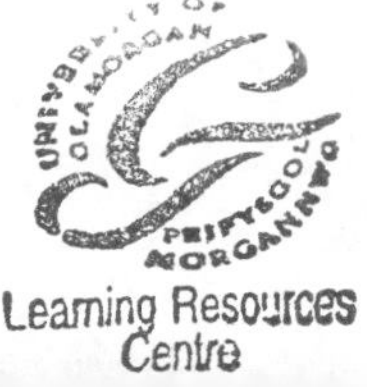

Continuous spinal anaesthesia

- This is not currently popular in the UK, although there are case reports which have described its successful use in some parturients, e.g with complex cardiac problems or severe scoliosis.
- It allows controlled and gradual development of a dense regional block while maintaining haemodynamic stability.
- Small incremental doses, i.e. 0.25mL of plain 0.5 or 0.25% bupivacaine, are titrated against the required height of the sensory block and maternal BP.

Further reading

Ng K *et al.* Spinal versus epidural anaesthesia for caesarean section. *Cochrane Database of Systematic Reviews* 2004; **4**: CD003765.

Husiani SW, Russell IF. Intrathecal diamorphine compared with morphine for postoperative analgesia after caesarean section under spinal anaesthesia. *British Journal of Anaesthesia* 1998; **81**: 135–139.

Vucevic M, Russell IF. Spinal anaesthesia for caesarean section: 0.125% plain bupivacaine 12ml compared with 0.5% plain bupivacaine 3ml. *British Journal of Anaesthesia* 1992; **68**: 590–595.

Russell IF. Effect of posture during the induction of subarachnoid analgesia for caesarean section. Right v. left lateral. *British Journal of Anaesthesia* 1987; **59**: 342–346.

Van Tuijl I *et al.* The effect of addition of intrathecal clonidine to hyperbaric bupivacaine on postoperative pain and morphine requirements after caesarean section: a randomized controlled trial. *British Journal of Anaesthesia* 2006; **97**: 365–370.

Parpaglioni R *et al.* Minimum local anaesthetic dose (MLAD) of intrathecal levobupivacaine and ropivacaine for caesarean section. *Anaesthesia* 2006; **61**: 110–115.

Saravanan S *et al.* Minimum dose of intrathecal diamorphine required to prevent intraoperative supplementation of spinal anaesthesia for caesarean section. *British Journal of Anaesthesia* 2003; **91**: 368–372.

Cowan CM *et al.* Comparison of intrathecal fentanyl and diamorphine in addition to bupivacaine for caesarean section under spinal anaesthesia. *British Journal of Anaesthesia* 2002; **89**: 452–458.

Ginosar Y *et al.* ED50 and ED95 of intrathecal hyperbaric bupivacaine coadministered with opioids for cesarean delivery. *Anesthesiology* 2004; **100**: 676–682.

Combined spinal–epidural (CSE)

The CSE technique is the technique of choice for anaesthesia for CS in an increasing number of clinical situations, in both the elective and emergency setting. It combines the speed of onset and reliability of a spinal anaesthetic with the flexibility to extend the sensory block by supplementation with slow boluses of LA via the epidural catheter. It allows a reduced dose of intrathecal LA to be injected when necessary, therefore minimizing many of the side effects frequently seen with a single-shot spinal technique.

Indications for CSE

The indications broadly fall into the following categories:

Minimizing hypotension

- When cardiovascular stability is paramount (e.g. valvular heart disease, complex congenital heart disease and severe PET), a low dose of intrathecal LA (1.5mL hyperbaric 0.5% bupivacaine) may be administered and the sensory block supplemented by incremental epidural top-ups, which are titrated against the BP. The CSE technique has significantly reduced the need to administer GA to mothers with severe cardiac disease.
- Increased uterine size (e.g. multiple pregnancies and polyhydramnios) are associated with increased aorto-caval compression and excessive cephalad spread of intrathecal LA, both contributing to increased hypotension and uterine hypoperfusion. A reduced spinal dose minimizes the associated symptoms and complications.

Unpredictability of block height

- When it is difficult to estimate the ideal intrathecal dose for the desired block height (e.g. short or tall stature), a CSE is beneficial.
- Prematurity is associated with less cephalad spread of LA and a less predictable sensory block; the presence of the epidural catheter to extend the block, if necessary, is useful.

Prolonged surgery

- If prolonged or technically difficult surgery is anticipated, the block may be extended via the epidural (e.g. placenta previa, previous CS, presence of adhesions from previous abdominal surgery or surgical access difficult due to morbid obesity).
- If additional surgery is planned at the same time (e.g. oophrectomy).

GA contraindicated

- When a GA is strongly contraindicated (e.g. malignant hyperpyrexia, suxamethonium apnoea or cases of previous failed intubation or anticipated difficult airway), a reduced dose of spinal may be administered and epidural top-ups given to extend the block. The presence of the epidural catheter should minimize the need to convert to GA.

Postoperative analgesia

When epidural analgesia is considered beneficial in the postoperative period (e.g. chronic pain conditions, allergy to opioids).

Advantages

- Rapid onset of anaesthesia.
- Good quality sensory block.
- Flexible and titratable to prevent rapid changes of BP.
- Allows rapid extension of the regional block.
- Reduces need for conversion to GA.
- Epidural may be used for postoperative analgesia.

Disadvantages

- More difficult technique to learn and perform.
- Higher rate of failure of spinal component.
- Rapid decrease in BP is still possible.
- Untested epidural catheter, therefore it cannot be totally relied upon to function as you would expect.
- Complications of both spinal and epidural techniques ever present.
- Possibility of increased infection rate.
- Possibility of conus damage.

See Chapter 7, p 214 for further details on the technique of insertion, contraindications and management of hypotension.

Choice of drugs

Local anaesthetics

- The dose of intrathecal LA administered will depend on the indication for CSE anaesthesia:
- *'Back-up' in the event of inadequate spinal anaesthesia or anticipated prolonged or difficult surgery.*
  - A standard dose of 10–12.5mg bupivacaine can be administered.
  - Care should be taken when flushing the epidural catheter with saline solution after insertion, as small volumes (2–3mL) of injectate can cause significant cephalad spread of LA and a high block will become quickly apparent.
- Minimize hypotension.
  - An intrathecal dose of 5–7.5mg bupivacaine can reduce the speed of onset and extent of the block.
  - It has been shown that reduced doses can produce the required sensory block for pain-free surgery, with less associated hypotension.
  - Extending the sensory block can be achieved by injecting 5–10mL of saline through the Tuohy needle before catheter insertion.
  - The epidural catheter can also be flushed with 5mL of saline to extend the block.
  - The sensory block produced by these small doses is adequate in ~50% of cases, depending on the exact dose used and opioids added.
  - The main drawback is the reduced surgical anaesthesia time of <1h following a reduced intrathecal dose.
  - The anaesthetist must be familiar with testing the intrathecal block and topping-up the epidural component before and during surgery before attempting a low dose technique.

- If additional supplementation of the sensory block is required, slow incremental top-ups should be given via the epidural catheter i.e. 3–5mL bupivacaine 0.5%, and the block re-assessed every 5min.

Opioids

- The addition of an intrathecal opioid, e.g. fentanyl 15–25 micrograms or sufentanil 2.5–10 micrograms, will enhance the quality of the sensory block and improve intraoperative analgesia, and must always be given if <10mg of bupivacaine is used.
- Long-acting opioids provide optimal postoperative analgesia and are strongly recommended, provided appropriate staff and facilities are available for monitoring of vital signs every 2h for the first 24h postoperatively.

Assessment of the block

- The extent of the sensory block should be mapped with great care, including assessment of the lower limit of the block. Bilateral motor block is expected from the spinal component.
- Re-assess the level of the block after each supplementary epidural bolus.
- The mother should be fully prepared for the sensation she may feel during surgery and warned of the possibility of intraoperative discomfort or pain, and how this will be dealt with.

Management of the failed block

Prior to surgery

- If there is no apparent sensory or motor block from the spinal component of the CSE, the two options are either to repeat the spinal using the same dose or to start topping-up the epidural *de novo* using slow incremental boluses of 5–10mL bupivacaine 0.5% or levobupivacaine 0.5%. If there were any difficulties siting the epidural catheter, it may be advisable to choose to repeat the entire CSE technique.
- If there is a degree of sensory block, further incremental dose of local anaesthetic should be administered via the epidural catheter, e.g. 5–10mL bupivacaine 0.5% or levobupivacaine 0.5%, titrated against the BP and the patient positioned appropriately.
- If the block remains inadequate, the CSE or just the epidural may be re-sited and further slow incremental epidural top-ups administered.
- Depending on the urgency of the clinical situation, a GA may be necessary. The obstetrician should be made aware if there are any unexpected difficulties or delays in performing the regional technique.

During surgery

- Remember that the epidural catheter may be untested until this stage.
- An inadequate block may become apparent after surgery has commenced, e.g. during peritoneal incision, exteriorization of the uterus or swabbing of paracolic gutters. At whatever stage of surgery pain becomes apparent, reassurance of the mother and partner that it will be dealt with is paramount, and any pain or discomfort should be communicated to the surgeon.

- If pain is apparent during peritoneal incision, i.e. before delivery of the baby, attempts can be made to improve the block with a further top-up of LA ± opioid. The surgeon should be asked to stop surgery and wait until the patient is comfortable and the administration of Entonox offered, and/or a short-acting supplementary opioid, e.g. 0.5–1mg alfentanil, until the 'top-up' is effective.
- If the supplemental epidural top-up is ineffective or the urgency of delivery is such that surgery cannot stop at this stage, conversion to GA is usually the only option.
- If pain becomes apparent after delivery of the baby, surgery should be stopped and similarly a supplemental epidural 'top-up' given and the administration of Entonox offered, and/or a short-acting supplementary opioid, e.g. 0.5–1mg alfentanil, until the 'top-up' is effective. IV ketamine in 10mg increments is an additional option. If this is ineffective, GA should be offered.
- If approaching the end of surgery, local infiltration of LA at the incision site should be offered.
- It is important to differentiate at every stage between pain and the sensation of pressure/tugging which can cause considerable discomfort. Verbal contact and support from the anaesthetic team are essential during a CS under regional anaesthesia. Give the mother an indication of the stage of surgery and an estimate of how long surgery will last.
- Symptoms of pain during a CS should never be dismissed. Appropriate action should always be taken, and any management offered or refused documented.
- All patients should be reviewed in the postdelivery period. Specific information about the proposed reasons for the inadequate block should be clearly explained.

Further reading

Rawal N *et al.* Combined spinal epidural technique. *Regional Anesthesia* 1997; **22**: 406–423.

Van de Velde M *et al.* Combined spinal–epidural anesthesia for cesarean delivery: dose-dependent effects of hyperbaric bupivacaine on maternal hemodynamics. *Anesthesia and Analgesia* 2006; **103**: 187–190.

Coppejans HC *et al.* The sitting versus right lateral position during combined spinal–epidural anesthesia for cesarean delivery: block characteristics and severity of hypotension. *Anesthesia and Analgesia* 2006; **102**: 243–247.

Choi DH *et al.* Combined low-dose spinal–epidural anesthesia versus single-shot spinal anesthesia for elective cesarean delivery. *International Journal of Obstetric Anesthesia* 2006; **15**: 13–17.

Beale N *et al.* Effect of epidural volume extension on dose requirement of intrathecal hyperbaric bupivacaine at caesarean section. *British Journal of Anaesthesia* 2005; **95**: 500–503.

HamLyn EL *et al.* Low-dose sequential combined spinal–epidural: an anaesthetic technique for caesarean section in patients with significant cardiac disease. *International Journal of Obstetric Anesthesia* 2005; **14**: 355–361.

James KS *et al.* Combined spinal–extradural anaesthesia for preterm and term caesarean section: is there a difference in local anaesthetic requirements? *British Journal of Anaesthesia* 1997; **78**: 498–501.

Common complications

The following complications are frequently seen when performing any regional technique for CS.

Hypotension

A fall is the systolic and diastolic BP is frequently seen within minutes of administering the regional technique, due to aorto-caval compression being unmasked by sudden autonomic blockade. (The autonomic system normally mitigates the haemodynamic effects of aorto-caval compression). Bradycardia <60/min is often associated with the sudden hypotension.

Manifestations

- Nausea and vomiting.
- Light-headedness.
- Pallor.

Management

- Increase left uterine displacement by ensuring a tilt of 20° or place in full left lateral position.
- Prompt treatment with vasopressors ± a vagolytic, e.g. glycopyrrolate 200–400mcg.
- Increase IV fluid infusion.
- Expedite surgical delivery if there is concern for fetal well-being.

Respiratory difficulty

It is not uncommon for mothers to complain of difficulty taking a deep breath or chest tightness as the block extends cephalad. This perceived difficulty in taking an adequate breath or cough is due to paralysis of the lower intercostal muscles, which contributes to forced expiration and the increased abdominal size, limiting diaphragmatic movement in the supine position. This always improves after delivery when diaphragmatic splinting is relieved.

Management

- Reassure mother and partner.
- Re-assess the upper limit of the block by assessing motor function in the hands.
- Place a pillow or wedge under the shoulders to the mid thorax. This improves diaphragmatic breathing.
- Monitor pulse oximetry and administer oxygen by face mask if SpO_2 <95%.

Headache

- The sudden onset of headache at the time of spinal insertion or immediately after lying down is thought to be due to air entering the intrathecal space and rising cranially. Reassurance should be offered.
- Headache in the days following a regional technique should always be investigated further.

- The PDPH rate associated with spinal anaesthesia when using atraumatic needles is ~1%. Features of the headache include:
  - Frontal pain, usually bilateral and posture-related.
  - Neck stiffness, again posture-related.
  - Nausea and vomiting.
  - Tinnitus.
  - Visual disturbance or photophobia.
- The headache that follows spinal dural puncture is often not as severe as that associated with an accidental dural puncture with a Tuohy needle. However, the symptoms should not be dismissed and all management options discussed, as detailed in Chapter 14, p 406. Other causes of headache postdelivery should also be excluded, e.g. dehydration, pre-eclampsia.
- Headache following an inadvertent dural puncture at the time of epidural or CSE insertion is frequently severe. Approximately 60–70% will require an epidural blood patch. See Chapter 14, p 408 details of management.

Chapter 11

Anaesthesia for caesarean section: general anaesthesia

Rachel Collis, Moira Evans, Claire Farley and Doddamanegowda Chethan

General anaesthesia and CEMACH

The number of obstetric GAs has fallen as the use of regional anaesthesia has increased. The recommendation that only 15% of caesareans should be performed under GA may decrease this further. This, coupled with the reduced training time available for trainees and reduced numbers of intubations in all areas of practice, has led to concerns about the ability of trainees to manage obstetric GA and intubation safely. The findings of the CEMACH 2000–2002 report revealed a number of problems.

- There were six deaths directly attributed to the conduct of GA in the triennium. One death as a late consequence of aspiration in the previous triennium was also reported.
- The authors estimated the risk of death following obstetric GA to be 1 in 20 000. Sadly, this is the same risk as in the 1980s.
- Five of the six direct deaths were related to substandard airway management:

Deaths related to airway management

- Unrecognized oesophageal intubations.
- Inadequately managed hypoventilation.
- Pulmonary aspiration of gastric contents which occurred after failed intubation.
- Inadequately managed extubation.

- Care was identified as substandard partly because of failure to adhere to national and local recommendations on:
  - Minimal monitoring standards.
  - Capnography was not used in two of the cases.
  - Checking equipment before each patient.
  - Competency training and assessment prior to independent practice.
  - Conduct of a failed intubation drill.
  - Administration of pulmonary aspiration prophylaxis.
  - Cardiopulmonary resuscitation.
- There were also many examples of failures of communication within multidisciplinary teams.
- There were also problems in early recognition of the severity of pathology and delays in obtaining senior anesthetic help.

Indications for general anaesthesia

Despite the identification of problems with GA, there will always be the need to give a GA quickly but safely to the pregnant woman; indeed it be may lifesaving.

Historically, some indications that were regarded as absolute may now be regarded as relative, particularly as the use of continuous spinal catheters and CSE anaesthesia has removed the need for GA in some cases. A clinical decision based on the risks and benefits of GA must be made for each patient.

- Category 1 CS, where there is immediate threat to the life of the mother or the baby and there is absolutely no time for a regional technique.
- Failure of regional anaesthesia. Either inability to establish a block or failure to provide adequate anaesthesia.
- Maternal refusal of regional technique, despite an adequate explanation of the options having been given by an experienced anaesthetist.
- Regional technique contraindicated.

Contraindications to regional anaesthesia

- Inadequate haemostasis pathological/pharmacological; platelet count $<70\times10^3$/L.
- Sepsis—global/focal.
- Allergy to LAs.
- Uncorrected hypovolaemia/ongoing haemorrhage.
- Fixed CO states, sympathetic-dependent pathology.
- Structural abnormalities of the lumbar spine/cord, e.g. spina bifida.
- Some spinal operations such as insertion of Harrington rods.
- Present or potential raised ICP.

Contraindications to general anaesthesia

There are very few contraindications to GA. If intubation has failed or has been very difficult in the past, the most senior anaesthetist available must be consulted about the need for further GA. If the appropriate equipment is not available, then induction of GA should not begin.

Airway assessment

Changes in maternal factors that increase the likelihood or consequences of airway management difficulties

Anatomical factors

- Increased chest diameter and enlarged breasts can make laryngoscopy with a standard Macintosh handle difficult.
- Respiratory tract mucosal oedema makes airway obstruction and bleeding more likely.
- Tongue enlargement may prohibit compression with the laryngoscope.

Physiological factors

- Increased oxygen consumption—this is increased 15–30% above normal and is mainly due to the demands of the fetoplacental unit and the uterus. This leads to an increased rate of desaturation.
- Decreased functional reserve capacity (FRC)—this is decreased by ~30% in the third trimester. During the last third of pregnancy, the diaphragm is displaced cephalad by the enlarging uterus. This reduces both the residual volume and expiratory reserve volume, such that the FRC is greatly reduced. This is more significant in the supine position and removes one of the largest stores of oxygen available to the body, making pregnant women very susceptible to hypoxia during anaesthesia.

Other factors

- Left lateral tilt used to minimize aorto-caval compression.
- Cricoid pressure applied excessively or inaccurately may make intubation difficult.

The airway must be assessed in all patients who receive an anaesthetic intervention. Even if a regional technique is planned, this may fail or the patient may develop one of the complications, e.g. a total spinal, that require intubation.

It is well recognized that there is a higher incidence of difficulty in the obstetric population. Work from the UK has shown for the period 1999–2003 in 4768 obstetric GA:

- Incidence of grade 3 view as 1 in 530.
- Incidence of grade 4 view as 1 in 1800.
- Incidence of failed intubation as 1 in 238 (1 in >2000 in non-obstetric).
- No cases of 'can't intubate, can't ventilate'.

Although anaesthesia-related deaths are a small proportion of the overall maternal mortality figures, GA-related deaths are usually due to lack of airway management skills and experience, and thus are preventable.

- Factors affecting this rate include:
  - Changes in maternal physiology during pregnancy.
  - The increasing incidence of obesity.
  - Increased use of regional techniques in the management of CS leading to a reduction in anaesthetists' experience of GA.

History

- Details of any previous difficulty must be sought. The patient may have been told of a problem. There may be a letter or medic alert bracelet, and any previous anaesthetic records available should be examined. Bear in mind that a previous successful intubation does not guarantee success this time!
- Pre-eclampsia, especially with concurrent upper respiratory tract infection (URTI), produces airway oedema and can increase the Mallampati score.
- Obstructive sleep apnoea increases the risk of difficult face mask ventilation as well as tracheal intubation, and a history of snoring should be sought.
- Obesity increases the risks of GA, and measurement of height and weight allows the BMI to be calculated.

Examination

Airway assessment is a basic skill and should always be undertaken regardless of the type of anaesthesia planned. Appropriate airway assessment should alert the anaesthetist to major anatomical abnormalities.

- Large breasts.
- Large tongue.
- Fixed head/neck flexion.
- Small jaw/receding mandible.
- Inability to bring lower incisors in front of the upper ones.
- Short neck.
- Short mandibulothyroid distance.
- Protruding maxillary incisors.
- Less than 5cm between incisors on mouth opening (3 fingers).
- Obesity >90kg booking.
- Mallampati score ≥3.
- Risk of airway oedema.

Note: Mallampati scores have been reported to increase during pregnancy and labour, and should be assessed immediately before GA.

- If two or more of the above are detected, senior help should be sought and considerations given to avoid GA. If the patient is thought to be difficult to manage under a GA, but refuses to have a regional anaesthetic, a senior anaesthetist with appropriate skills should be present and awake fibreoptic intubation considered.
- Scoring systems are not good at predicting the difficult airway, in part due to its rarity. However, the combination of decreased neck extension, Mallampati grade 3 or 4 and decreased mouth opening is associated with a high incidence of difficult intubation.

Communication and preparation

Rapid effective communication of the likelihood of a GA CS allows time for an airway assessment to be made and an appropriate management plan to be instituted. If difficulties with intubation are considered likely, senior/additional help should be sought as early as possible, although lack of abnormality of the airway assessment does not exclude an airway problem developing later. A GA should only be induced in the presence of a properly checked anaesthetic machine and equipment, with minimum monitoring established and with the help of a dedicated trained anaesthetic assistant.

Equipment

The intubation trolley/cart should contain the following equipment and should be available immediately in case of any difficulties with intubation:

- Face masks of various sizes.
- Oropharyngeal and nasopharyngeal airways.
- Short- and long-bladed Macintosh laryngoscopes.
- Short-handled laryngoscope.
- McCoy (or other flexible-tipped) laryngoscope.
- Gum elastic bougie/tube introducer.
- Selection of tracheal tubes—6.5 to 8mm (including microlaryngeal tube).
- Laryngeal mask airway (size 3 and 4), Proseal™ LMA size 3 and 4.
- A device for cricothyroidotomy and equipment for ventilation (anaesthetists working on the labour ward should be familiar with the connections).

Although fibreoptic intubation by the inexperienced has no place during a failed intubation, it should be available to the experienced practitioner who is skilled at asleep, fibreoptic intubation (with cricoid pressure).

Intubation

Positioning the mother

- Before induction of anaesthesia, the patient should first be positioned supine with a left lateral tilt on the operating table in theatre to avoid aorto-caval occlusion.
- To aid airway manipulation, the head position should be that described as 'sniffing the morning air', neck flexed, head extended, ensuring that the mouth can be maximally opened. This can only be achieved with a pillow placed away from the shoulders (neck flexion) and plumped up behind the head with the patient's chin raised (head extension).
- Braided, tied and knotted hair on the occiput is an additional problem that prevents neck extension. Hair should be untied and spread across the pillow.
- Knotted scarves around the head are a similar hazard, as they can hide knotted hair and should be removed. Headscarves can be loosely applied around the head for religious purposes.
- Encourage the patient to extend her head (raise her chin) during preoxygenation. This improves the overall position of the head and allows accurate inspection of the neck before application of cricoid pressure.

Optimizing laryngoscopy in the obese

- Position the head using the 'ramped' position (see Figs. 11.1 and 11.2) for the obese, which brings the tragus and sternum onto the same horizontal plane. This improves the view at laryngoscopy and makes intubation easier.
- Careful choice of laryngoscope blade and handle.
- Use arm boards if necessary to ensure the patient's breasts are not going to interfere with laryngscope manipulation.
- Some functions of the operating table may not work if the patient's weight is above a certain threshold, which can cause difficulty in safe positioning.
- Adequate dose of suxamethonium.
- Adequate time for full relaxation to occur, even with increased rate of oxygen desaturation.

Cricoid pressure

- Badly applied cricoid pressure has been implicated during intubation difficulties.
- Ensure cricoid pressure is applied correctly and not altered by table tilt; often best achieved if applied from the patient's left side.
- Single-handed cricoid pressure can flatten the neck on the pillow, reducing neck extension.
- Two-handed cricoid pressure can improve intubation position but reduces help to the anaesthetist, unless there is a second assistant.
- Excessive backward and poorly directed pressure can obliterate the laryngeal opening (no greater than 30N).
- Only trained and regularly updated anaesthetic assistants should apply cricoid pressure.

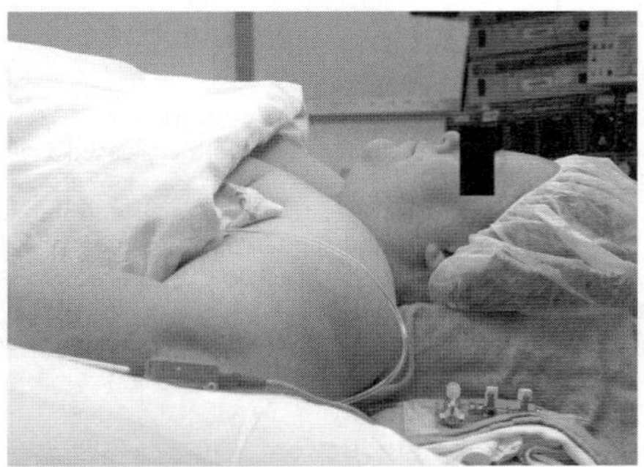

Fig. 11.1 The 'sniff' head position.

Reproduced with permission from Laryngoscopy and morbid obesity: a comparison of the 'sniff' and 'ramped' positions. *Obesity Surgery* 2004; **14**: 1171–1175.

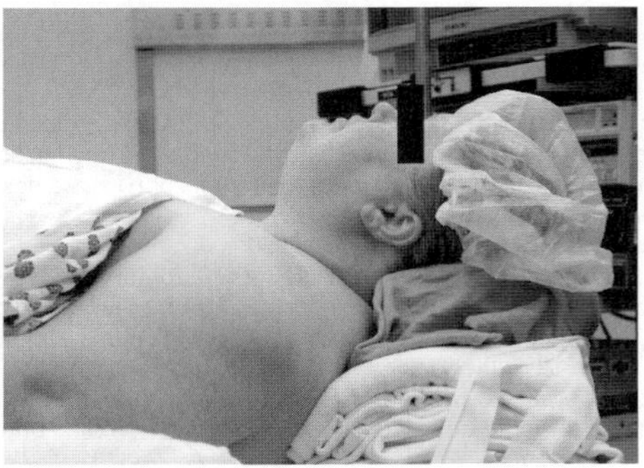

Fig. 11.2 The 'ramped' head position.

Reproduced with permission from Laryngoscopy and morbid obesity: a comparison of the 'sniff' and 'ramped' positions. *Obesity Surgery* 2004; **14**: 1171–1175.

Preoxygenation

- There is an increase in oxygen consumption of up to 12–16% at term, compared with non-pregnant controls.
- In early labour, oxygen consumption may further increase up to a total of 30% of the non-pregnant state.
- A healthy, non-pregnant patient will sustain up to 3min of apnoea before desaturating. A pregnant woman with her increased oxygen requirement and decreased functional residual capacity will desaturate much faster, particularly if she is obese. A realistic time may be as short as 60–90s before desaturation occurs.

- There are three different methods of preoxygenation.
  - High flow oxygen for 3min.
  - Eight vital capacity breaths.
  - Awaiting a fractional end-tidal O_2 measurement of >0.9. The last is probably more accurate and practical with increased availability of end-tidal monitoring.
- A tight-fitting mask should be used to minimize air entrainment. The mother may be very anxious and repeatedly push the mask away from her face. She must be persuaded not to do this as preoxygenation must start again if she does so.

The advantage of preoxygenating for 3min is that it allows the anaesthetist to make visual checks before induction of anaesthesia.

Final check list prior to induction

- Head in best position.
- IV infusion working.
- Appropriate drugs drawn up and available.
- Visual check of anaesthetic machine.
- Suction under the pillow.

Induction, paralysis and intubation

- It is important that the first intubation is the best intubation attempt.
- An adequate dose of induction agent (thiopental 4–7mg/kg) should be followed by 100mg of suxamethonium (an appropriate dose should be used in the very obese, e.g. 1–1.5mg/kg).
- An adequate time must be allowed for the suxamethonium to work. In the pregnant woman, this is usually ~30s. Attempts to place the laryngoscope in the mouth before full relaxation may lead to dental damage and mucosal bleeding (both of which will increase the likelihood of intubation difficulties).
- After the drugs have worked, laryngoscopy and intubation should be performed. It would be reasonable to use the gum elastic bougie for the initial attempt.
- Depending on individual circumstances, a long-blade, short-handled laryngoscope or a McCoy blade may be used for the first intubation.

Assessing tracheal tube position

- Capnography is the gold standard to confirm correct tracheal palcement.
- Bilateral auscultation of the chest is important, particularly if laryngoscopy is >grade 2.
- It is probably wise to have a back-up test to confirm tracheal intubation in the event of a failure or malfunction of the capnography (e.g. Wee oesophageal detector or a disposable CO_2 detector).
- The cuff should be placed below the vocal cords and inflated gradually until the air leak with manual ventilation stops and the pressure in the cuff is between 20 and 30cmH_2O.

Failed intubation

There are currently no national obstetric airway guidelines. If intubation is anticipated to be difficult, any contraindications to regional anaesthesia must be reconsidered.

In order to ensure maximum safety, it is essential that every anaesthetist has a clear plan for airway management. The use of a simple protocol is preferable in which the only requirement is the competent use of a small number of airway adjuncts Fig. 11.3.

Failure to intubate must be acknowledged without delay

The priorities are:

- Call for help.
- Oxygenate the patient.
- Do not give further muscle relaxant.
- Optimize the patient's head position.
- Do not turn the patient into the lateral position as this will hinder ongoing airway manoeuvres.

- Oxygenation is most likely to be successful if a four-hand ventilation technique is used with an oropharyngeal airway.
- It is important that the jaw thrust is properly applied to ensure that three primary areas of airway obstruction (tongue, epiglottis, soft palate) are bypassed, allowing oxygenation and ventilation to continue.
- With the above manoeuvres, oxygenation should be possible in most cases, but cricoid pressure may need to be removed or adjusted to improve the airway.

The second attempt

If a second attempt at intubation is considered, a 'left molar approach' may be successful where conventional laryngoscopy is not.

- This is described as inserting the laryngoscope directly down the left side of the mouth above the molar teeth to access the larynx. It is thought to improve the view because the tongue does not need to be compressed in order to see the larynx.
- This particular technique should be practised on an intubation mannequin or on elective non-obstetric cases before being used in the emergency situation.
- If the larynx can be seen but not intubated, a smaller tracheal tube may be needed; using a bougie or Magill's forceps may aid intubation.

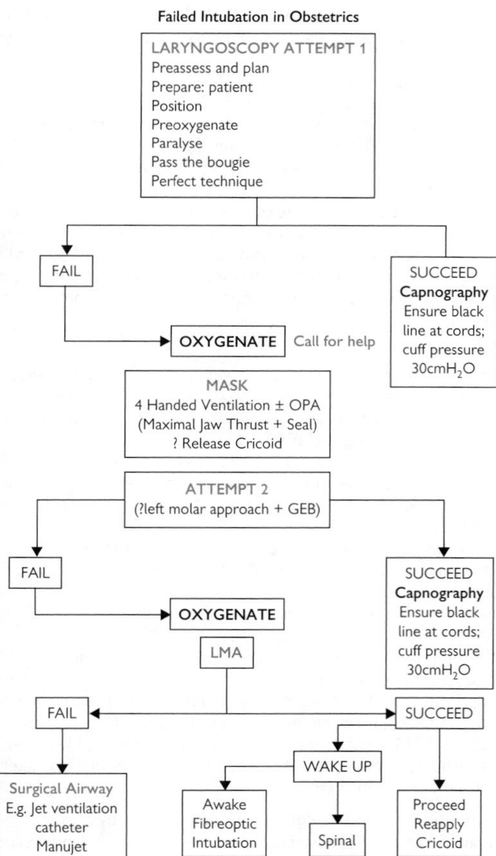

Fig. 11.3 Failed intubation algorithm.

Reproduced with permission of Dr M.R. Stacey, DAME, Cardiff.

Airway rescue techniques

- It is important to decide on a rescue technique before induction of anaesthesia, as a failed intubation and ventilation situation is not the time to be making such a decision. The question of whether to continue the anaesthetic with an unprotected airway or to risk death of the fetus and allow the mother to wake is a difficult one. It depends on the indication for CS and the experience of the anaesthetist.

- In practice, the primary duty of the anaesthetist is to the mother, and there are only two absolute indications to continue with surgery:
  - Maternal cardiac arrest.
  - Life-threatening haemorrhage.
- A GA for a CS using spontaneous ventilation and an unprotected airway is such a difficult and unfamiliar anaesthetic technique, it requires expertise, but may be the only option in these cases. Trainees should be careful in taking such decisions, and senior help should be sought urgently.
- In a maternal cardiac arrest, the uterus must be evacuated in order for cardiopulmonary resuscitation to have any chance of success. In massive obstetric haemorrhage, bleeding is unlikely to be controlled until the placenta has separated. In other situations, such as fetal distress, it may be sensible to wake up the patient and consider other methods of anaesthesia.

Laryngeal mask

- If the second attempt at laryngoscopy is unsuccessful and oxygenation is difficult, consider insertion of a classic laryngeal mask airway (cLMA).
- It may be necessary to ease the degree of cricoid pressure to allow proper positioning of the cLMA.
- If the cLMA insertion is successful and oxygenation is possible, the safest decision is to wake up the mother. Additional help can then be used to provide anaesthesia, e.g. using either a regional technique or awake fibreoptic intubation.
- If surgery has to proceed, oxygenation and anaesthesia can be continued with spontaneous ventilation through the cLMA and cricoid pressure reapplied.
- It may be worth considering fibreoptic tracheal intubation through the LMA to provide a more secure airway.
- Volatile agents may have to be used to deepen anaesthesia, and this can lead to reduced uterine tone with increased risk of bleeding.
- Although the obstetric situation is exempted from the Difficult Airway Society guidelines, it recommends the intubating LMA (Fastrach LMA) or ProSeal™ LMA as alternatives for failed intubation. However, both devices are larger than the cLMA, and anaesthetists are less likely to have experience with them.

Failed intubation, failed ventilation: the surgical airway

- When all the above methods fail, a purpose-designed cricothyroidotomy kit or jet ventilation catheter with a jet ventilator should be used to provide a surgical airway.
- All anaesthetists covering the maternity unit should be trained to put the equipment together and to jet-ventilate a dummy before they are faced with a GA on a patient.

Training and assistance

- Training, using simulator-based scenarios, can be useful for practising failed intubation/ventilation. This will allow skills, knowledge of equipment, flexibility of thinking and team-work to be taught.

- In the operating theatres, the skill of managing an airway with a mask and oropharyngeal airway needs a raised profile and should be practised on non-obstetric patients.
- Any elective obstetric GA should be used as a training opportunity to teach a rapid sequence induction, providing there are no concerns regarding the airway. Appropriate seniority should always be available for training and managing more difficult patients.
- A skilled assistant is part of the successful management of GA and must be available at all times. It is important that assistants are also trained in and practise failed and difficult intubation drills with the team so that they clearly understand the principles of their management.

Awake fibreoptic intubation

Indications

The indications for awake fibreoptic intubation in obstetric practice are limited to:

- An elective or semi-urgent caesaran section where there is concern that intubation may/will be difficult.
- After a failed intubation when the mother is woken and regional anaesthesia is still not possible.

Unless the anaesthetist is considered an expert in the technique of awake fibreoptic intubation, it is considered best practice NEVER to attempt the technique as part of a failed intubation with the mother anaesthetized.

Options available if difficulty anticipated

- Regional anesthesia.
- CSE or spinal catheter offers lowest risk of unexpectedly high block.
- Secure airway with patient awake.
- Fibreoptic intubation—the technique of choice.
- Avoid intubation and use alternative airway.
- LMA used in 1067 selected elective cases in Korea.
- ProSeal™ LMA has been used in cases of failed intubation in obstetrics.
- CS under local infiltration only.

Technique of awake fibreoptic intubation

- Both oral and nasal routes have been successfully used.
- Careful preoperative explanation is needed.
- Glycopyrrolate (5mcg/kg) IM to reduce secretions.
- Oxymetazoline to shrink the nasal mucosa and produce vasoconstriction.
- Maximize airway space by sitting up and avoiding sedation.
- Multiple techniques have been described for anaesthetizing the airway; choose the one you are most familiar with.
- Smaller tubes than usual should be selected (size 6mm) armoured or tapered tip (as provided with the intubating LMA) and preloaded on the fibrescope.
- GA is only induced when tube placement has been confirmed by capnography.
- Direct laryngoscopy should be performed to give an impression of the ease of intubation.
- Extubation should be performed awake when protective airway reflexes have returned.

A survey in one UK region showed that 91.4% would choose awake intubation if regional was contraindicated or had failed in a patient with a known difficult airway. However, only 6/74 choosing awake fibreoptic intubation had obstetric experience of this.

- It is important to involve colleagues experienced in fibreoptic intubation as recommended in the CEMACH 2000–2002 report.

Drugs for general anaesthesia

Preventing awareness

- The incidence of awareness is said to be higher than in the non-obstetric population and could be between 0.4 and 1.3%.
- This high incidence is probably caused by:
  - Anxious, unpremedicated patient.
  - Reduced dose of anaesthetic agents because of fear of increased sedation in the baby.
  - Start of surgery when the mother is asleep under the affects of thiopental rather than the inhalational agents.
  - A reduced dose of inhalational agent because of fear of uterine relaxation.
- These problems can be reduced by:
  - Giving an adequate dose of thiopental.
  - Using nitrous oxide with oxygen.
  - Using an over-MAC technique at the start of surgery guided by end-tidle vapour analysis.
  - Using agents with low blood/gas partition coefficients such as sevoflurane, isoflurane or desflurane.

Although an adequate dose and concentration of anaesthetic agents must be used, pregnancy is also associated with a reduction in MAC requirement. This can be seen from the first trimester. MAC requirements may be reduced by 30%.

Induction agents

Thiopental

- Remains the gold standard.
- Rapid predictable sleep with eye closing makes it the easiest drug to use when suxamethonium must be administered quickly.
- There is reliable anaesthesia for 5–7min, which allows the brain concentration of inhalational agent to come up to a sleep dose.
- At a dose of 4mg/kg, sedation at birth of the baby is minimal.
- At higher doses (8mg/kg), fetal depression will occur.
- Rapid redistribution in the maternal and fetal circulation allows the baby to be born in a vigorous condition.

Propofol

- Although very popular in non-obstetric practice, it is not considered first choice in obstetrics.
- Lack of a clear induction end-point and an unreliable sleep dose make it a difficult drug to use for rapid sequence induction.
- At 2.5mg/kg, the baby is born in a vigorous condition. In higher doses it is associated with neonatal sedation.
- Rapid wakening may be associated with an increased risk of maternal awareness.
- Total IV anaesthesia has been described, but at doses >6mg/kg/h it is associated with neonatal sedation. At this dose, it may lead to maternal awareness, especially if opioids have not been used as a co-agent.

Ketamine

- Has been described for induction of the severely haemodynamically compromised mother.
- It is not an ideal agent as induction is slow and an end-point difficult to detect.
- It causes hallucinations and delirium, especially in the unpremedicated mother.
- At 1mg/kg the condition of the neonate is comparable with thiopental.
- At 2mg/kg (probably a better dose for the mother) neonatal depression can be expected.

Etomidate

- Has been described for induction of the severely haemodynamically compromised mother.
- In a dose of 0.3mg/kg the baby is born in a vigorous condition.
- The drug is associated with pain on injection, myoclonic rigidity and involuntary movements, making it a difficult drug to use as part of a rapid sequence induction.
- Its use in GA practice is associated with lower cortisol levels and adverse outcomes in ICU patients.
- Lower cortisol is also seen in the neonate after its use, the significance of which is uncertain.

Benzodiazepines

- Their slow onset make these less appropriate under normal circumstances than the other agents, with increased risk of aspiration.
- Midazolam at an induction dose of 0.2mg/kg is associated with prolonged sedation in the neonate and doubling of the time to sustained respiration compared with thiopental.
- Are also associated with poor feeding, neonatal hypothermia, hypotonia and neonatal jaundice.

Neuromuscular agents

Suxamethonium

- At the present time, it remains the drug of choice in obstetric practice because of giving rapid ideal intubating conditions and rapid reversal of effect.
- Is given in a dose of 1–1.5mg/kg.
- Spontaneous respiration returns in 1–5min.
- Time to neuromuscular reversal may be slightly prolonged in pregnancy due to the physiological dilution of plasma pseudocholineserase.
- Suxamethonium does not cross the placenta so the neonate is not affected.
- There is a case description of neonatal paralysis in a pseudocholinestease-deficient neonate born to a deficient mother.
- The neuromuscular blocking effect is not altered by magnesium sulphate, but fasciculations are attenuated and therefore difficult to see.

Contraindications to suxamethonium are the same as for the non-pregnant population.

Non-depolarizing neuromuscular blockers

- An intermediate acting agent is required to maintain paralysis during CS after neuromuscular recovery from suxamethonium.
- Vecuronium, atracurium and rocuronium have been extensively investigated.
- They do not cross the placenta.
- Rocuronium has been extensively described to facilitate a rapid sequence induction when suxamethonium is contraindicated.
- It can be used in a dose of 0.6–0.8mg/kg, with good intubating conditions within 70s.
- This dose will cause paralysis for 45min.
- All the non-depolarizing agents are attenuated by magnesium sulphate, and neuromuscular function must be closely observed in the mother at reversal and into the postoperative period if she is on this drug.

Inhalational agents

Nitrous oxide

- Is a useful carrier gas with oxygen.
- It freely crosses the placenta, and concentrations will continue to increase in the neonate for 15min during maternal administration.
- Concentrations >50% are associated with neonatal depression.
- The use of nitrous oxide and oxygen alone will cause light anaesthesia, increased maternal catecholamines, adverse acid-base status in the baby and an increased risk of awareness.
- Its main advantage is that it does not cause uterine relaxation and can be used to reduce the concentration of the volatile agents required.

Volatile agents

- All cause dose- and time-dependent neonatal depression.
- Induction to delivery time should be <11min.
- All cause dose-dependent uterine relaxation and their use should be restricted to 0.5 MAC. Nitrous oxide should be used to supplement anaesthesia.
- Agents such as sevoflurane, isoflurane and desflurane have the advantage of a low blood gas solubility, allowing rapid induction and recovery.
- Sevoflurane should ideally be available as it is the best agent should anaesthesia with spontaneous ventilation be required.

Opioids

- Are not usually given as part of a rapid sequence induction in obstetric practice.
- They cause neonatal depression and delayed recovery of spontaneous respiration in the mother should there be a failed intubation.
- 100–200 micrograms of fentanyl or 10mg morphine should be given after delivery of the baby.
- 1mg of alfentanil or 100 micrograms fentanyl will help obtund the intubation response and can be given at induction if hypertension or tachycardia must be avoided.

Conduct of general anaesthesia

- Drugs for rapid sequence induction must be permanently available, ready drawn up and renewed daily.
- A trolley containing equipment for routine airway management as well as difficult/failed intubation must be available and checked with each shift.
- Capnography must be used for all GAs and, if not available, the patient or the equipment moved.
- An assistant with experience in obstetric anaesthesia must be available.
- A separate oxygen source should be used for supplementary oxygen for the patient receiving regional anaesthesia to avoid the need to disconnect the circuit from the fresh gas flow outlet.

Preoperative preparation

- Reduce gastric pH and volume.
  - Ranitidine 150mg, 6hly orally in labour if high risk.
  - Ranitidine 50mg IV if not previously given orally.
  - Metoclopramide 10mg IV.
  - 30mL sodium citrate 0.3M immediately prior to induction.
- Explain what will happen to the mother.
- In emergencies, continue active fetal resuscitation measures:
  - Stop oxytocin infusion.
  - Place mother in the full left lateral postion during transfer to theatre.
  - Give oxygen.
  - IV infusion of crystalloid.
  - Hypotension should be corrected by the use of IV vasopressor.
  - Tocolysis.
- A plan should be made in the event of a failed intubation.
- Recheck equipment.

Induction

- Place mother supine with left lateral tilt with head in optimal postion.
- Preoxygenation to an end-tidal O_2 fraction >0.9 with 100% oxygen and a tightly fitted face mask: either 3min of tidal volume breathing or in the emergency situation 8 deep breaths within 1min with an oxygen flow of 15L/min.
- Cricoid pressure is applied.
- Rapid sequence induction of anaesthesia is performed with:
  - Thiopentone 5–7mg/kg.
  - Suxamethonium 1.5mg/kg.
  - (Rocuronium 0.6–0.8mg/kg if the patient has a contraindication to suxamethonium).
- If required, obtund sympathetic response to intubation with, e.g. alfentanil 20 micrograms/kg. Consider a 60mg/kg bolus of magnesium sulphate in patients with pre-eclampsia.

Maintenance

Predelivery

- Ventilate to normocapnia of pregnancy (4.0–4.5kPa) with 50:50 mixture of O_2 and N_2O. Use overpressure to ensure >0.75 MAC of volatile is delivered. Any less increases the risk of awareness.
- Use a nerve stimulator to confirm the offset of suxamethonium. Then use small doses of a non-depolarizing agent to maintain neuromuscular blockade.

Postdelivery

- Level the table to improve surgical access.
- Reduce O_2 to 30%, if maternal SpO_2 will allow with 70% N_2O.
- Give oxytocin 5IU IV slowly.
- Antibiotic prophylaxis according to local protocols.
- Give IV opiate analgesia:
  - Fentanyl 100 micrograms.
  - Morphine 10mg in titrated aliquots.
  - Or administer morphine 4mg or diamorphine 2.5mg epidurally if catheter is *in situ* but there was no time for topping-up.
- Diclofenac 100mg rectally if consent obtained previously, or diclofenac 75mg diluted in 100mL normal saline IV.
- Paracetamol 1g IV.
- Consider bilateral illioinguinal nerve blocks.

Local anaesthetic techniques

- Local wound infiltration by surgeons.
- Bilateral ilioinguinal nerve blocks, subfascial or subrectus infiltrations are all viable adjuncts or alternatives to systemic analgesia.

Postoperative analgesia

Aims

- To allow early mobilization of the mother.
- Minimal maternal side effects.
- Minimal fetal side effects.
- Minimal secretion in breast milk.
- To allow normal maternal bonding with the newborn.
- To allow early discharge from hospital.

Undoubtedly balanced analgesia using multimodal analgesic therapy is the ideal (see Chapter 12, p 340).

Extubation and postoperative care

- If the patient was difficult to intubate, extreme care should be taken at extubation.
- There is debate as to whether extubation should be done in the left lateral position or the upright position.
  - The left lateral position is used by radiologists to encourage stomach emptying, will facilitate forward jaw thrust and is an optimal position should the patient regurgitate or vomit.
  - The sitting upright position allows free excursion of the diaphragm, which is particularly relevant in the obese patient. If the intra-abdominal pressure is high, it is still possible to regurgitate in the sitting or reclining position.
- Laryngeal competence is impaired for some hours after anaesthesia, so the patient is at risk of aspiration of gastric contents during recovery.
- Postoperative care should be in an HDU environment, and with midwifery staff trained to assess and manage airway obstruction.
- If there have been any intubation difficulties the mother must be fully informed of the problem. Patients should be given a letter to keep, clearly describing the problem and management; a copy should be kept in the notes and the GP informed.

Further reading

Lipman S *et al.* The demise of general anesthesia in obstetrics revisited: prescription for a cure. *International Journal of Obstetric Anesthesia* 2005; **14**: 2–4.

Rahman K *et al.* Failed tracheal intubation in obstetrics: no more frequent but still managed badly. *Anaesthesia* 2005; **60**: 168–171.

Han TH *et al.* The laryngeal mask airway is effective (and probably safe) in selected healthy parturients for elective Cesarean section: a prospective study of 1067 cases. *Canadian Journal of Anaesthesia* 2001; **48**: 1117–1121.

Popat MT. Awake fibreoptic intubation skills in obstetric patients: a survey of anaesthetists in the Oxford region. *International Journal of Obstetric Anesthesia* 2000; **9**: 78–82.

Collins JS *et al.* Laryngoscopy and morbid obesity: a comparison of the 'sniff' and 'ramped' positions. *Obesity Surgery* 2004; **14**: 1171–1175.

Thurlow JA *et al.* Intrauterine resuscitation: active management of fetal distress. *International Journal of Obstetric Anesthesia* 2002; **11**: 105–116.

Chiron B *et al.* Standard preoxygenation technique versus two rapid techniques in pregnant patients. *International Journal of Obstetric Anesthesia* 2004; **13**: 11–14.

Hart EM, Owen H. Errors and omissions in anesthesia: a pilot study using a pilot's checklist. *Anesthesia and Analgesia* 2005; **101**: 246–250.

Russell R. Failed intubation in obstetrics: a self-fulfilling prophecy? *International Journal of Obstetric Anesthesia* 2007; **16**: 1–3.

Stacey M. General anaesthesia and failure to ventilate. In Dob D, Cooper G, Holdcroft A, ed. *Crises in Childbirth*. 2007.

Yamamoto K *et al.* Left-molar approach improves the laryngeal view in patients with difficult laryngoscopy. *Anesthesiology* 2000; **92**: 70–74.

Chapter 12

Postdelivery symptom control

Sarah Harries, Dan Redfern,
Jon Hughes and Viju Varadarajan

Analgesia after vaginal delivery

The severity of pain and analgesia required after delivery usually depend on the mode of delivery. However, accurate pain scoring is essential when determining the strength of analgesics that may be required. A verbal rating scale (0–3) is recommended, aiming for a pain score of <2, i.e. no pain (0) or mild pain (1), on movement.

Analgesia after vaginal delivery

Normal vaginal delivery

- A normal vaginal delivery may not require any analgesics postdelivery or simple analgesia such as paracetamol 1g and an NSAID, e.g. diclofenac 50mg as required.

Vaginal delivery with episiotomy or vaginal tear

- The pain following a difficult vaginal delivery often requires REGULAR PRESCRIPTION of paracetamol 1g 6 hourly and an NSAID, e.g. diclofenac 50mg 8 hourly.
- Moderate strength opioids, e.g. tramadol 50–100mg or codeine 30–60mg, may also be needed in addition, and should be prescribed as required.

Analgesia after caesarean delivery

General recommendations

- A balanced analgesia approach is highly recommended.
- Paracetamol with an NSAID and an opioid have been extensively investigated, and this combination is safe and efficacious.
- Intrathecal and epidural opioids have been extensively shown to be safe, highly acceptable to the mother and provide excellent analgesia.
- Breastfeeding is safe when ordinary therapeutic doses are used.
- NSAIDs are contraindicated in a number of situations, and care should be exercised when prescribing them. However, they are not contraindicated in all asthmatics; if the patient has taken them without problem previously, they may be used normally.
- A small number of studies have shown that an epidural infusion or PCEA, if an epidural catheter is *in situ*, provides excellent postcaesarean delivery.
- If surgery is complicated or other adjuncts contraindicated, this approach may be very beneficial.
- There is no evidence that epidural analgesia produces superior maternal satisfaction or outcomes after routine surgery.
- Early mobilization is strongly recommended after delivery, and continuing epidural analgesia into the postdelivery period may impede this.

General anaesthesia

- *Intraoperative*: Paracetamol 1g IV and an NSAID, e.g. 100mg diclofenac PR or 75mg diluted IV after delivery of the baby, plus titrated morphine IV boluses.
- Consider bilateral ilioinguinal blocks or wound infiltration with 20mL 0.5% bupivacaine or levobupivacaine.
- *Postoperative*:
  - IV morphine via a PCA device.
  - Paracetamol 1g 6 hourly PO/PR/IV.
  - Diclofenac 100mg 12 hourly for 4 doses, followed by 50mg 8 hourly, thereafter PO/PR.
  - Moderate strength opioids, e.g. tramadol 50–100mg PO/IV or codeine 30–60mg PO may be required for break through pain or step-down analgesia after 24 hours.

Spinal anaesthesia

- *Intraoperative*: Intrathecal morphine 100 micrograms and intrathecal fentanyl 10–20 micrograms or intrathecal diamorphine 250 micrograms before delivery, with paracetamol 1g IV or PR and diclofenac 100mg PR after delivery.
- *Postoperative*:
  - Paracetamol 1g 6 hourly PO/PR.
  - Diclofenac 100mg 12 hourly for 4 doses, followed by 50mg 8 hourly thereafter PO/PR.
  - Moderate strength opioids, e.g. tramadol 50–100mg PO/IV or codeine 30–60mg PO may be used for breakthrough pain.

Epidural top-up

- *Intraoperative*: Epidural fentanyl 50–100 micrograms before delivery followed by epidural morphine 4mg or epidural diamorphine 2.5mg, with paracetamol 1g IV or PR and diclofenac 100mg PR after delivery.
- *Postoperative*:
  - As for after spinal anaesthesia.

Combined spinal–epidural

- *Intraoperative*: Either as for single-shot spinal anaesthesia (see above) or intrathecal fentanyl 20 micrograms before delivery, followed by epidural morphine 4mg or epidural diamorphine 2.5mg, with paracetamol 1g IV or PR and diclofenac 100mg PR after delivery.
- *Postoperative*:
  - As for after spinal anaesthesia.

Additional notes

- Always prescribe a laxative, e.g. lactulose 15mL, 12 hourly, with IV or PO opioid prescription.
- All mothers receiving morphine or diamorphine via the intrathecal, epidural or IV route should be monitored closely for the first 24 hours, i.e. pulse, BP, respiratory rate and oxygen saturation should be measured and documented every 30min for the first 2h, followed by 2 hourly intervals up to 24 hours.
- Regular prescription of codeine and other opioids should be avoided for at least 24 hours after intrathecal morphine because of the risk of late respiratory depression.
- All the drugs mentioned above have been safely used in mothers who are breastfeeding; however, the manufacturer of tramadol advise avoiding its use during lactation.
- Caution must be exercised in using any NSAID in mothers with moderate to severe pre-eclampsia, and any other contraindications for NSAID use.

Management of nausea and vomiting

Postdelivery nausea and vomiting is multifactorial, therefore all underlying causes should be considered to prevent maternal morbidity.

Causes

- Opioids.
- Pain.
- Ergometrine.
- Antibiotic use.
- Postoperative ileus.
- Postdural puncture headache (PDPH).
- Postpartum eclampsia.
- Intracranial pathology, e.g. cerebral venous thrombosis.

Treatment

- Antiemetics:
  - Cyclizine 50mg IV 8 hourly is safe to use during lactation.
  - Ondansetron is excreted in small amounts in the breast milk and has no clinical effects on the baby and is safe to use, but the manufacturers advise avoiding it. No data are available for the new generation 5-hydroxytryptamine 3 antagonists.
- If nausea and vomiting is persistent or has an atypical presentation, uncommon causes should be considered early.

Pruritus

- Pruritus is a common complaint in the postpartum period when the mother has received an epidural or spinal opioid in labour or for operative delivery.
- The mechanism of pruritus is complex and has recently been explained:
  - A specialized subpopulation of unmyelinated chemonociceptors and dedicated spinal neurons responsible for the itch sensation have been identified.
  - Pruritus can be caused by many other mechanisms, and pertinent to obstetric anaesthesia is μ-opioid receptor agonism.
- Spinal opioids can cause segmental analgesia and also segmental pruritus.
- Pruritus can be reduced by the painful sensation caused by scratching.
- Conversely, good analgesia can reduce this inhibition and increase the sensation of itching.
- Avoiding opioids can prevent pruritus, but this is impractical after operative delivery.

Treatment

- There are many treatments for pruritus; however, many are ineffective and may incur side effects.
- The following IV treatments are in the order of decreasing efficacy:
  - Naloxone 50 micrograms IV increments (higher doses will reverse analgesia effect).
  - Droperidol 1.25–2.5mg (higher doses are ineffective).
  - Propofol 20mg.
  - Alizapride 100mg.
  - Nalbuphine 3mg.
  - 5-Hydroxytryptamine antagonists, e.g. ondansetron (the evidence is conflicting).
- Naloxone has also been used as an IV infusion with effect.
- Droperidol has also been used as a bolus dose epidurally.
- Histamine receptor antagonists are ineffective in opioid-induced pruritus, as these receptors are not involved in the mechanism. Antihistamines are frequently prescribed, but any improvements in symptoms are probably related to a sedative or placebo effect.
- Better understanding of the receptors and mechanisms of pruritus will probably lead to more effective treatment options in the future.

Chapter 13

Anaesthesia and analgesia for specific obstetric indications

Sarah Harries, Stuart Davies,
Martin Garry, Felicity Howard
and Dave Watkins

Feticide

Definition

A therapeutic feticide involves the injection of potassium chloride into the fetal heart under ultrasound control when severe fetal abnormalities are present and the decision has been made to terminate the pregnancy. This is in line with recommendations from the Royal College of Obstetricians and Gynaecologists, which state that the decision to terminate a pregnancy after 21 weeks and 6 days gestation should ensure that the fetus is born dead.

Key issues

- The feticide procedure and the delivery that follows are always conducted in difficult circumstances. The mother and partner must be approached in a sensitive and understanding manner.
- The feticide may be performed in the fetal medicine unit or on the labour ward.
- If asked to administer analgesia, anxiolysis or sedation for the procedure in whatever setting, check that the necessary monitoring and resuscitation equipment are readily available.
- Following the feticide, labour is induced with prostaglandins.
- The onset of labour may be prolonged, with an increased risk of retained products following delivery.

Management

- The anaesthetist may be requested to administer analgesia ± sedation routinely for such procedures, or only for the very anxious patient.
- Oral analgesia and sedation, e.g. tramadol 100mg or pethidine 100mg, with lorazepam 2mg, are effective if administered prior to the procedure.
- IV midazolam in 1mg increments ± IV fentanyl/alfentanil may be safely administered during the feticide for the anxious patient provided appropriate monitoring is applied.
- Following induction with prostaglandins, labour usually proceeds rapidly.
- Analgesia should be offered, either systemic opioids or regional techniques, in the usual way.
- If anaesthesia for retained products of conception is required, an assessment of the risks and benefits of general vs regional anaesthesia should be done. Rapid sequence induction and tracheal intubation are recommended following mid-trimester terminations.
- If an anaesthetist considers for religious or cultural reasons that they are unable to manage a women undergoing a feticide, they should communicate this to a senior anaesthetist as early as possible.

Intrauterine death

Definition

Unexpected death of the fetus after 20 weeks gestation occurs in <1% of pregnancies, and frequently no specific maternal or fetal cause can be found. It may be detected by a prolonged period of absent fetal movements and confirmed by the absent of a fetal heart beat on ultrasound scanning.

Key issues

- Intrauterine death is a devastating event for parents, and the management of the subsequent delivery is emotionally difficult and stressful for all staff involved.
- There are major obstetric consequences:
  - Deranged clotting leading to DIC.
  - Sepsis.
  - PPH.
  - Retained products of conception.
- Tissue thromboplastin, the stimulus for DIC, is released from the fetus 3–5 weeks following fetal death; however, it may be released from the placenta much earlier if placental separation has occurred.
- Labour is usually induced as soon as feasible after the diagnosis has been confirmed, with the aim to deliver the fetus vaginally.
- Labour may be prolonged and difficult, especially if the fetus is near term gestation, and may require assisted delivery, e.g. forceps extraction or hysterotomy.

Management

- The situation always demands sympathy and sensitivity from all staff.
- The mother should be assessed for signs of a coagulopathy or sepsis prior to discussion about the methods of analgesia available for delivery.
  - Check FBC, clotting screen, serial temperature, pulse rate and BP.
  - Clotting abnormalities should be corrected with FFP or cryoprecipitate. Discussion with the haematologist is helpful.
  - Any signs of infection should be treated with broad-spectrum antibiotics, e.g. IV penicillins and metronidazole, as untreated sepsis can trigger a coagulopathy.
- Analgesic options for labour should be discussed early:
  - Systemic opioids, e.g. IV PCA fentanyl or morphine are often used as first-line analgesics and provide a degree of sedation for the mother.
  - Adjuvant sedatives. e.g. incremental IV midazolam are helpful to distract from the delivery process and will provide a degree of amnesia if this is the mother's wish.
  - Epidural analgesia will provide effective analgesia and allow the mother to remain more lucid and in control. Epidural analgesia is contraindicated if a coagulopathy is present or uncorrected.

Complications

- Uterine rupture should always be considered in a mother with a previous uterine scar.
- PPH is a risk in multiparous women.
- Intrauterine death of one twin is a recognized complication in a monochorionic twin pregnancy. Management is usually conservative, and the pregnancy is allowed to continue with the viable remaining twin.

Breech presentation and abnormal lie

Definition

The position of the fetus at term is defined by its lie, i.e. the relationship of the longitudinal axis of the fetus to that of the mother, and the nature of the presenting part foremost in the pelvis, e.g. cephalic (head), breech (buttock) or compound.

Breech presentation

The fetus lies longitudinally with its buttocks in the lower pole of the uterus. The presenting part may be buttocks with hips flexed and knees extended (frank breech), buttocks with hips and knees flexed (complete breech) or a foot or knee presenting before the buttocks (footling breech). It occurs in 3–4% of singleton term pregnancies.

Abnormal (transverse) lie

The fetus lies across the uterine cavity, not along the longitudinal axis, with a variable presenting part. The fetus must be converted to a longitudinal lie for a vaginal delivery to be successful. It occurs in 0.3% of term pregnancies.

Key issues

- An antenatal diagnosis of a breech presentation or abnormal lie is not absolute as the fetus frequently turns in the final weeks prior to delivery. This should be confirmed with ultrasound.
- Fetal presentation is dependent on several factors: uterine tone, the tone and pressure of surrounding structures including the maternal abdominal wall, fetal mobility and the amount of amniotic fluid present.
- Breech presentation and abnormal lie are both associated with grand multiparity, polyhydramnios, placenta praevia and other obstructive lesions in the pelvis, e.g. large uterine fibroids.
- Both breech presentation and abnormal lie are associated with an increased risk of cord prolapse and consequently fetal compromise.
- If a mother presents to delivery suite with a malpresentation, early anaesthetic assessment of the mother is important because of the high incidence of intervention. The anaesthetic assessment should be documented and handed over to subsequent shifts of staff.
- Effective team-work between obstetrician, anaesthetist and midwife is essential to ensure a safe delivery and best outcome for mother and baby.

Management

Breech presentation

- Several antenatal management options are possible, provided there is no evidence of an obstructing structure in the pelvis:
  - Vaginal breech delivery.
  - Planned CS.
  - External cephalic version (ECV).

- The Term Breech Trial demonstrated that perinatal mortality, neonatal mortality and serious neonatal morbidity are significantly lower following a planned CS compared with a planned vaginal breech delivery. As a result of this trial, many women opt for a planned CS if breech presentation persists. Consequently, obstetricians and midwives skilled at performing vaginal breech deliveries are likely to be less readily available in the future.
- Vaginal breech delivery has been shown to be associated with greater intrapartum hypoxia than a vaginal cephalic delivery, due to prolonged compression of the umbilical cord during the second stage of labour.

External cephalic version

- An ECV is performed for breech presentation at ≥37 weeks gestation, with the aim of turning the fetus around to a cephalic position to facilitate a vaginal birth.
- ECV has been shown to reduce the incidence of breech presentation at term and the incidence of CS for non-cephalic births.
- Obstetricians trained and skilled in the procedure should perform it.
- Routine tocolysis to relax the uterine muscles is recommended to improve the success of ECV.
- Routine CTG recording should be undertaken before and after an ECV.
- Suggested tocolytic agents:
  - β sympathomimetic agents, e.g. inhaled salbutamol, IV infusion of ritodrine, have demonstrated increased success of ECV.
  - Nitroglycerin, e.g. sublingual GTN spray.
  - No significant difference between these different agents has been found in terms of success rate.
- Epidural anaesthesia has been shown to have a positive effect on the success rate of ECV but not to the extent where it is wholly recommended.
- A spinal injection of 2.5mg bupivacaine and 10 micrograms sufentanil has been used in the USA to provide analgesia for the procedure, which can be painful, and some mothers do not tolerate it. However, it does not improve the success and may mask the pain associated with complications, e.g. abruption. If this treatment was to be translated to UK practice, 15 micrograms fentanyl with bupivacaine would be a suitable alternative to the sufentanil.
- Significant maternal hypotension, requiring aggressive management with vasopressors, can occur with ECV under spinal block.
- Contraindications to ECV include: previous CS or uterine surgery, oligohydramnios, compromised or premature fetus, antepartum haemorrhage, pre-eclampsia or maternal refusal.
- Risks associated with the procedure include: uterine rupture and placental abruption; thus it should only be performed where there is a dedicated obstetric team available to manage these complications.
- In the UK, it is unusual for anaesthetic teams to participate in this procedure, other than to be on 'stand-by' in the event of any complications requiring immediate delivery by CS.

- However, there are some institutions where the administration of epidural or general anaesthesia is advocated for ECV.
- Fetal scanning following the ECV will confirm the new position and fetal well-being.

Labour management

- Quite frequently presents when the mother presents in advanced labour with an undiagnosed breech presentation. Some mothers at this stage will opt for a vaginal birth, although an emergency caesarean is an option.
- Continuous fetal monitoring is essential throughout labour, with the facilities available to proceed to emergency CS if required.
- Adequate analgesia should be offered and maintained for the duration of labour and delivery, as the mother wishes. Perineal analgesia and anaesthesia are essential for the second stage.
- There are clear benefits to effective epidural or CSE analgesia for the delivery; however, there is a lack of definitive evidence to substantiate this.
- **Effective epidural analgesia**:
  - Prevents premature 'pushing' prior to full dilatation, which can be associated with a breech presentation. Involuntary maternal pushing can result in the small breech presenting part being pushed through a cervix which is not fully dilated. This can lead to head entrapment.
  - Provides sacral analgesia for an extended episiotomy or the application of forceps to the after-coming head.
  - Can be extended rapidly in the event of fetal distress and the need for an emergency CS.
- After the insertion of an epidural, usual delivery suite protocols for top-up regimes, infusions or PCEA should be followed.
- The anaesthetist should remain in close proximity to the delivery room to deal swiftly with any complications.

Caesarean section

- There are many situations when a CS may be required for breech presentation:
  - Planned CS.
  - Emergency CS following a known or undiagnosed breech presenting in labour.
  - Category 1 CS if fetal distress occurs during planned vaginal breech delivery.
- Regional anaesthesia confers significant benefits over GA for CS, and should be attempted provided time allows.
- If an epidural is sited for labour analgesia, it should be checked frequently to ensure an adequate sensory block is present and the block can be extended rapidly for an emergency CS, e.g. 20mL 0.5% bupivacaine or levo-bupivacaine + 50–100 micrograms fentanyl.
- If an emergency CS is required during the second stage of labour, extraction of the fetus may be extremely difficult. Additional uterine relaxation may be required, e.g. 50–100 micrograms IV GTN or sublingual GTN spray.
- Elective CSs are usually straightforward, although difficulties in extracting the fetus can occur.

Abnormal lie

- The management options include:
  - Planned CS.
  - Stabilization of fetal head in the pelvis, followed by immediate induction of labour, usually with a controlled artificial rupture of membranes.

Caesarean section

- A planned CS is indicated if the reason for the abnormal lie is due to an obstruction in the pelvis preventing descent of the fetal head, e.g. placenta praevia.
- Hypotension may be difficult to manage as the fetus lies across the venocava, and usual lateral tilt may not relieve the obstruction.
- Emergency CS may be indicated if during or following induction of labour, the umbilical cord prolapses into the pelvis, causing fetal distress.
- The anaesthetic technique will depend wholly on the situation and the time available. Regional anaesthesia confers significant benefits over GA for CS, and should be attempted provided time allows.

Stabilization of fetal position

- Abnormal lie is associated with grand-multiparity and polyhydramnios.
- It may be possible to turn the fetus of these women to a cephalic position and induce labour immediately, usually by controlled artificial rupture of membranes in the obstetric operating theatre.
- The major risk of this procedure is cord prolapse, precipitating the need for an immediate caesarean delivery.
- There are a number of possible management options for this procedure and will ultimately depend on applying a risk–benefit analysis for each individual situation. Discussion with the obstetrician regarding the risks of immediate delivery is essential.
- Management options include:
  - CSE anaesthesia—the spinal component should be sufficient to allow an immediate CS to be performed if necessary, whilst the epidural component could be used for labour analgesia if no complications occurred.
  - Spinal anaesthesia—an intrathecal dose for immediate CS and management of labour analgesia, as required, thereafter.
  - Anaesthetist 'on-standby' in the operating theatre ready to administer a GA if required for immediate delivery. This option is not recommended in certain situations, e.g. the morbidly obese patient or an anticipated difficult airway.

Further reading

Hannah ME *et al.* Planned Caesarean section versus planned vaginal birth for breech presentation at term: a randomized multicentre trial. Term Breech Trial Collaborative Group. *Lancet* 2000; **356**: 1375–1383.

Hofmeyr GJ. Interventions to help external cephalic version for breech presentation at term. *Cochrane Database of Systematic Reviews* 2004; **1**: CD000184.

Breeson AJ *et al.* Extradural analgesia—the preferred method of analgesia for vaginal breech delivery. *British Journal of Anaesthesia* 1978; **50**: 1227–1230.

Chadha YC *et al.* Breech delivery and epidural analgesia. *British Journal of Obstetric Gynaecology* 1992; **99**: 96–100.

Twins and other multiple pregnancies

Definition

Multiple gestations have become a more common occurrence with the increasing success of *in vitro* fertilization (IVF). However, certain restrictions now apply which limit the number of embryos that can be implanted at any one time, which should decrease the number of extreme multiple births. The incidence of twin pregnancies is 1 in 80, triplets 1 in 8000 and quads 1 in 800 000 after natural conceptions.

Key issues

- Multiple pregnancies are associated with a number of major obstetric complications, placing them at increased risk during pregnancy and delivery:
  - Pre-eclampsia.
  - Anaemia.
  - IUGR.
  - Intrauterine death.
  - Malpresentations.
  - Premature labour.
  - Prolonged labour.
  - Malpresentation of second twin following delivery of first twin.
  - PPH secondary to uterine atony.
- Many of the minor complaints of pregnancy, e.g. heartburn, exertional breathlessness, backache, pelvic-related pain, will be present in excess.
- Aorto-caval compression is much more severe. Mothers suffer symptoms of supine hypotension in the third trimester and particularly so following sympathetic blockade during regional anaesthesia.
- The anaesthetist has a key role to play in the safe management of these mothers during their delivery.

Management

- In a twin pregnancy, if the first twin is cephalic presentation and there is no evidence of other co-existing problems, there is usually no reason why these women cannot labour, although some may not wish to do so.
- In triplet and quadruplet pregnancies, a planned CS between 34 and 36 weeks gestation is the preferred mode of delivery, before preterm labour is threatened.

Labour

- The labour may be long, and the second fetus may present abnormally, necessitating instrumental delivery, cephalic version or immediate CS.
- The early insertion of an effective epidural is beneficial in a twin pregnancy as it allows rapid top-up for a trial of instrumental delivery, external or internal version of the second twin or CS if there are problems.

- The anaesthetist should be aware at all times of the progress of labour in twin births, and be present during the second stage of labour to respond and treat appropriately if the decision is made to transfer to theatre or for emergency CS.
- Elective epidural top-up with 10mL bupivacaine or levobupivacaine 0.5% for the delivery of the second twin will facilitate intrauterine manipulation, instrumental delivery and rapid extension of the epidural block for CS. The mother will have successfully delivered her first twin at this stage, and this stronger top-up will not impede her effort.

Caesarean section

The usual choices for anaesthetic technique apply. Points to consider:
- Engorged epidural veins may increase the risk of a bloody tap.
- Compressed epidural and subarachnoid spaces increase the risk of a high regional block, so the dose of LA injected intrathecally should be reduced.
- Aorto-caval compression is likely to be more severe; therefore, maintain left lateral position for as long as possible following establishment of the regional block.
- Surgery for triplet or quadruplet deliveries may be prolonged. A CSE technique may be preferable by allowing modification of the spinal dose and minimizing the risk of hypotension from aorto-caval compression.

Complications

- The incidence of pre-eclampsia and preterm labour is increased, often necessitating early delivery.
- The risk of a PPH is increased following both vaginal delivery and CS, due to the large uterus and atony following delivery. Close observation, large-bore venous access and additional oxytocic drugs, e.g. IV/IM ergometrine and a continuous oxytocin infusion are recommended.

Further reading

Weekes AR *et al.* Lumbar epidural analgesia in labour in twin pregnancy. *British Medical Journal* 1977; **2**: 730–732.

Vaginal delivery after CS (VBAC)

Definition

If a woman has undergone a transverse incision CS for a previous delivery, subsequent vaginal delivery is possible provided a risk assessment is undertaken by the responsible obstetrician and no obvious contraindications exist. It is often termed 'trial of labour' (TOL) or VBAC (vaginal birth after caesarean section).

Key issues

- The alarming rise in CS rate over the last 20yrs has driven the need to reconsider vaginal delivery after a previous CS.
- VBAC is safe and effective in carefully selected mothers and has a success rate of 72–76%. Repeat elective CS is also safe, but does carry additional risks, e.g. haemorrhage, thromboembolism, bladder damage, adhesions.
- Contraindications to VBAC are:
  - Previous classical incision CS.
  - Extensive uterine surgery.
  - Previous rupture.
  - ≥3 CSs.
- Caution is recommended prior to advising VBAC:
  - Twin pregnancy.
  - Fetal macrosomia.
  - 2 previous CSs.
  - Short interdelivery time period <18 months between delivery.
- The main risk is uterine dehiscence or rupture during labour. Induction agents, e.g. prostaglandins and oxytocics, should be used cautiously.
- Epidural analgesia for labour is not contraindicated and may be beneficial if extension of the block is required for CS. In the past, there has been concern about epidural analgesia masking the pain of uterine rupture. Provided close observations of mother and continuous fetal monitoring is performed, early signs of uterine dehiscence will be detected.
- A low dose epidural analgesia regime as per usual labour ward protocols is recommended.

Management

- A low dose epidural is beneficial.
- Continuous CTG monitoring is mandatory.
- The mother and the epidural should be frequently assessed by the anaesthetist.
- Low dose epidural techniques do not usually mask the pain of uterine rupture and therefore breakthrough pain in a well-functioning epidural must be taken seriously.
- The epidural should be topped-up frequently so it can be rapidly converted to a block suitable for an emergency CS.

Complications

- The main complication is uterine scar rupture, which can present with:
  - Severe abdominal pain, continuous in nature.
  - Intrapartum bleeding.
  - Maternal tachycardia, hypotension or collapse.
  - Fetal distress or demise.
- Management includes immediate delivery by CS and prompt resuscitation of the mother.

Further reading

Royal College of Obstetricians and Gynaecologists. *Birth after Previous Caesarean Section. Royal College of Obstetricians and Gynaecologists Guidelines*. No. 45. February 2007.

Premature fetus

Definition

The premature fetus is defined as a delivery between 20 and 37 weeks gestation. Its incidence in the UK is ~10% of all pregnancies. Delivery of the premature fetus usually follows spontaneous onset of preterm labour or premature rupture of membranes, but may be necessary due to obstetric complications, e.g. pre-eclampsia or IUGR.

Key issues

- Risk factors for preterm delivery include:
  - Previous preterm delivery.
  - Multiple pregnancy.
  - Infection, e.g. chorioamnionitis, pyelonephritis.
  - Abnormal placentation, e.g. placenta praevia.
  - Cervical incompetence.
  - Smoking.
  - Extremes of age <15 and >40yrs.
- In many cases, no apparent risk factors are found.
- Delivery prior to 32 weeks gestation is associated with major morbidity and mortality for the baby. Neonates have a higher incidence of respiratory distress syndrome, acidosis and intracranial haemorrhage.
- Once the diagnosis of preterm labour has been confirmed, the obstetrician must decide if tocolysis is appropriate to stop the labour or to allow spontaneous labour to continue.
- Tocolytic drugs include β-sympathomimetics, e.g. salbutamol or terbutaline, calcium antagonists, e.g. nifedipine, nitroglycerin, and the oxytocin receptor antagonist—atosiban.
- The greatest benefit of tocolysis is to delay delivery and allow sufficient time for corticosteroid therapy to aid fetal lung maturity.
- Two doses of steroid, e.g. betamethasone, 12h apart, are beneficial if administered to the mother when the gestational age is <34 weeks. Delivery should be delayed until 24h following the first dose if possible.
- The method of delivery of the premature infant <30 weeks is controversial. Some obstetricians would advocate a CS, as labour is too great a stress for the fetus, particularly a growth-restricted fetus.
- There is a higher incidence of operative delivery with the premature fetus; early anaesthetic assessment of the mother and optimization of any co-existing systemic disease is essential.
- If pre-eclampsia is present, request an up-to-date FBC and clotting studies if a regional technique is planned for delivery.
- A woman faced with premature delivery is often very frightened and distressed. Take time to explain the anaesthetic plan of management and answer her concerns.

Management

Labour

- If time permits, an epidural for labour analgesia can be beneficial. It will prevent the early sensation to push prior to full dilatation and a precipitous delivery of the premature baby, which can increase the risk of intracranial haemorrhage.

Caesarean section

- A 'classical' CS with a vertical incision in the uterus may be necessary if the gestational age is <28 weeks. The lower segment of the uterus has not developed at this stage.
- A regional anaesthetic technique is appropriate for either a classical or lower segment CS; however, the dose of LA required to provide an adequate block will be greater than that required for a term CS.
- As the uterus is smaller, due to the preterm fetus and reduced liquor volume, compression of the epidural and subarachnoid spaces will not be as pronounced and therefore will not assist in the cephalad spread of LA to the same degree. **The usual intrathecal dose for a term CS may result in an inadequate block.**
- Surgery and extraction of the fetus is often more difficult and the mother and partner are extremely anxious; therefore, an adequate block is essential.
- A CSE technique has the advantage of extending the block, if the intrathecal component if found to be inadequate on assessment.
- In the extreme preterm situation, syntocinon may not be fully effective in promoting uterine contraction as the receptors are not fully developed. Ergometrine should be considered postdelivery to prevent uterine atony.
- GA is acceptable, but the mother will not see the baby after delivery 'however brief' and sometimes the baby will die before the mother has recovered sufficiently to see her baby.

Placenta praevia

Definition

Placenta praevia occurs when the placenta either completely or partially covers the internal cervical os, or is implanted at its margin. It is associated with considerable morbidity and mortality. The incidence is ~1 in 200 pregnancies, but is higher with previous uterine scars, multiparity and increasing maternal age.

Grading of placenta praevia

- **I**—placenta extends into the lower uterine segment but does not reach the internal cervical os.
- **II**—placenta extends into the lower uterine segment and reaches but does not cover the internal cervical os.
- **III**—placenta eccentrically covers the internal cervical os.
- **IV**—placenta covers the internal cervical os centrally.

I and **II** are considered minor praevia, and **III** and **IV** major praevia
The grading can be further divided into anterior and posterior praevia.

Key issues

- Placenta praevia can present with painless insidious vaginal bleeding, catastrophic obstetric haemorrhage or be asymptomatic.
- The management of a patient with placenta praevia will depend on the grading of the praevia at abdominal ultrasound. However, many grading systems have been superseded by ultrasonic techniques relating the leading edge of the placenta to the cervical os.
- Clinical suspicion often follows antepartum bleeding, but is raised in any woman with vaginal bleeding and a high presenting part or abnormal lie, irrespective of previous imaging.
- The differential diagnosis is placental abruption, which is usually associated with abdominal pain and uterine tenderness or irritability. An ultrasound will differentiate these two diagnoses.

Management

Initial resuscitation

- Following presentation with a vaginal bleed, an urgent ultrasound will confirm the diagnosis and the position of the praevia.
- In the event of major haemorrhage, two large-bore cannulae should be inserted and fluid resuscitation commenced.
- Blood should be sent for FBC, clotting studies, and 4–6 units of cross-matched blood requested.

Vaginal delivery

- It is possible for a minor praevia, i.e. the leading edge of the placenta must be >2cm away from the os, to have a successful vaginal delivery.
- Epidural analgesia should be encouraged for labour as it may be rapidly extended if a CS is required.
- Continuous fetal monitoring in labour is essential.

Elective caesarean section

- Women with major placenta praevia who have bled are usually admitted and managed as an in-patient from the time of their first major bleed. They may have repeat episodes of bleeding, each time being managed with resuscitation, sometimes requiring blood transfusion, and close observation of mother and fetus.
- Whenever possible, elective CS is delayed until 38 weeks to minimize neonatal morbidity.
- Traditionally, regional anaesthesia has been relatively contraindicated for an elective CS for major praevias.
- This is of particular concern with an anterior placenta praevia as the placenta is frequently incised prior to delivery and considerable haemorrhage can occur before it is possible to give uterotonics. GA has been advocated by some because of the risk of uncontrolled bleeding.
- However, it is possible for an experienced anaesthetist to manage a major anterior placenta praevia successfully with a regional technique, either a single-shot spinal or preferably a CSE technique.
- CSE has the advantage of extending the regional blockade if surgery becomes prolonged.
- A senior anaesthetist and obstetrician should be present for the CS.
- Two large-bore cannulae should be inserted prior to commencing surgery, and invasive BP monitoring is recommended for a major anterior praevia.
- Major haemorrhage during surgery should be anticipated. Cross-matched blood should be available in theatre or in the delivery suite fridge prior to surgery.
- Resuscitation of the mother will be optimized by the use of rapid infusion devices, with the facility to warm all infusion fluids, and the use of cell salvage is encouraged.

Emergency caesarean section

- GA should be performed in any mother with:
  - uncontrolled bleeding despite resuscitation.
  - cardiovascular instability.
  - coagulopathy.
  - fetal distress.
- As above, a senior anaesthetist and obstetrician should take responsibility for surgery.
- Resuscitation should continue throughout transfer to theatre and preparation for GA.
- It is not advisable to start surgery before blood is available for rapid infusion at the time of uterine incision.

Complications

- PPH is a major risk, due to atony of the lower uterine segment and bleeding from the raw placental bed. Discuss with the obstetrician before starting surgery the plan for additional oxytocics following the first IV dose of oxytocin 5IU.
- Early use of ergometrine, continuous syntocinon infusion, misoprostol PR and carboprost should be considered.
- The lower segment of the uterus is less responsive to uterotonics, and be very much less effective than expected.
- If bleeding is uncontrolled following delivery, early use of a B-Lynch suture or intrauterine balloon tamponade may avoid the need for a caesarean hysterectomy.

Further reading

Fredericksen MC *et al.* Placenta previa: a 22-year analysis. *American Journal of Obstetrics and Gynecology* 1999; **180**: 1432–1437.

Parekh N *et al.* Caesarean section for placenta praevia: a retrospective study of anaesthetic management. *British Journal of Anaesthesia* 2000; **84**: 725–730.

Placenta accreta

Definition

Placenta accreta occurs when a placenta praevia implants over a previous uterine scar, following either previous CS or uterine surgery. The normal cleavage plane between placenta and myometrium is lost, and following delivery it becomes impossible to separate the placenta from the uterus, resulting in potentially life-threatening haemorrhage.

Classification

Dependent upon the extent of infiltration:

- **Placenta accreta vera**—placenta grows through the endometrium to the myometrium.
- **Placenta increta**—placenta grows into the myometrium.
- **Placenta percreta**—placenta grows through the myometrium to the uterine serosa and on into surrounding structures, e.g. bladder or broad ligament.

Key issues

- The incidence of placenta accreta is rising due to an increase in deliveries by CS, with an incidence of 20–30% in mothers with a placenta praevia and one previous scar, and 40–50% with a placenta praevia and two or more previous CS scars.
- Placenta increta and percreta are both rare but more severe.
- CS is the only possible mode of delivery. This should be planned in advance with a senior anaesthetist and senior obstetrician.
- Preoperative MRI scanning should be performed in those women considered to be at high risk, as the anaesthetic technique and surgical procedure may be influenced by the degree of risk.
- Bleeding at the time of delivery can be catastrophic.

Management

Anaesthetic management

- The anaesthetic management is dictated by the likelihood of major haemorrhage, maternal preference and the level of obstetric and anaesthetic experience of dealing with such cases.
- The risk of haemorrhage, transfusion and hysterectomy should be discussed with the patient as part of the consent procedure, and a minimum of 6 units of blood available in theatre prior to surgery.
- The facility for rapid infusion of warmed fluids and blood is essential, and cell salvage is strongly recommended.
- Invasive BP monitoring is essential.
- There is increasing evidence to support the safety of regional anaesthesia provided the patient is normovolaemic before neuroaxial techniques are employed.

- CSE would be the regional technique of choice, as the block can be extended if surgery is prolonged.
- In cases of significant haemorrhage and hypovolaemia, fluid resuscitation and conversion to GA is advised.
- Many experienced anaesthetists would still choose to perform an elective CS for a placenta accreta under GA.
- Resuscitation should follow guidance on major obstetric haemorrhage (see Chapter 16).

Surgical management

- Surgery should be performed by a senior obstetrician with skilled surgical assistance, and the equipment to proceed to a hysterectomy readily available.
- The placenta may have to be divided to facilitate delivery.
- Poor contraction of the lower uterine segment causes continued bleeding following delivery.
- A plan for the use of additional oxytocic agents should be decided prior to surgery commencing.
- Haemorrhage may be controlled by:
  - Bimanual compression of the uterus.
  - B-Lynch suture.
  - Ligation, embolization or balloon occlusion of the internal iliac arteries.
  - Temporary aortic compression, either manual with the operator's fist or arterial clamp or with an intra-aortic occlusion balloon.
  - Hysterectomy.

Interventional radiology

- Interventional radiology has an increasing role in the management of women with a diagnosed placenta accreta.
- Consideration should be given to preoperative insertion of bilateral internal iliac balloons under radiological control. If uncontrolled bleeding occurred, the balloons could be inflated to occlude the uterine blood supply.
- This has been successfully achieved in many units in the UK and usually necessitates the CS being conducted within the radiology department, which requires advanced planning.
- Uterine embolization may be performed in the emergency situation, provided the mother is cardiovascularly stable for transfer.

Complications

- Continued observation throughout the postnatal period is vital as haemorrhage may be delayed.
- Any ongoing coagulopathy should be corrected.
- Damage to the bladder, ureters and other surrounding structures may result from surgery.

Further reading

O'Rourke *et al.* Cesarean delivery in the interventional radiology suite: a novel approach to obstetric hemostasis. *Anesthesia and Analgesia* 2007; **104**: 1193–1194.

Harnett MJ *et al.* Anesthesia for interventional radiology in parturients at risk of major hemorrhage at cesarean section delivery. *Anesthesia and Analgesia* 2006; **103**: 1329–1330.

Controlled rupture of membranes

Definition

Artificial rupture of membranes (ARM) is a method commonly employed to induce labour, provided the cervix is favourable. A controlled ARM is required when the fetal head is high and not fully engaged in the pelvis. The main danger during a controlled ARM is the cord prolapsing into the birth canal in front of the presenting part and causing severe fetal distress.

Key issues

- Due to the high risk of cord prolapse, a controlled ARM should be performed in the obstetric theatre with facilities and staff fully prepared to proceed to a category 1 CS if necessary.
- Mothers suitable for controlled ARM include those with abnormal lie following stabilization of the fetal head position, polyhydramnios or multiparous women.

Management

- There are a number of possible management options for this procedure and these will ultimately depend on applying a risk–benefit analysis for each individual situation.
- Discussion with the obstetrician regarding the risks of immediate delivery is essential.
- A full explanation of the regional technique, including the possible complications, should be given to the mother and documented.
- An assessment for GA should be made.

Combined spinal–epidural anaesthesia

- A CSE technique will cover all eventual obstetric possibilities.
- The spinal component should be an intrathecal dose sufficient to allow an immediate CS to be performed, e.g. 12.5mg 0.5% heavy bupivacaine + 20 micrograms fentanyl.
- The epidural component can be used for labour analgesia if no complications occur at the time of the ARM.
- In addition, a long-acting opioid can be administered into the epidural space for postoperative analgesia if a CS is required.

Spinal anaesthesia

- Insertion of a single-shot spinal with a sufficient intrathecal dose for CS would cover the immediate concerns of a cord prolapse at the time of ARM.
- If the ARM is uneventful, labour analgesia can be offered, depending on what the mother requests when labour is established,
- This option for regional anaesthesia should be taken if the mother presents any risks for a possible CS under GA, e.g. difficult airway, obesity, malignant hyperpyrexia.

Anaesthetist 'on-standby'

- Instead of choosing to administer a regional technique, which may not be ultimately used, the anaesthetist can be 'on standby' in the operating theatre.
- Some mothers may not want a regional technique.
- If an immediate CS is required due to a prolapsed cord, a GA would be required for delivery.
- This option is not be recommended in a mother with significant risks of GA, e.g. the obese patient or an anticipated difficult airway.

Complications

- The major risk of this procedure is cord prolapse, precipitating immediate caesarean delivery by GA, if a regional technique has not been administered.

Fetal distress

Definition

- The most important thing to appreciate when dealing with cases of 'fetal distress' is that the term covers a wide range of degrees of risk to the fetus.
- The diagnosis may be made on a variety of criteria, either antenatally or intrapartum, and encountered in numerous different modes of fetal assessment, e.g. CTG, fetal blood sampling, fetal ECG ST analysis (STAN).
- The diagnosis of intrapartum fetal distress usually indicates that the obstetrician considers that the fetus needs early or immediate delivery, and the timing of delivery is graded according to the following categories for CS:
  - Category 1: threat to life of mother or baby that requires immediate delivery.
  - Category 2: compromise to mother or baby that requires early delivery.
  - Category 3: early delivery where neither the baby nor mother is compromised.
  - Category 4: elective CS.
- However, there are very few precise methods of diagnosing fetal distress which strongly correlate with measures of poor fetal outcome, either biochemical or clinical.

Key issues

- Effective team-work and communication is essential. Discuss the patient with the obstetrician, midwives and obstetric theatre team.
- Ascertain the degree of urgency immediately and ask for a review if you feel the situation has changed.
- The mother is your first priority and, as her anaesthetist, her safety is your prime concern. In difficult situations, everyone else will be focused on the baby and you may be the sole voice for the mother. Don't be afraid to speak up for her.
- During transfer to theatre, every effort should be made to improve the fetal condition and provide 'intrauterine resuscitation', which includes:
  - Position the mother in full left lateral to reduce aorto-caval compression.
  - Administer oxygen by face mask.
  - Treat hypotension with increments of vasopressor, e.g. IV ephedrine or phenylephrine.
  - Stop oxytocic drug infusions.
  - Consider tocolytic drugs, e.g. IV terbutaline 100–250 micrograms, IV GTN 50 micrograms or sublingual GTN 200–400 micrograms.
- Always reassess the situation with the obstetrician after transfer to theatre. Reapply the CTG monitor—if the fetal heart is more reassuring, the options for the anaesthetic technique for delivery should be discussed again.

Management of delivery

- The management of 'fetal distress' depends on the stage of labour and the degree of concern. It is essential to establish immediately with the obstetrician the required 'decision to delivery' time.
- A neonatologist should be contacted as soon as the diagnosis of fetal distress is made to attend the delivery and provide emergency resuscitation of the newborn.

First stage of labour

- 'Fetal distress' during first stage almost always necessitates delivery by emergency CS.
- GA is usually required for a category 1 section when the mother's life is in danger or the 'decision to delivery' time is <15min. In extreme urgency, most anaesthetists would accept that they could achieve anaesthesia more rapidly and reliably with GA.
- There is an increasing trend to perform a 'rapid sequence spinal' for category 1 sections, where the mother's life is not in danger, although the fetus may be significantly distressed. An experienced anaesthetist may decide to have ONE attempt inserting a spinal, whilst the woman is being preoxygenated via a tight-fitting mask and the fetus monitored continuously. If the attempt is successful, the CS may proceed; however, there should be a low threshold for stopping and no time is lost before converting to a GA. There must be no compromise in standards of monitoring or sterile technique.
- The degree of urgency following the decision for CS can change in either direction, therefore it is vital that the fetal heart is monitored continuously. In some cases, a category 1 CS is rapidly moved to theatre assuming that a GA is necessary, but as the fetal condition stabilizes, perhaps as a result of intrauterine resuscitation, it becomes apparent that there is sufficient time to perform a regional technique or no CS is necessary at all.
- Alternatively, the initial assessment may indicate sufficient time for a regional technique; however, during transfer, deterioration in the fetal condition necessitates a change of plan to a GA.

> In every situation, prompt and effective communication between anaesthetists, midwives and obstetricians is vital.
>
> It is important for all professionals involved to know their own roles clearly and understand the factors affecting the decision-making of other disciplines.

Further information on the details of each technique is provided in Chapters 10 and 11.

Second stage of labour

- Fetal distress in the second stage occurs quite frequently when the vertex is visible. This is often successfully managed with experienced midwifery care. The mother should be encouraged to push as effectively as possible to ensure rapid delivery.

- If fetal distress occurs in the second stage of labour, when the presenting part is below the ischial spines, an emergency assisted ventouse or outlet forceps delivery in the delivery room may be appropriate. This may be performed under a pudendal nerve block—10mL of 1% lidocaine is injected just below and medial to the ischial spines bilaterally, and it should be supplemented with perineal infiltration for the episiotomy.
- If the obstetrician considers a 'trial of instrumental delivery' to be appropriate, the woman should be transferred rapidly to the obstetric theatre with continuous fetal monitoring in place. This usually occurs when the fetal head is still in the mid-cavity of the pelvis or malpresented. Stay with the mother and, if a good working epidural is *in situ*, start topping up the epidural block immediately.
- If the decision to delivery time is <15min, the most appropriate decision is an emergency CS. It is essential that the degree of urgency for CS is discussed before deciding on a particular anaesthetic technique. Again, stay with the mother and, if a good working epidural is *in situ*, start topping up the epidural block immediately.

Further information on the anaesthetic technique is detailed in Chapters 10 and 11.

Recognition of the 'at risk' fetus

- Regular communication with the midwives and obstetricians while working on the delivery suite is of paramount importance to enable you to spot the 'at risk' fetus and form an early management plan of 'what to do if…' in your mind.
- It is good practice to attend all staff handover rounds and have regular updates on new admissions and each woman's progress in labour.

***At risk labours include*:**

Maternal factors

- Slow labour, induced or augmented with syntocinon.
- Induction for >2 weeks postdates.
- Pre-eclampsia.

Fetal factors

- IUGR ('small for dates').
- Meconium staining of liquor.
- Poor biophysical profile.
- Fetal Doppler studies showing absent or reversed end-diastolic flow in the umbilical arteries.
- Fetal abnormalities.
- Twins.

Identification of any of these conditions in early labour allows time for an early epidural block to be established in the usual way, which could then be topped-up for all but the most immediate of CS.

Further reading

Lucas D *et al.* Urgency of caesarean section: a new classification. *Journal of the Royal Society of Medicine* 2000; **93**: 346–350.

Cord prolapse

Definition

Cord prolapse occurs when the umbilical cord lies in front of or beside the presenting part, in the presence of ruptured membranes. The incidence of cord prolapse is 0.2–0.4% with a cephalic presentation; however, this increases to 2–4% with multiple pregnancies and malpresentations.

Key issues

- Cord prolapse is an obstetric emergency, as compression of the umbilical cord will severely compromise the fetal blood supply and precipitate immediate fetal distress.
- Delivery by category 1 CS must be performed extremely quickly, i.e. within minutes, to ensure no hypoxic damage to the fetus.
- Predisposing factors include:
  - High/ill-fitting presenting part.
  - High parity.
  - Prematurity.
  - Multiple pregnancy.
  - Polyhydramnios.
  - High head at the time of either spontaneous or artificial membrane rupture.

Management

- Although speed is essential, the situation should not prevent a rapid preoperative assessment prior to CS.
- Reassurance and an explanation of the problem must be given to the mother and partner.
- Antacid prophylaxis—IV ranitidine 50mg and 30mL 0.3M sodium citrate, should be given.
- Oxygen 15L/min should be administered via a tight-fitting face mask.
- There are two possible positions suggested for transfer to theatre:
  - Knee–chest.
  - Exaggerated Simm's—left lateral.
- In addition, the presenting part must be pushed out of the pelvis with manual upward pressure by the obstetrician or midwife. This must continue until surgery is commenced.
- Alternatively, the presenting part can be pushed out of the pelvis by filling the bladder with 400–700mL of saline via a catheter, which often also inhibits uterine contractions.
- If time allows, tocolytic drugs are used to stop labour, as uterine contractions make it difficult to prevent excessive cord pressure, e.g. IV salbutamol or terbutaline 100–250 micrograms, or IV GTN 50–100 micrograms.
- If fetal blood supply remains compromised, GA is the only option and a standard technique is applied with the usual safety precautions.
- The drugs required for a GA should always be prepared in advance and refrigerated, in the event of a category 1 CS for cord prolapse.

- Regional anaesthesia may be considered by an experienced anaesthetist only if the cord is free from compression and there is no evidence of fetal compromise, which is more likely with bladder filling.
- Standard spinal anaesthesia in the lateral position is the regional technique of choice.
- Topping-up an *in situ* epidural should only be used if it is working well and the anaesthetist is very confident that anaesthesia will be satisfactory.
- There is no place for siting an epidural *de novo*.
- Simulated drills of cord prolapse involving the delivery suite and theatre teams should be performed regularly, and any weak points from the drills addressed.

Placental abruption

Definition

Placental abruption is defined as premature separation of a normally implanted placenta. There may be a complete or partial separation and it occurs in ~1% of pregnancies.

Key issues

- There are many associated risk factors:
  - Pre-eclampsia, eclampsia or chronic hypertension.
  - Premature rupture of membranes.
  - Increased uterine size, e.g. multiple pregnancy, polyhydramnios.
  - Increasing parity.
  - Previous history of abruption.
  - Amniocentesis.
- Classical signs include: abdominal pain, haemorrhage, uterine tenderness or irritability, coagulopathy or fetal distress or demise.
- The presence of abdominal pain often differentiates an abruption from bleeding secondary to a placenta praevia.
- It may present with either profound revealed or concealed bleeding, requiring rapid resuscitation of the mother. Blood loss with a concealed retroplacental haemtoma is frequently underestimated.
- Close observation of the mother is required as cardiovascular stability is often maintained until >40% of circulating blood volume is lost.
- Clotting abnormalities occur early following an abruption with very low platelet numbers and fibrinogen <1g/L. Urgent correction of a coagulopathy is necessary to minimize further maternal bleeding.
- Stabilization of the mother and immediate delivery can be life saving for the mother and fetus.
- The perinatal mortality rate following a major placental abruption is as high as 50%.

Management

- Establish IV access with two large-bore cannulae and commence fluid resuscitation, administer oxygen by face mask and send blood for urgent FBC, clotting studies and cross-match 4–6 units of blood, depending on the degree of concern.
- Early administration of platelets and clotting products can be life saving to the mother.
- Rapid assessment of the cardiovascular status of the mother and viability and gestational age of the fetus is important, as this will determine the ultimate obstetric management of delivery.

Viable fetus

- If bleeding is minimal or has stopped, the mother is haemodynamically stable and the fetus not compromised, it may be appropriate to adopt a watch and wait policy, particularly if the gestational age is <34 weeks. The mother should be given β-methasone to aid fetal lung maturity. The mother should stay on the delivery suite for close maternal and fetal monitoring, and the decision for delivery reviewed regularly.
- If bleeding continues and/or the fetus demonstrates signs of distress, immediate delivery by CS is indicated.
- CS should **not** be delayed until blood results, cross-matched blood or blood products are available, if the mother or fetus remain compromised in any way.

Choice of anaesthetic technique

- GA is the technique of choice for the mother who is cardiovascularly compromised, or coagulopathy is present.
  - Resuscitation of the mother will be optimized by the use of rapid infusion devices with the facility to warm all infusion fluids.
  - Invasive BP and CVP monitoring should be instituted if the mother remains cardiovascularly unstable or if there is evidence of co-existing pre-eclampsia.
  - Regular checks on platelet count and clotting studies should be performed.
- Regional anaesthesia is not contraindicated provided the mother is normovolaemic and there is no evidence of clotting abnormalities.
  - A single-shot spinal technique would be appropriate.
  - If an abruption becomes apparent during labour and the mother has a working epidural *in situ*, it may be safely 'topped-up' for the CS.
- Despite the urgency of the situation, it is important to complete a rapid preoperative anaesthetic assessment and not forget to administer antacid prophylaxis.

Dead fetus

- If the placental separation has caused intrauterine death, vaginal delivery is the preferred mode, provided there is no ongoing catastrophic maternal haemorrhage.
- The uterus frequently becomes irritable, and precipitous delivery is characteristic.
- Following resuscitation, any coagulopathy should be corrected and platelet and clotting studies re-checked regularly.
- Epidural analgesia is not contraindicated for labour, provided the clotting results are entirely normal and platelet count >100.

Complications

- Always exclude co-existing pre-eclampsia when faced with a placental abruption. Effective fluid management can be difficult and the mother can rapidly develop pulmonary oedema.

- The risk of uterine atony following delivery is increased, particularly if blood has extravasated into the uterine musculature (Couvelaire uterus). At CS, all blood clots should be fully evacuated from the uterus and the uterus massaged to aid contraction. Additional oxytocics may be required to maintain uterine contraction, e.g. IV/IM ergometrine, IV oxytocin infusion or misoprostol PR.
- DIC complicates ~10% of all abruptions but is more common if fetal death has occurred. DIC causes consumption of factors I, II, V and VIII and platelets. DIC is reversed by transfusion of FFP, cryoprecipitate, fibrinogen concentrate and platelets, under the guidance of the haematologist.
- Acute renal failure may result if DIC or hypovolaemia remains uncorrected.

Instrumental vaginal delivery

Definition

An instrumental delivery facilitates successful vaginal delivery and may be performed with either a suction device (ventouse) or forceps. The type of forceps can be further subdivided into outlet (Wrigleys), non-rotational (Neville–Barnes) or rotational (Keillands) forceps.

Key issues

- The reason for instrumental delivery should be clarified with the obstetrician at the time the decision is made, together with an assessment of the likelihood of success.
- Reasons include:
  - Failure to progress in the second stage of labour (usually >2h).
  - Maternal exhaustion.
  - Presence of significant cardiac disease.
  - Fetal distress.
- These factors guide any decisions about the most appropriate place to conduct the delivery, i.e. the delivery room or theatre, and the type of anaesthetic that will be required.
- If there is any doubt regarding the estimation of success of an instrumental delivery, the mother should be transferred to theatre for the procedure.
- Anything other than a simple 'lift-out' technique will require the mother to be prepared to proceed for emergency CS if the instrumental delivery is unsuccessful.

Management

Simple 'lift-out'

- This may be appropriate if the fetal head is very low and there is a very high likelihood of successful vaginal delivery.
- Perineal anaesthesia, S2–S5, is essential for any assisted vaginal delivery.
- In patients without a working epidural, the obstetrician may choose to perform a pudendal nerve block, for a simple 'lift-out' procedure with either a ventouse or outlet forceps in the delivery room. Further local anaesthetic should be infiltrated for the episiotomy.
- If the patient has a working epidural *in situ*, a light 'top-up' of ~10mL of 0.25% bupivacaine or levobupivacaine can be given, preferably with the mother in a sitting position to ensure a dense sacral block.
- Care should be taken to ensure that all appropriate monitoring and emergency drugs are readily available, whenever an epidural is 'topped-up' in the delivery room.

Trial of instrumental delivery

- If the obstetrician considers a 'trial of instrumental delivery' to be appropriate, the woman should be transferred to the obstetric theatre. This usually occurs when the fetal head is still in the mid-cavity of the pelvis or malpresented. If there is no fetal compromise, transfer the

mother before topping-up an epidural. If there is fetal compromise, stay with the mother and, if a good working epidural is *in situ*, start topping-up the epidural block immediately.
- A 'trial of instrumental delivery' should always be performed in the operating theatre with the equipment and staff to proceed to immediate CS.
- A GA is not usually indicated for a vaginal delivery, as the mother cannot bear down and it is likely to fail.

Prior to transfer to theatre
- A thorough preoperative assessment should be completed, followed by an explanation of the anaesthetic technique and delivery plan, including the possibility and consequences of proceeding to CS.
- FBC and a request for blood group and save should be sent to the laboratory immediately. However, it is often necessary to proceed to theatre before the results are available.
- Make it your responsibility to ensure prompt transfer to a well-prepared theatre.
- Assess the sensory and motor block if an epidural is *in situ*, review the timing of last top-up and consider commencing a further epidural top-up if it has worked well for labour analgesia.
- Stay with the mother and ensure regular BP measurements are performed and hypotension promptly treated.
- Review need for further antacid prophylaxis.

Anaesthetic techniques
- A dense sensory sacral block extending to T10 will be required for the instrumental delivery, with the facility to extend the sensory block rapidly to light touch to T5 if the instrumental delivery fails.
- When deciding on the anaesthetic technique, a balance must be struck between ensuring the woman is able to push as effectively as possible and providing the ideal conditions for rapid conversion to a CS.
- The anaesthetic technique will depend on whether an epidural has been sited for labour analgesia and its efficacy. If no epidural is in place, the decision between a single-shot spinal and a CSE technique is often determined by the time available.

Epidural top-up
- If an epidural is *in situ*, review how it has performed in labour and the timing of the last top-up, and assess the sensory block prior to commencing with further incremental top-ups.
- If there is a high likelihood of successful vaginal delivery and the epidural has been functioning well, 10mL of 0.5% bupivacaine or levobupivacaine + 50–100 micrograms fentanyl should be given and the block re-assessed. Anaesthetists sometimes favour lidocaine or the addition of adrenaline and bicarbonate, believing it to be faster acting.
- Ensure evidence of sacral anaesthesia prior to starting the instrumental extraction.
- Incremental epidural top-ups in this way will still allow effective maternal effort for pushing, without causing intercostal motor block.

- If attempted instrumental delivery is unsuccessful, a further 10–15mL of 0.5% bupivacaine or levobupivacaine +/– 50–100 micrograms of fentanyl should be given and the sensory and motor block re-assessed for CS.
- Epidural diamorphine or morphine may be administered for postoperative analgesia if a CS becomes necessary.

Spinal anaesthesia

- If a spinal is inserted, the dose MUST be sufficient for delivery to proceed to a CS.
- The woman's ability to push will be reduced by intercostal motor blockade.
- The addition of a long-acting opioid, e.g. intrathecal morphine, may prove to be unnecessary if the trial is successful, but postdelivery monitoring for late respiratory depression must be the same as after a caesarean delivery.
- Alternatively, the decision to omit a long-acting opioid from the intrathecal mixture will increase postoperative pain scores if a CS is necessary, and parenteral opioids will be required.

Combined spinal–epidural

- This is the gold standard technique if a *de novo* regional technique is required.
- A low dose spinal technique, e.g. 5mg bupivacaine and 10–20 micrograms fentanyl, will facilitate a pain-free instrumental delivery. However, if vaginal delivery is unsuccessful, the epidural may be topped-up incrementally with 5–10mL aliquots of 0.5% bupivacaine or levobupivacaine until an adequate sensory block for CS is achieved.

It is essential that the anaesthetist fully understands all obstetric possibilities when proceeding with a trial of instrumental delivery. Failure of instrumental delivery may necessitate an immediate and often very difficult CS; the lower the fetal head, the more difficult the CS will be. Inadequate regional anaesthesia will require conversion to GA.

Complications

- Following a prolonged labour, difficult or failed instrumental vaginal delivery, the mother is at risk of major PPH either due to uterine atony or following trauma of the structures within the birth canal.
- An infusion of oxytocin should be continued following delivery, with close observation of the mother in the immediate postpartum period for bleeding.
- Bleeding is often underestimated, particularly if a prolonged repair of the perineum is required or the instrumental delivery fails. Weigh all swabs to assess blood loss accurately or observe for continued bleeding from the vagina during surgery.
- A difficult instrumental delivery will be painful in the postnatal period. Ensure adequate analgesia is prescribed regularly, with a laxative to prevent constipation.

Uterine inversion

Definition

Puerperal uterine inversion is the displacement of the fundus of the uterus, usually occurring during the third stage of labour, and is a serious but infrequent complication of childbirth. Although rare, it can be a life-threatening emergency due to associated blood loss and cardiovascular instability.

Key issues

- The reported incidence of uterine inversion varies considerably in the literature and is quoted to be between 1 in 2000 and 1 in 40 000 births.
- It may be classified as:
  - Complete—the fundus passes through the cervix.
  - Incomplete—the fundus remains above the cervix.
- The contributing causal factors include:
  - Fundal implantation of the placenta.
  - Excessive cord traction or pulling on the placenta prior to the beginning of placental separation.
  - Poor uterine tone.
  - Abnormal adherence of the placenta.
  - Coughing or vomiting during third stage.
- The classical presentation of uterine inversion is an obviously displaced uterus during placental delivery, which is commonly associated with PPH, severe pain and clinical shock that appears out of proportion to the blood loss.
- Shock is thought to be due, in part, to the parasympathetic response to traction on the uterine suspensory ligaments, and may be associated with profound bradycardia.
- This is an obstetric emergency and there should be no delay in instituting treatment.

Management

- Treatment of haemorrhagic shock, i.e. high flow oxygen, aggressive IV fluid resuscitation, atropine to treat any bradycardia and replacement of the uterus must occur simultaneously.
- Any delay in replacement of the uterus will increase uterine oedema, impeding later replacement, and may exacerbate cardiovascular instability.
- Immediate GA is usually required to facilitate uterine replacement unless a recently topped-up epidural is already *in situ*.

Replacement of uterus

This may be achieved by:

- Manual replacement—the uterus is pushed back through the cervix to its normal position.

- Hydrostatic correction—the woman is placed in a steep Trendelenberg position, warm normal saline is delivered to the posterior fornix of the vagina which causes gradual stretching of the orifice, aiding correction of the inversion.
- If unsuccessful, tocolytic drugs can be given to increase cervical relaxation:
  - β_2 receptor agonists—salbutamol 250 micrograms IV bolus.
  - Magnesium sulphate—4g IV over 10min.
  - GTN—50–100 micrograms IV bolus.
- The halogenated vapour of GA agents will cause uterine and cervical relaxation.
- Severe cases may require laparotomy and combined abdominal–vaginal correction.

Complications

- Severe PPH is the most frequent consequence of uterine inversion.

Intrauterine fetal surgery

Definition

Surgery on the fetus while still *in utero* is a rapidly growing and evolving area of medicine. Advances in high-resolution ultrasound scanning allow accurate and relatively early diagnosis of many congenital malformations. An increasing number are amenable to intrauterine fetal surgery, which successfully modify or optimize the outcome at delivery. It is predicted that the treatment of congenital malformations *in utero*, prior to development of secondary morbidity, will become routine in the future.

Key issues

- Surgery is considered appropriate only when the risk of death or severe injury to the fetus is greater than with no intervention, and the risk to the mother is low.
- Intrauterine surgery has been successfully completed for many complex congenital heart disorders, e.g. transposition of the great vessels, upper airway problems, congenital diaphragmatic herniae and renal disorders.
- Fetal anomalies resulting in hydrops fetalis and an almost certain fetal demise are also considered for surgical intervention.
- Contraindications include lethal or disabling genetic disease in the fetus and serious medical disease in the mother.
- Many of the anaesthetic considerations for fetal procedures and surgery are the same as those for non-obstetric surgery during pregnancy, including avoidance of teratogenic drugs, concern for maternal safety and prevention of preterm labour and delivery.
- Fetal surgery involves either an open procedure requiring a maternal hysterotomy, or a minimally invasive fetal procedure involving a fetoscope and ultrasound.
- GA or regional anaesthesia, usually a CSE technique, is administered to the mother for intrauterine fetal surgery to be performed.
- Anaesthesia and relaxation of the fetus is given by the operating surgeon by the instillation of a benzodiazepine and opioid mixture with a muscle relaxant either IM to the fetus or via the umbilical vessels.

Complications

- The main complications of intrauterine surgery are preterm labour, premature rupture of membranes and chorioamnionitis, which may have significant consequences for both the mother and fetus.

Further reading

Myer LB *et al.* Anaesthesia for fetal sugery. *Paediatric Anaesthesia* 2002; **12**: 569–578.

EXIT procedures

Definition

Ex utero intrapartum treatment (EXIT) procedures offer the advantage of performing life-saving upper airway surgery on a newborn baby at the time of CS, before the umbilical cord is severed and therefore maintaining uteroplacental gas exchange until an airway can be secured.

Key issues

- The range of indications for EXIT procedures include:
  - Congenital high airway obstruction syndrome.
  - Reversal of tracheal balloon occlusion when managing severe congenital diaphragmatic hernia.
  - Giant fetal neck masses.
  - Lung or mediastinal tumours.
  - Transfer from EXIT to ECMO (extracorporeal membrane oxygenation).
- The advantage of EXIT procedures is that they allow for intubation and ventilation at birth.
- If intubation is not possible, fetal tracheostomy can be performed, or any lung or neck masses causing anatomical distortion can be resected on placental support.
- The mother usually requires GA for the CS, with increased volatile concentration (2–3 MAC) to facilitate prolonged uterine relaxation.
- Uterine relaxation and placental circulation have been maintained for as long as 2–3h to enable secure airway management prior to delivery of the fetus.

Management

- The key aims of management are:
  - Partial delivery of the fetus.
  - Prolonged uterine relaxation.
  - Preservation of the uteroplacental circulation.
  - Delayed uteroplacental separation.

Procedure

- Preoperative indomethacin 50mg rectally is given prophylactically as a tocolytic, and routine antacid prophylaxis.
- A lumbar epidural catheter may be sited for intraoperative and postoperative pain relief.
- Rapid sequence induction of anaesthesia is performed, with left lateral tilt.
- High doses (2–3 MAC) of inhalational agents are used to maintain uterine relaxation.
- IV GTN or terbutaline may also be administered to reduce uterine tone.
- Maternal BP must be maintained in order to continue perfusion through the placenta.

- Administration of agents causing smooth muscle relaxation is balanced against vasopressors and fluid administration as necessary.
- Using ultrasound, the placental edges are mapped and the hysterotomy performed avoiding the placenta.
- The fetal head is exposed and intubation can be attempted.
- The indication for the EXIT procedure will determine the fetal exposure necessary; this should be kept to a minimum in order to reduce heat loss and the risk of umbilical cord compromise or premature placental detachment.

The key to successful outcome of EXIT procedures is the co-ordination of multiple personnel from various disciplines including anaesthesia, paediatric surgery, obstetrics, radiology, neonatology and midwifery.

Further reading

Dahlgren G *et al.* Four cases of the ex-utero intrapartum treatment (EXIT) procedure: anaesthetic implications. *International Journal of Obstetrics and Anesthesia* 2004; **13**: 178–182.

Retained placenta

Definition

The third stage of labour involves the separation, descent and delivery of the placenta. The retroplacental myometrium must contract, allowing the placenta to come away from its bed and be expelled. The placenta is considered retained if it fails to deliver within 60min of birth.

Key issues

- Retained placenta is a common cause of PPH with an incidence of ~2% worldwide, and is a significant cause of maternal morbidity and mortality.
- The reasons may be broadly divided into:
  - Failed separation due to poor or absent uterine contraction.
  - Failed separation due to morbid adherence, e.g. to a fibroid, uterine scar or in the presence of placenta accreta.
  - Successful separation but retained by a contracted uterus and closed cervical os.
- Risk factors for a retained placenta include:
  - Previous retained placenta.
  - Previous injury to or scarring of uterus.
  - Preterm delivery.
  - Induced labour.
  - Multiparity.

Management

Early management

- Initial management may be conservative, e.g. bladder emptying and waiting for signs of spontaneous separation and delivery of the placenta.
- Early initiation of breastfeeding may assist placental separation.
- Active management of the third stage involves use of IM oxytocin and ergometrine mixture (syntometrine) or oxytocin alone, with controlled cord traction after uterine contraction.
- A second dose of syntometrine should be given, followed by a oxytocin infusion at 10IU/h to aid separation.
- Blood loss may be concealed, and close observation for maternal pallor, tachycardia and hypotension must be maintained:
  - Establish IV access with a large-bore cannula.
  - Estimate amount and rate of blood loss and cardiovascular stability.
  - Check FBC ± clotting studies, and send sample for group and save or cross-match depending on blood loss.
- Alternative non-surgical therapies include umbilical venous injection of saline, plasma expanders or prostaglandins.
- If the placenta has not been expelled after 1h of oxytocin infusion or there is significant bleeding ± haemodynamic instability, the placenta must be removed manually.

Manual removal of placenta

- Manual removal of placenta should be performed in the theatre environment, preferably under regional anaesthesia, provided no contraindications exist, e.g. uncorrected hypovolaemia, coagulopathy.
- A sensory (temperature) block to T6 is required for pain-free manual removal of placenta as the uterine fundus is often manipulated.
- Always assess the sacral component of the block before surgery starts.
- Regional anaesthesia may be established by:

Epidural top-up

- 15–20mL 0.5% bupivacaine ± short-acting opioid should be administered if there is an indwelling epidural catheter.
- Short-acting opioids are beneficial to supplement the LA block during difficult removal.
- Continuous monitoring of ECG and pulse oximetry, and intermittent BP should be performed.

Spinal anaesthesia

- 2.0–2.5mL heavy 0.5% bupivacaine ± short-acting opioid should be injected into the intrathecal space.
- Short-acting opioids are beneficial to supplement the LA block during difficult removal.
- Site the spinal with the mother in the lateral position if she is uncomfortable.
- The postpartum uterus does not augment the extent of cephalad spread of LA to the same degree as the pregnant uterus, therefore a full CS dose of intrathecal LA should be used.

General anaesthesia

- GA may be required for the haemodynamically unstable mother or if a coagulopathy prevents a regional technique.
- Antacid prophylaxis should be given and a standard rapid sequence induction performed.
- The halogenated volatile agents will assist placenta removal by providing greater uterine relaxation; however, they may precipitate increased postpartum bleeding.

Additional uterine relaxants

- GTN.
  - During regional anaesthesia, aliquots of GTN are effective, i.e. sublingual spray or 50–100 micrograms IV as required.
  - Either route of administration may cause hypotension.
- β-sympathomimetics, e.g. salbutamol or terbutaline, will assist uterine relaxation.

On placental delivery, administer 5IU syntocinon IV bolus (caution if patient is hypotensive) and commence an infusion of 40IU syntocinon in 500mL normal saline over 4h.

Complications

Potential complications include:

- Primary PPH.
- Secondary (delayed) PPH, due to retained placental fragments.
- 'Cervical shock—profound bradycardia and hypotension, precipitated by increased vagal tone, when the placenta sits in the open cervix .
- Uterine inversion.
- Postpartum sepsis. Prophylactic antibiotics are usually administered.

Suturing the perineum

Definition

Perineal trauma may occur spontaneously during vaginal birth or by surgical incision, i.e. episiotomy, where an incision is intentionally made to increase the diameter of the vulval outlet to facilitate delivery.

- Episiotomy rates vary considerably according to individual practices and policies of staff and institutions.
- In the UK, an estimated 85% of women having a vaginal birth will sustain some degree of perineal trauma and, of these, 60–70% will require suturing.

Clinical classification of spontaneous tears

- 1st degree—injury to the skin only.
- 2nd degree—injury to the perineum involving perineal muscles but not the anal sphincter.
- 3rd degree—injury to perineum involving the anal sphincter.
- 4th degree—injury to the perineum involving the anal sphincter and anal epithelium.

Key issues

- There are a number of recognized risk factors for perineal trauma:
  - Primiparity.
  - Fetal birth weight >4000g.
  - Prolonged second stage of labour.
  - Instrumental delivery.
  - Direct occipito-posterior position.
  - Maternal factors: age, nutritional status.
- Perineal trauma can be associated with significant postdelivery haemorrhage, which is often underestimated. Continuing vaginal bleeding should always be investigated. High vaginal or cervical lacerations may be missed and continuing bleeding falsely attributed to uterine atony.
- Perineal trauma causes significant pain and discomfort in the immediate postdelivery period and in the longer term.
- Examination and suturing should be performed as soon as possible to reduce bleeding, pain and the risk of infection

Management

- Assess the mother for signs of hypovolaemia, establish IV access, check FBC ± clotting studies and send blood for group and save or cross-match 2–4 units depending on estimated blood loss.
- Perineal trauma is conventionally repaired in three layers; deep and superficial perineal muscle layers, vaginal tissue and skin.

First- and second-degree tears

- Superficial suturing of the perineum is usually performed with local infiltration instilled by the obstetrician or midwife, or an epidural top-up should be given if an indwelling epidural catheter is present, e.g. 10mL 0.1–0.25% bupivacaine to establish a perineal block.

Third- and fourth-degree tears

- More extensive suturing of the perineum usually requires transfer to the operating theatre for further assessment, and both anaesthetic and surgical management.
- To facilitate adequate anaesthesia of the sacral dermatomes, the anaesthetic options for management are:

Epidural top-up

- 10mL 0.5% bupivacaine ± short-acting opioid may be administered via an indwelling epidural catheter, preferably with the mother sitting up or with 45° head-up tilt.
- Always assess the sacral component of the sensory block prior to allowing suturing to commence.

Spinal anaesthesia

- 1.5–2mL heavy 0.5% bupivacaine ± short-acting opioid should be injected into the intrathecal space.
- Site the spinal with the mother in the lateral position if she is uncomfortable, and sit her up or with 45° head-up tilt as soon as possible thereafter.
- The postpartum uterus does not augment the extent of cephalad spread of LA to the same degree as the pregnant uterus.

General anaesthesia

- GA may be necessary to achieve adequate muscle relaxation and visualization for surgical repair of severe or complex lacerations, or for delayed or revision of suturing.
- GA may be required for the haemodynamically unstable mother or if a coagulopathy prevents a regional technique.
- Antacid prophylaxis should be given and a rapid sequence induction performed on all mothers requiring GA within 24h of delivery.

Complications

- Perineal trauma can cause significant PPH. Check FBC following the repair.
- Significant pain and discomfort can follow perineal tears or an episiotomy. Prescribe balanced analgesia regularly for the postpartum period.
- Beware of opioid analgesia causing constipation and straining at defaecation. A regular laxative should be prescribed with all opioids.
- Urinary and faecal incontinence may be apparent in the early postpartum period.
- Urinary retention. A catheter is frequently left *in situ* for the first 24h. If this is not the case, then specific observations should be mandatory.

Chapter 14

Postpartum review and problems

Sarah Harries, Raman Sivasankar, Alun Rees and Dan Redfern

Postdelivery ward round and documentation

- Documentation of all anaesthetic procedures performed in the delivery suite and obstetric theatre should be completed both in the patient's medical notes and as a separate anaesthetic register of work. This may be kept in a paper-based or computer-based format.
- The surgical procedure, anaesthetic technique, obstetric indication and urgency, relevant medical history and any complications should all be documented.

The anaesthetic register is an essential tool in maintaining continuity of care and effective communication between the doctors at handover times and during postdelivery ward rounds.

The postdelivery ward round should be informal, respecting the mother's privacy, and happen at least once a day.

The following can be reviewed:

- Maternal satisfaction.
- Any difficulties during the anaesthetic procedure.
- Consequences of problems encountered, e.g. inadequate analgesia, dural tap, etc.
- Time interval between request and labour analgesia.
- Postdelivery analgesia.
- Fluid balance, blood transfusion and postdelivery haemoglobin.
- Mobilization.
- Pruritis.
- Micturition.
- Neurological recovery and deficits.
- Thromboprophylaxis.

The outcome of the postdelivery ward round and any action taken must be documented. The community midwife should be informed of ongoing problems (e.g. headache), with written information in the mother's handheld notes. More serious problems can in addition be communicated via the local community midwifery office.

- The ward round gives the anaesthetist an opportunity to continue care in the postdelivery phase and to address any concerns the mother may have.
- It is an excellent time for formal and informal feedback between a senior and trainee anaesthetist about techniques used.
- Information and feedback from the mother can be used as part of the anaesthetic trainee's appraisal.
- Documentation of appropriate levels of monitoring after operative delivery or administration of opioids can be checked.
- Adequacy of postdelivery analgesia, both caesarean and vaginal, can be verified.

Early identification of dissatisfaction

- It is an ideal time for a senior anaesthetist to identify and talk to the mother who has been less than satisfied with her anaesthetic care.
- Addressing issues at this early stage can avoid potential complaints or litigation later.
- The incidence of litigation is high in obstetric practice and is most frequently due to inadequate analgesia, but delay in providing analgesia is also a problem.
- Patients can expect an accurate and honest explanation of events, with an apology if there are shortcomings.
- All discussions with the mother should be formally documented.
- Some mothers may need more than one follow-up, and the anaesthetic register can be used to continue their follow-up care, e.g. persistent headache, neurological symptoms or signs.
- All documentation should be legible and complete, with a signature and surname in capitals.
- It is not uncommon for complaints to be received many months or years following the delivery, when reference to accurate documentation is essential.
- In addition, the anaesthetic register can also be used for purposes of clinical audit or as a reference guide for the anaesthetic management of rare medical disorders complicating pregnancy.
- The postdelivery ward round and accompanying documentation should form part of the anaesthetic care and be given the same importance as intrapartum care.

Maternal satisfaction

- Maternal satisfaction about the experience of childbirth is mentioned frequently, but poorly defined.
- Maternal satisfaction has many dimensions and is a complex, multifactorial psychological response to childbirth.
- Different methods have been used to quantify maternal satisfaction, e.g. postdelivery interviews, self-completed questionnaires with visual analogue scales, verbal numerical scales, and question and answers.
- COMFORTS (Care in Obstetrics Measure for Testing Satisfaction) has been used recently to measure satisfaction, but needs to be validated further.
- Studies of maternal satisfaction have traditionally assumed good analgesia as the most important factor, but this view has been dispelled in many surveys. In some surveys, the mothers with epidurals and the best analgesia were less satisfied, probably because of the complexity of their labour.

Factors that improve maternal satisfaction

- Support in labour.
- Listening to the woman's concern.
- Kindness and compassion of staff.
- Continuity of care.
- Antenatal class attendance.
- Vaginal delivery.
- Privacy.
- Requested and expected labour analgesia.

- Information and support are considered to be the most important factors for mothers.
- Labour analgesia is placed low on the indicators for maternal satisfaction.
- Excessive maternal education and expectation are also associated with less satisfaction.
- Women having a CS found the lack of control a less fulfilling experience.
- Maternal age, social class, income, marital status, support of the partner, planned vs unplanned pregnancy, previous terminations, depression and ethnicity are other factors which influence maternal satisfaction greatly.
- Epidural analgesia for labour has been the focus for anaesthetists with regards to maternal satisfaction.
- Low dose epidurals have improved the quality and safety of anaesthesia, and retaining motor power improves satisfaction.
- PCEA confers no advantage over an intermittent bolus regimen in relation to maternal satisfaction.
- During elective CS, lower preoperative anxiety is associated with greater maternal satisfaction and better recovery.
- Information provided by the anaesthetist and perceived emotional support is also of importance.

- It may be possible to identify women with high anxiety and facilitate satisfaction and recovery through additional support.
- The time of assessment of satisfaction is also very important as maternal satisfaction alters with time.
- The ideal time for satisfaction assessment is not known.
- Maternal satisfaction is multifactorial, therefore it is difficult to draw conclusions solely from anaesthetic studies as they usually concentrate on the dimension of pain relief.
- Effective pain relief may be the top priority for the anaesthetist, but not necessarily the priority of the mother.

Further reading

Janssen PA, Dennis CL, Reime B. Development of psychometric testing of the Care of Obstetrics Measure for Testing Satisfaction (COMFORTS) scale. *Research in Nursing and Health* 2006; **29**: 51–60.

Advice on drugs and breastfeeding

- The administration of drugs to breastfeeding mothers can cause harm to the nursing infant.
- Drugs can inhibit lactation or cause direct harmful effects to the infant due to excretion in breast milk.
- For many medications, there is insufficient evidence available to provide accurate guidance on drug safety during breastfeeding. Therefore, for this reason alone, manufacturers often advise avoiding medications that are probably quite safe.
- See p 152 for further information.

General principles for prescribing drugs to lactating women

- Is the medication really necessary?
- Choose the safest drug available.
- Minimize drug exposure by administering medications just after breastfeeding or before the infant is due to have a lengthy sleep period.
- Breastfeeding is the gold standard in infant nutrition. The risks of a potentially harmful drug being excreted in milk have to be balanced with the advantages of continued breastfeeding.

Analgesics

Considered to be safe

- Paracetamol.
- Diclofenac.
- Morphine (in therapeutic doses).
- Codeine.

Advised to avoid by manufacturers (however, safely used by many mothers)

- Tramadol.
- Ibuprofen.
- Sumatriptan (advised to withhold breastfeeding for 24h).

Avoid

- Aspirin should be avoided due to risk of Reye's syndrome. Regular use of high doses may impair platelet function. It is probably safe to give in low dose <100mg/day.

Local anaesthetics

- Bupivacaine and lidocaine—the amounts in breast milk are too small to be harmful.

Antiemetics

- Ondansetron—manufacturer advises avoid.
- Cyclizine—no information available.

- Metoclopramide—small amount in breast milk, manufacturers advise avoid.

Induction agents

- Propofol—amount present in milk probably too small to be harmful.
- Thiopental—no adverse effects reported.
- Etomidate—avoid breastfeeding for 24h after administration.

Neuromuscular-blocking drugs

Breastfeeding is unlikely to be harmful after maternal recovery from neuromuscular block.

- Suxamethonium—no information available.
- Atracurium—some manufacturers advise avoiding breastfeeding for 24h after administration.

Antibiotics

- Most antibiotics (including the penicillins, clavulanic acid, erythromycin and the cephalosporins) are considered to be safe.
- Metronidazole—significant amount in breast milk; manufacturers advise avoiding large single doses.
- Quinolones, e.g. ciprofloxacin, should be avoided as secreted in high concentrations in the breast milk.
- Clarithromycin—manufacturers advise avoid unless potential benefit outweighs risk.

Miscellaneous drugs

Avoid

- Amiodarone—present in significant amounts in breast milk and may cause neonatal hypothroidism.
- Ergotamine used for treatment of migraines—may cause vomiting, diarrhoea and convulsions.

Further reading

British National Formulary Appendix 5: Breastfeeding.

Backache in pregnancy

Simple backache assessment and advice

Background

- Back pain affects ~50% of women during pregnancy and 40% of women postpartum.
- One-third of pregnant women report that it is a severe problem, interfering with normal daily life and their ability to work.
- Back pain in pregnancy is usually most troublesome between week 12 and week 28.
- A multidisciplinary approach to management should be adopted.
- Advice and the treatment options provided by experienced obstetric physiotherapists are invaluable.

Postulated causes of back pain during pregnancy

- Rapid postural changes and altered biomechanics.
- Endocrine changes (relaxin) soften ligaments around the pelvis and increase joint laxity.
- Engorgement of epidural veins. There are case reports of distended epidural and paravertebral veins causing nerve root compression.
- Weight gain (conflicting evidence).

Risk factors

- Previous back pain (especially during pregnancy).
- Increasing parity.
- Physically strenuous and unrewarding employment.
- Repetitive lifting and bending.
- Young age.

Management of back pain

Prevention

- Maintaining a good level of fitness prior to pregnancy.
- Patient education early in pregnancy.
- Back care (correct posture, rolling and lifting techniques).
- Cessation of smoking is thought to reduce the severity of back pain and the risk of intervertebral disc prolapse.

Good back care

- **Lying**. Ensure comfortable sleeping and resting positions. May require extra pillows for support. Avoid positions of unsupported rotation.
- **Rolling techniques**. Roll with legs adducted and knees flexed. Turn head in direction of roll. Lead with top arm across chest and lay outside knee on inside leg (to facilitate rolling of the mid and lower trunk, respectively).
- **Sitting**. Maintain good posture. Buttocks well back on seat, thighs fully supported for most of their length and hips and knees at 90°. Feet supported flat on floor. Spine fully supported allowing natural curvature.
- **Standing**. Weight evenly distributed over both feet. Feet apart and slightly angled, knees off stretch. Avoid trunk on hip flexion and twisting movements (particularly when load bearing).

- **Lifting**. Avoid heavy lifting. Hold load close to the centre of mass. Bend at the knees.

Analgesia options
- See (Chapter 5, p 138).

Advice on long-term backache following epidurals
- It is very common to have localized tenderness and bruising at the site of epidural insertion, particularly if there were multiple attempts with the Tuohy needle.
- This will resolve spontaneously over a few days and is not a cause for concern.
- Simple analgesics such as paracetamol and NSAIDs should be prescribed in the postpartum period.
- Patients can be reassured that there is no association between epidural analgesia and long-term backache.
- Epidurals were implicated in the development of chronic backache in two retrospective studies in the early 1990s. These studies were criticised as the reported antenatal backache rates were much lower than expected.
- Multiple prospective studies have since failed to show an association between long-term backache and epidural analgesia.

Assessment of back pain
- If back pain presents during pregnancy or following delivery, a thorough history and neurological examination is essential before deciding whether further investigations or referral is appropriate.
- There are many causes of back pain that may be unrelated to pregnancy, delivery or anaesthetic procedure and which must not be missed.

'Red flags'—when to ask for help/further investigations
- Bladder or bowel dysfunction.
- Saddle anaesthesia.
- Progressive neurological deficit.
- Back pain associated with fever (especially in immunocompromised or diabetic patients).
- History of IV drug abuse.
- Suspected pyelonephritis.
- Suspected abscess/haematoma following epidural or spinal anaesthesia, usually indicated by severe deep-seated back pain (see p 416, 419).
- Recent significant trauma.
- Unexplained weight loss/systemic illness.
- Previous malignancy.

Investigations

- Plain radiographs are unlikely to be of diagnostic benefit in the investigation of lower back pain (with the exceptions of malignancy and trauma) and will expose antenatal mother and baby to ionizing radiation.
- If imaging is required the investigation of choice is MRI. If backache is associated with **ANY** neurological deficit, an urgent MRI should be requested.
- If there is a suggestion of an infective source, serial WCC, C-reactive protein and blood cultures should be taken.

Further reading

Russell R, Reynolds F. Back pain, pregnancy and childbirth. *British Medical Journal* 1997; **314**: 1062–1063.

Reynolds F. Epidurals and backache: again? *British Medical Journal* 2002; **325**: 1037.

Howell CJ *et al.* Randomised study of long term outcome after epidural versus non-epidural analgesia during labour. *British Medical Journal* 2002; **325**: 357–359.

Headache

Headache is a common complaint in the postpartum period and there are many causes. It resolves spontaneously in the majority of cases; however, there is potential for considerable morbidity.

Differential diagnosis

- PDPH is one of the most common causes of headache in the postpartum period.
- In women receiving epidural analgesia, the incidence of dural puncture ranges from 0 to 2.6% and is largely dependent on operator experience.
- 30% of dural punctures are not recognized at the time of epidural insertion and first present in the postpartum period with a classical postural headache.
- After a dural puncture with 16G Tuohy needle, up to 70% of women will report symptoms of PDPH.
- It is always important to consider other causes of headache to avoid serious morbidity.
- Surveys have reported that 39% of women suffer symptoms of headache unrelated to dural puncture following delivery.

Other causes of headache

- Non-specific (tension) headache frequently associated with fatigue.
- Pre-eclampsia (30% of eclampsia occurs in the postpartum period).
- Dehydration.
- Migraine.
- Sinus headache.
- Viral, bacterial or chemical meningitis.
- Intracranial haemorrhage.
- Cerebral venous thrombosis.
- Intracranial tumour.
- Cerebral infarction.
- Drugs.
- Benign intracranial hypertension.

Aetiology of PDPH

- Following a dural tap, there is a leak of CSF and a lowering of CSF pressure.
- There are two possible explanations for the headache:
    - The lowering of the CSF pressure causes traction on the pain-sensitive intracranial structures in the upright position and causes the classical postural headache.
    - Monro–Kellie hypothesis states that the sum of volumes of the brain, CSF and blood is constant. When the CSF volume decreases there is a compensatory increase in blood volume. The subsequent venodilatation stretches pain receptors in the vessel wall and causes the headache. There is radiological evidence for this and forms the basis for some of the therapeutic drug treatments.

Diagnosis of PDPH

Clinical

- Headache is the predominant complaint; it is usually distributed over the frontal and occipital areas, radiating to the neck and shoulders, sometimes associated with neck stiffness.
- It can start almost immediately and is usually present within 72h of dural puncture.
- Headaches in the temporal, vertex and nuchal areas are less commonly reported.
- The headache is exacerbated by an upright posture and relieved by lying down.
- Pressure over the upper abdomen can cause very temporary relief of PDPH and aid in diagnosis.
- Other associated symptoms are nausea, vomiting, hearing loss, tinnitus, vertigo, dizziness, paraesthesia of scalp, visual disturbances, light intolerance and cranial nerve palsies.
- Subdural haematoma, cerebral herniation and death have been reported as a consequence of dural puncture.
- If the headache is not posture related, a diagnosis of PDPH should be questioned and other serious intracranial causes of headache excluded.

Risk factors associated with PDPH

- Female.
- Young.
- Lesser BMI.
- History of chronic or recurrent headache.
- Previous PDPH.
- Large needle.
- Quincke (cutting tip) spinal needles.

Investigations

- When a clinical diagnosis of PDPH cannot be made with certainty, additional tests may be used.
- MRI may demonstrate diffuse dural enhancement, evidence of a sagging brain and enlargement of the pituitary gland.
- CT myelography or thin section MRI can be used to locate the CSF leak in severe persistent cases.

Management of PDPH

Prevention

The size of the dural perforation is the most important factor for the development of the headache.

- Needle size.
  - A fine gauge spinal needle, 29G, produces a small dural perforation with a lower incidence of headache and a higher failure rate.
  - A 25G probably represents the optimum balance between the risk of headache and technical failure.

- Needle orientation.
  - A needle orientated with the cutting tip parallel to the dural fibres may reduce the incidence of PDPH (relevant to Tuohy and Quincke needles only).
- Needle design.
  - Pencil point (atraumatic needles) needles produce fewer headaches than medium bevel cutting needles (Quincke). However, an increased incidence of paraesthesia has been observed with pencil point needles.
- Operator skill and fatigue.
  - An inexperienced operator and fatigue may increase the incidence of inadvertent dural puncture.

Treatment

After diagnosis of a PDPH is made, a rational approach to management must be adopted. The severity of the headache should be assessed and a full explanation of the problem given to the mother. The natural history of most PDPHs is that they will resolve with time, with anticipated improvement over 5–10 days. Some headaches if left untreated may become chronic. An epidural blood patch (EBP) is considered the optimal treatment for severe PDPH. However, other treatment options can be considered before an EBP is performed:

- Simple.
  - Rehydration.
  - Paracetamol, NSAIDs.
  - Opioids and antiemetics.
- Comfortable posture—supine posture is not mandatory.
- Caffeine.
  - Acts by vasoconstriction of the dilated cerebral vessels.
  - Dose: 300–500mg oral or IV.
  - One cup of coffee contains 50–100mg.
  - Therapeutic doses may cause atrial fibrillation or seizures.
- Sumatriptan, desmopressin.
  - Some small case series demonstrating benefit, but no strong evidence for use.
- Synthetic ACTH.
  - Was popular but recent evidence showed it to be ineffective.
- Psychological support. Reassure the mother that in most cases the headache is not harmful.

Epidural blood patch

The option of an EBP should be offered to women 24h after suspected dural puncture when other measures have failed. The benefits of delaying EPB for the first 24h are:

- Clarification of nature of headache.
- Observe for signs of maternal infection.
- Increased success rate after the first 24h. (A hypothesis for this is that local anaesthetic has a very small antiplatelet action and may inhibit clot formation over the dural hole).

Contraindications

- Patient refusal.
- Fever associated with a raised WCC.
- Coagulopathy.
- Infection on skin of lower back.
- HIV-positive patients with other active bacterial or viral illness (blood patch has been safely reported in HIV patients without active signs of other infection).

Technique

- Two operators, strict asepsis with hat, gloves, mask and gown for both.
- A clean spacious environment is required.
- The lateral position is usually recommended, but the procedure can be carried out in the sitting position if technical difficulties are encountered in the lateral position or the mother finds it more comfortable.
- The Tuohy needle should be inserted into the same intervertebral space as the dural puncture, or the one below. Look carefully for puncture marks on skin rather than estimate the intervertebral level.
- Blood should be drawn from the antecubital vein under strict asepsis and handed directly to the epidural operator.
- Inject up to 30mL of blood into the epidural space slowly over several minutes. Stop when the mother feels that further injection is painful. Pain can be felt as a deep-seated fullness in the back or as a radiculopathy-type pain in her legs. Less than 10mL of blood can cause these symptoms, and the ability to inject less blood is not associated with a greater failure rate.
- Send remaining blood for culture and sensitivity.
- Bed rest for 1h, then try to mobilize as usual.
- There have been occasional reports of haemodynamic disturbance with EBP.

Mechanism of action of blood patch

- Initially, there is compression of the dural sac and an increase in CSF pressure. A dramatic rapid improvement in symptoms is characteristically seen.
- Clot formation follows in minutes to hours. The failure of clot formation over the dural puncture is thought to be the mechanism of secondary failure when the headache returns over hours to days.
- By 7 days, there is fibroblastic activity and collagen formation.
- There is no evidence of axonal oedema, necrosis or demyelination.

Outcome

- There is a 70% complete and further 20–25% partial success rate if carried out >24h after the dural puncture.
- Further blood patches may be repeated with increasing success.

Complications

- Repeat accidental dural puncture.
- Immediate exacerbation of symptoms and radicular pain.
- Long-term complications are very rare.

Prophylactic blood patch

- Prophylactic blood patch has been performed when blood is given into a resited epidural catheter before removal.
- It cannot be performed if the epidural catheter has been placed intrathecally.
- It is an unnecessary intervention in the 20–30% of women who would not get a headache.
- It is generally thought to be less effective than a deferred blood patch, but the evidence is conflicting.

Additional treatment options

- Epidural saline, dextran 40 and fibrin glue have been advocated, but there is inadequate evidence to support their use.
- In unresponsive patients, surgical closure of the dural perforation may be required.

When to ask for further help

- Severe non-posture headache.
- Atypical presentation of symptoms and signs, especially if sudden and late.
- Other associated symptoms.
  - Neurological symptoms or signs.
  - Evidence of systemic infection with true meningism.
  - Altered level of consciousness.
  - Seizures.
- Headache persisting after two epidural blood patches.

Further reading

Turnbull DK, Shepherd DB. Post-dural puncture headache: pathogenesis, prevention and treatment. *British Journal of Anaesthesia* 2003; **91**: 718–729.

Evans RW, Mathew NT, ed. *Handbook of Headache*. Lippincott Williams and Wilkins, 2000; 216–220.

Neurological complications

Neurological deficit after delivery

- Neurological deficit is well recognized after delivery. The overall incidence is between 11.0 and 27.9 patients per 10 000.
- Maternal obstetric palsy, often termed neuropraxia, is caused by compression or stretching of nerves and nerve roots by the fetal presenting part or abnormal posture adopted by the mother. It most commonly improves after ~72h, but can take months to resolve or be permanent.
- Maternal obstetric palsies are more common in primiparous women of short stature, a large baby, persistent posterior or transverse position of the fetal head and in those requiring instrumental delivery, particularly following a prolonged labour.
- The incidence of neurological symptoms following regional anaesthesia has been quoted as 0–36 per 10 000 procedures after epidural and 35 per 10 000 procedures after spinal anaesthesia.
- Neurological deficits caused by acute prolapsed intervertebral discs are associated with pregnancy and childbirth and are a reversible cause of injury. They are usually associated with pain, but not invariably.

Maternal obstetric palsies

- Lumbosacral plexus injury—L4/5, S1/5. Caused by compression of the lumbosacral trunk against the sacrum by the head of the fetus.
  - The classic injury is an L5 compression injury of the nerve root as it passes over the pelvic brim.
  - The more posterior L5 root fibres eventually form the common peroneal nerve and are more readily damaged.
  - The distribution of the injury results in a foot drop and numbness on the lateral aspect of the lower leg and foot crossing to the great toe.
  - It can be clinically difficult to differentiate from a more distal injury.
  - The injury most commonly presents on the side of the fetal occiput with a persistent occipital-posterior presentation.
  - All forms of rotational delivery are associated with lumbosacral damage.
  - Damage by forceps blades can result in injury on the opposite side to the occiput.
- Common peroneal neuropathy—L4/5, S1/2.
  - Caused by compression of the common peroneal nerve as it turns around the head of the fibular.
  - Is associated with lithotomy position but can be caused by persistent flexion of the knee and prolonged resting of the leg against a hard surface.
- Femoral neuropathy—L2/4. Forced flexion of the hips causes the femoral nerve to be compressed under the inguinal ligament.
- Obturator neuropathy—L2/4. Damaged by the fetal head or forceps.
- Perineal nerve injury—S3/5 caused by deep arrest of the fetal head. Presents with saddle anaesthesia and bladder disturbance.

- Sciatic nerve injury—L4–S1. Occasional reports of damage possibly at the sciatic notch. May be related to prolonged periods of sitting or the supine position with tilt.
- Meralgia paraesthetica—L2/3. Compression of the lateral cutaneous nerve of the thigh. Probably present in late pregnancy, but may be first noted after delivery.
- Obstetric palsies can present with a very mixed picture, making accurate location of the site of injury difficult.
- Motor and sensory fibres may be differently affected within a single nerve.
- Reflexes may or may not be affected.
- Conventional nerve conduction studies can be difficult to perform and interpret because of the proximal site of some nerve injuries.
- In servere or persistent cases, an early neurology opinion is important.
- The neuropathy can be painful and will not respond to conventional analgesia. Neuropathic pain strategies may have to be used.

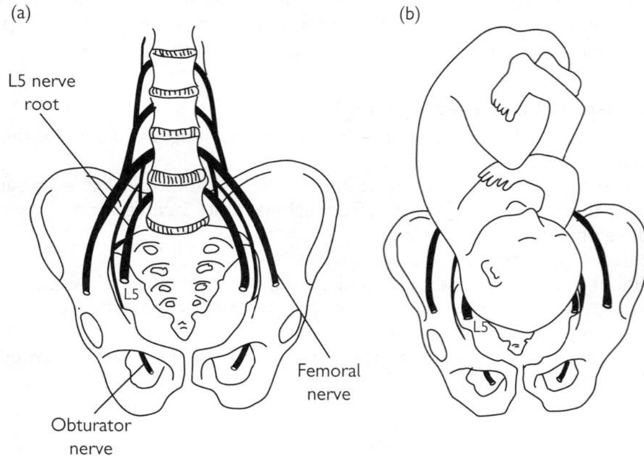

Fig. 14.1 Postpartum neuropathy. (a) The L5 nerve root is especially vulnerable as it emerges over the sacroiliac junction. (b) This is especially so when the fetus is in a persistent occipital-posterior postition. The resulting neuropathy is nearly always on the side of the occiput.

Injuries related to regional anaesthesia

- Nerve root damage—due to direct needle or catheter trauma or due to injection of local anaesthetic into the nerve.
  - Pain or paraesthesia is felt at time of insertion.
  - Frequently over the L3 dermatone across the front of the thigh.
  - Persistent paraesthesia should never be dismissed.
  - The needle should be removed.
  - If severe or persistent pain is felt on inserting an epidural catheter, the catheter and needle should be removed.

- Spinal cord damage—direct damage to the conus medullaris.
  - High placement of spinal needle.
  - Abnormally low conus.
  - Dural puncture during high epidural placement.
- Cranial nerve palsy—usually due to CSF leak following dural puncture; most common lesion is VIth nerve palsy (owing to its long intracranial path).
- Epidural/spinal haematoma.
- Epidural/spinal abscess.
- Meningitis—bacterial or aseptic.
- Anterior spinal artery syndrome.
- Cauda equina syndrome.
- Arachnoiditis.

The spinal cord usually terminates at the level of L1 and becomes the cauda equina below this. In up to 20% of the population, it may extend to the lower border of L2. It is therefore advisable to use the lowest possible intervertebral space for regional, especially spinal anaesthesia, particularly as Tuffier's line is an unreliable landmark.

Assessment and management

- Full history, with particular attention to pre-existing problems and the progress of labour and delivery.
- Careful documentation of paraesthesia at the time of spinal or epidural.
- Was there return of function after regional block before the development of symptoms?
- Have the symptoms and signs progressed?
- Full neurological examination and careful documentation of deficit, including both sensory and motor signs by a senior anaesthetist.
- No symptoms should be dismissed.
- Serial temperature recordings, blood for WCC and C-reactive protein if infection suspected.

Signs of serious pathology must be sought:

- Pain, redness or swelling at the site of injection.
- Pyrexia, raised WCC.
- Evidence of meningism.
- Persistent or progressive neurological deficit.
- Bladder or bowel dysfunction.
- Saddle anaesthesia.
- Back pain associated with fever (especially in immunocompromised or diabetic patients).
- Bilateral signs.

- Close observation and reassurance may be adequate as symptoms often resolve within 72h postdelivery.
- Small areas of numbness across the buttocks after an apparently uncomplicated spinal anaesthetic is relatively common. If there are no associated bladder symptoms or other nerve injuries then the mother can usually be reassured that normal skin sensation will return.
- Urgent neurology opinion and MRI must be considered in all cases of suspected spinal injury, epidural and spinal abscess or haematoma.
- If nerve injury is suspected, nerve conduction studies and out-patient neurological referral at 6 weeks postdelivery is appropriate. Many cases of nerve injury (obstetric and anaesthetic related) will become the subject of a complaint. Early and close liaison with a neurologist may be helpful.

Further reading

Holdcroft A *et al.* Neurological complications associated with pregnancy. *British Journal of Anaesthesia* 1995; **75**: 522–526.

Loo CC, Dahlgren G, Irestedt L. Neurological complications in obstetric regional anaesthesia. *International Journal of Obstetric Anesthesia* 2000; **9**: 99–124.

Haematoma

An epidural or spinal haematoma is rare, but potentially catastrophic if missed.

- It may occur spontaneously or after regional anaesthesia, particularly in patients with evidence of clotting dysfunction.
- Clotting dysfunction may be intrinsic, e.g. thrombocytopaenia or haemophilia, or acquired, e.g. thromboprophylaxis.
- All obstetric units should have guidelines for the safe timing of regional anaesthesia and anticoagulation (see p 181 for further guidance).

Signs

- Prolonged (>8h) effect of anaesthesia, with back pain and localized tenderness.
- Bilateral motor and sensory loss combined with disturbance of bowel or bladder function.
- Return of function followed by progression of deficit.

Management

- Always follow-up regional blocks which appear to last longer than expected.
- Urgent MRI if signs are suggestive of spinal haematoma.
- If epidural or spinal haematoma evident, emergency neurosurgical decompression is indicated to prevent permanent disability.
- Prognosis is poor if neurological deficit is >12h old.

Meningitis

The incidence of meningitis following regional anaesthetic techniques ranges from 1 to 15 in 100 000 in spinal anaesthetics.

Septic meningitis

- Septic meningitis may be secondary to bacterial or viral infection.
- Bacterial infection, often due to *Streptococcus pneumoniae* or *Neisseria meningitides*, may be secondary to a bacteraemia and not related to regional anaesthesia.
- If secondary to spinal anaesthesia, *Streptococcus viridans* is frequently the causative organism.
- The causative organism is most probably a contaminant from the patient's own skin.
- For meningitis to occur following regional anaesthesia, there may have been a breech in the aseptic field.
- CSE technique has been associated with an increase in reported cases of meningitis and epidural abscess. The true incidence is not known, as there may be reporting bias.
- The breakdown in the protective barrier offered by the dura and introduction of the epidural catheter, which is continuous with the skin as part of the CSE technique, are the possible contributory factors.
- Viral meningitis may occur following regional anaesthesia in women with herpes simplex or herpes zoster infection.

Signs

- Fever.
- Headache.
- Neck stiffness.
- Photophobia.

Management

- Lumbar puncture to identify the causative organism.
- Aggressive antimicrobial treatment.
- Referral to neurology or general medicine.
- The prognosis for recovery is better following meningitis than an epidural abscess.

Aseptic meningitis

- Rare consequence of disinfectant from the skin preparation or contaminated syringes being introduced into the epidural or intrathecal space.
- Features mimic septic meningitis.

Arachnoiditis

- Rare inflammatory disorder where the membranes around the spinal cord and cauda equina become fibrotic.
- This causes constriction of the cauda equina with progressive painful neurology.
- Cause is unknown.
- Spinal and epidural anaesthesia has been implicated, but there is no proved association, and most cases are not linked with regional anaesthesia.
- Preservatives within local anaesthetic solutions have been blamed.

Further reading

Rice I, Wee MY, Thomson K. Obstetric epidurals and chronic adhesive arachnoiditis (Review). *British Journal of Anaesthesia* 2004; **92**: 109–120.

Epidural abscess

- A rare but serious complication of regional anaesthesia.
- Incidence is 0.2–3.7 cases per 100 000 obstetric epidurals.
- May occur spontaneously or following a breech in sterile conditions during epidural or spinal anaesthesia.
- CSE technique has been associated with an increase in reported cases.
- The most common organism involved is *Staphylococcus aureus* (57%).

Signs

- Classically presents with severe deep-seated backache ± localized tenderness.
- Pyrexia and signs of systemic sepsis occur late in the presentation.
- Localizing nerve root pain and sudden onset of weakness may follow after 2–3 days.
- It is a neurosurgical emergency.

Management

- Aggressive treatment with IV antibiotics and urgent neurosurgical decompression is paramount.
- If neurological symptoms present, prognosis for full recovery is poor.

Further reading

Grewel S, Hocking G, Wildsmith J. Epidural abscesses. *British Journal of Anaesthesia* 2006; **96**: 292–302.

Reynolds F. Infection as a complication of neuraxial blockade. *International Journal of Obstetric Anesthesia* 2005; **14**: 183–188.

Cauda equina syndrome

- Caused by damage to the sacral nerve roots (S2–S4) either due to direct needle trauma or after injection of large volumes of LA causing root compression.
- Continuous spinal infusions via a spinal microcatheter and high concentration lidocaine have also been implicated.

Signs

- Bowel and bladder dysfunction.
- Saddle anaesthesia.
- Residual sensory loss.
- Lower limb paralysis (varying degrees).

Management

- Urgent MRI to exclude a reversible cause, e.g. haematoma, abscess, prolapsed intervertbral disc.
- Neurological referral for assessment of signs.
- Ongoing management is largely supportive.

Further reading

Loo CC, Dahlgren G, Irested L. Neurological complications in obstetric regional anaesthesia. *International Journal of Obstetric Anesthesia* 2000; **9**: 99–124.

Brooks H, May A. Neurological complications following regional anaesthesia in obstetrics. *British Journal of Anaesthesia CEPD Reviews* 2003; **3**: 111–114.

Dealing with a complaint

- Complaints against health service staff are increasing year on year, and the field of obstetric anaesthesia is no exception.
- Complaints are a source of great anxiety to all healthcare staff who may be implicated.
- If a complaint is being made against you, it is essential that you understand your hospital or Trust's process for dealing with it.
- There are broadly three stages at which a complaint may be resolved:
  - Local Trust response.
  - Independent Review Panel.
  - Health Service Commissioner or Ombudsman.
- Many complaints relevant to childbirth are not forwarded for many months or sometimes up to 2yrs following delivery.
- It is essential that accurate, contemporaneous documentation is maintained at all times.
- If a woman indicates in the immediate postnatal period that a complaint is likely, documentation in the contemporary notes should be reviewed. They must NOT be changed in any way, but supplementary comment is appropriate as long as it is absolutely clear when the additional notes were made.

Local response

- Written complaints are normally sent directly to the Trust Chief Executive and passed to a complaints team or department for further action.
- If a complaint is received directly, do not respond personally. It should be forwarded to the Chief Executive via the Clinical Director or the Directorate Manager.
- Complaints are handled by a team of experienced co-ordinators, who will request a response from all staff involved in the woman's care.
- The complainant is entitled to the following:
  - A full, detailed and honest explanation of what happened, when and why.
  - An apology if there was an error or omission in their care.
  - If an error or omission occurred, they should be advised about the Trust's action, or proposed action, to prevent a recurrence.
- Many complaints are resolved with a clear explanation and a timely apology, with the assurance that any failures will be rectified for the future.
- An open and sympathetic approach is recommended.
- A hostile and defensive reaction is more likely to lead to attempted litigation challenges later.
- A written response, signed by the Chief Executive, will be compiled based on the statements from all staff implicated, and forwarded to the complainant.
- The majority of written complaints are concluded with local resolution.

- A meeting with the complainant is sometimes arranged at an early stage. This involves a group discussion with senior doctors and managers involved in the case. The Trust's complaints manager usually chairs the meeting and is responsible for taking minutes. The complainant usually comes with an advocate (often from a patients advocate group). Any doctor who is asked to attend such a meeting is also entitled to an advocate (frequently a senior colleague).

The Independent Review Panel

- If the local response does not satisfy the complainant, referral for independent review is considered by a Convener.
- The independent review panel comprises the Convener, an independent lay chairman, a third lay person and usually two independent clinical assessors to advise the panel.
- Its purpose is to establish the facts and make recommendations to improve the effectiveness of the service.
- Following review of all documentation, all parties are interviewed by the panel, and recommendations are sent to the parties concerned.

Health Service Commissioner

- If the complainant remains dissatisfied after receiving the report from the independent review, she has the right to take the matter to the Health Service Commissioner (Ombudsman).
- The Ombudsman is independent of the NHS and the government.

Legal action

- If a woman explicitly indicates an intention to take legal action, the complaints process should stop immediately.
- Legal action is taken out against the Trust not individual doctors.
- The Trust's legal department take over the case and request their own expert views.

Chapter 15

Anaesthesia for non-obstetric surgery

Martin Garry and Shilpa Rawat

General principles

- Up to 2% of pregnant women undergo surgery unrelated to pregnancy each year.
- The most common procedure during the first trimester is laparoscopy.
- Appendicectomy and cholecystectomy are the most commonly performed open abdominal procedures during pregnancy.
- Surgery during pregnancy has been associated with premature labour and fetal loss.
- The incidence is higher during lower abdominal and pelvic surgery.

Anaesthetic concerns

A thorough knowledge of physiological changes of pregnancy and of placental transfer of drugs is essential.

Major anaesthetic concerns are:
- Maternal risk resulting from anatomical and physiological changes of pregnancy.
- Maintenance of adequate uteroplacental blood flow.
- Teratogenic effects on the fetus of drugs administered to the mother.

Surgical concerns

- The changes of pregnancy can often modify the disease process and make diagnosis difficult.
- Patients may therefore present late with advanced or complicated disease.
- Surgical management is also more complicated than in non-pregnant patients.

Timing

- Whenever possible, elective surgery should be delayed until 6 weeks postpartum.
- More urgent surgery should be delayed until after the period of organogenesis of the first trimester, unless there is an immediate threat to the mother.
- If surgery is needed, make sure the obstetric team are informed.

Preparation

- Thorough preoperative evaluation including airway assessment should be performed and gestational age noted.
- The mother should be counselled about the relative risks of surgery to the pregnancy.
- Premedication may be necessary to allay maternal anxiety, as excess maternal catecholamines are harmful to fetal well-being.
- All women >14 weeks pregnant should have antacid prophylaxis, as hormonal changes at the lower oesophageal sphincter increase the risk of regurgitation and aspiration.

Anaesthetic principles

- Where possible, a regional technique should be used. It has the benefits of the woman maintaining her own airway and providing good analgesia. However, hypotension should be aggressively treated to maintain uteroplacental circulation.
- Ensure correct positioning for all women >20 weeks gestation whatever surgery is being performed. Aorto-caval compression must be avoided by placing a wedge under the right hip and manual uterine displacement. Even when aorto-caval compression does not cause maternal hypotension, it can reduce placental perfusion and cause fetal compromise.
- In addition to routine monitoring for the mother, the FHR and uterine activity should also be monitored perioperatively.
- Maternal FRC is reduced and oxygen requirement increases in pregnancy. Preoxygenate for at least 3min prior to GA.
- Avoid hypoxia, hypotension, hypercarbia and hyperventilation regardless of the anaesthetic technique used.
- If a GA is used, adequate depth of anaesthesia should be maintained. Light anaesthesia increases maternal catecholamine release and reduces uteroplacental perfusion. In addition, the tocolytic effect of volatile anaesthetics is beneficial.
- Treat blood loss early and vigorously. Physiological changes of pregnancy mask early signs of blood loss, and subclinical hypovolaemia will compromise placental perfusion. Hypotension from hypovolaemia in a pregnant woman may not be evident until 25–30% of blood volume is lost.

Postoperative considerations

- Consider DVT prophylaxis for all pregnant women, e.g. clexane 20mg SC. Pregnant women are hypercoaguable, with increased levels of fibrinogen, factors VII, VIII, X and XII and fibrin degradation products.
- Give adequate postoperative analgesia. The sympathetic response from pain and stress increases maternal catecholamine levels, which causes vasoconstriction of all blood vessels, including those of the uteroplacental circulation.
- External tocodynamometry should be used whenever possible intra- and postoperatively. It can detect the onset of preterm labour, so that tocolysis can be started early. Prophylactic tocolysis is controversial.
- Continuous FHR monitoring using transabdominal Doppler is possible from 16 weeks of gestation.

Fetal considerations

Teratogenicity has been defined as any significant postnatal change in function or form in an offspring after prenatal treatment.

- Causes of teratogenicity are diverse, and include infection, pyrexia, hypoxia and acidosis as well as the better recognized hazards of drugs and radiation.
- It is estimated that drug/chemical exposure is the cause of 2–3% of birth defects.
- Ionizing radiation is a known human teratogen. Exposure below 5–10rads is safe. Fetal exposure from a chest radiograph is ~8mrads.
- The teratogenic potential of drugs is influenced by genetic predisposition, dose, duration and timing of exposure.
- The fetus can be affected at three stages.
    - During the first 2 weeks of intrauterine life, the teratogens have either a lethal effect or none at all on the fetus.
    - The 3rd to 8th week is the most vital period for organogenesis. Drug exposure during this period would cause most teratogenic effects and subsequent organ abnormalities.
    - From the 8th week onwards, the organ formation is completed and then organ growth takes place. Drug exposure after 8 weeks gestation should not cause major organ abnormalities, but can cause fetal growth retardation.

Fetal monitoring

- Prior to 24 weeks gestation the fetus is generally not usually considered viable and confirmation of fetal well-being should be performed at an appropriate time in the postoperative period.
- If urgent surgery is required after the fetus is viable
    - Neonatologists should be informed.
    - Continuous CTG monitoring should be performed if practical in the peri- and postoperative period.
    - The CTG can be difficult to interpret in the presence of GA drugs.

Anaesthetic drugs

During pregnancy, the response to anaesthetic drugs is altered:

- MAC for inhalational anaesthetics is decreased.
- Neuronal block from spinal and epidural anaesthesia is more extensive.
- Enhanced block from peripheral nerve blocks.
- Plasma cholinesterase levels decrease by >25% and the effect of suxamethonium may be prolonged.
- Albumin concentration is reduced and thus plasma binding of drugs decreases, resulting in a greater fraction of unbound drug. This explains the increased toxicity of bupivacaine during pregnancy.

No anaesthetic drugs, with the exception of cocaine, have been associated with proven teratogenic effects.

Premedication

Antacids

- Sodium citrate is safe.
- Ranitidine and cimetidine are usually safe, but caution with chronic exposure to cimetidine because of known androgenic effects in adults.

Anxiolytics

- Although animal studies have shown an association of benzodiazepines with cleft lip and cleft palate, effects on humans are still controversial. A single dose has never been shown to be teratogenic. Long-term exposure should be avoided, as it can cause neonatal withdrawal symptoms following delivery; exposure just before delivery can cause neonatal drowsiness and hypotonia.

Anticholinergics

- Glycopyrronium bromide is preferred to atropine if an anticholinergic is required. It does not readily cross the placenta and is a better antisialogogue.
- Atropine crosses the placenta and can cause fetal tachycardia and loss of FHR variability when given in large doses.

IV induction agents

It should be remembered that, opioids and IV induction agents decrease FHR variability, and this should not be a cause of concern.

Thiopental

- Clinical experience shows that this is a very safe drug to use, although formal studies have not been conducted.
- Ideal if rapid sequence induction is planned.

Propofol

- It is not teratogenic in animal studies.
- Its use in early human pregnancy is not formally investigated. However, it is safe to use during CS at term.

Etomidate

- Is a potent corticosteroid inhibitor and, when used during CS, neonates have reduced cortisol levels.
- Its use in early pregnancy has not been formally investigated.

Ketamine

- Should be avoided during early pregnancy, as it increases intrauterine pressure and can cause fetal asphyxia. This effect is not seen in the third trimester of pregnancy.

Inhalational anaesthetic agents

All volatile anaesthetic agents decrease the uterine tone, dilate uterine arteries and increase uterine blood flow up to a MAC of 1.5. However, at higher concentrations, the uterine blood flow decreases secondary to falls in maternal BP and CO.

- Halothane and isoflurane have been used extensively in pregnancy and are safe. The halogenated vapours also cause uterine relaxation, which may be beneficial for surgery during pregnancy.
- Since nitrous oxide inhibits methionine synthetase, there is a concern that it can affect DNA synthesis in a developing fetus. It has been shown to be consistently teratogenic during the peak organogenic period in animal studies, but there is no evidence of such an effect in humans. However, given that anaesthesia can be safely delivered without nitrous oxide, it is sensible to avoid this agent.

Analgesics

- Opioids are highly fat-soluble and readily cross the placenta. Although brief exposure is safe, long-term exposure will cause symptoms of withdrawal when the fetus is delivered. Animal studies show possible fetal teratogenicity if prolonged hypercapnia or impaired feeding develop as side effects of opioid exposure.
- Paracetamol and codeine are the safest analgesics for minor surgery during pregnancy.
- NSAIDs are contraindicated in the third trimester and especially shortly before delivery as they may prevent closure of the neonate's ductus arteriosis at delivery.

Anaesthetic management

General principles

- The mother should be counselled and reassured whenever possible about the risks to the pregnancy.
- The obstetric team should be involved.
- Regional is preferable to general anaesthesia.

- Meticulous anaesthesia is required with attention to
  - good oxygenation.
  - normal CO_2 (for pregnancy).
  - normotension and normovolaemia.

First trimester

- Ideally avoid surgery or at least delay to second trimester if possible.
- Care with potential teratogenic drugs.
- Avoid N_2O.
- Consider the possibility of undiagnosed pregnancy in all women of reproductive age.

Second trimester

- This is the optimum time for surgery.
- Care with positioning to avoid/minimize aorto-caval compression.
- At risk of aspiration:
  - Ranitidine 150mg, 12 and 1h (or similar) before surgery.
  - Sodium citrate 20mL immediately before induction.
  - Rapid sequence induction with cricoid pressure.
- Monitor uterine activity during and postsurgery. Treat with tocolytic agents if necessary.
- Monitor FHR during and postsurgery.

Third trimester

- As for second trimester regarding:
  - Positioning.
  - Fetal and uterine monitoring.
- At particular risk of premature induction of labour, so that intra- and postoperative uterine monitoring is essential.
- Consider the use of prophylactic tocolysis.

Further reading

Kuczkowski KM. Nonobstetric surgery during pregnancy: what are the risks of anaesthesia. *Obstetrical and Gynecological Survey* 2004; **59**: 52–56.

Goodman S. Anesthesia for nonobstetric surgery in the pregnant patient. *Seminars in Pernatology* 2002; **26**: 136–145.

Rosen MA. Management of anesthesia for the pregnant surgical patient. *Anesthesiology* 1999; **179**: 1643–1653.

Chapter 16

Major obstetric haemorrhage

Sue Catling

Definition, incidence and impact

The CEMACH reports that 14 women in the UK died directly from obstetric haemorrhage in the period 2003–2005, i.e. 6.6 deaths per million maternities. Haemorrhage is the third most common cause of direct maternal deaths after thromboembolism, and pre-eclampsia. It is salutary to realize that not only is the current death rate more than twice that of the triennium 1997–1999, when there were 7 deaths, i.e. 3.3 deaths per million maternities, but the latest figures have returned to that of 20 years ago. CEMACH also highlights that 58% of the deaths involved 'substandard care'—these women may well have survived with optimal management.

Major obstetric haemorrhage is variously defined as:
- Single blood loss of 1000–1500mL.
- Continuing blood loss of 150mL/min.
- Transfusion requirement of 4 units of red cells.

It has been estimated that major obstetric haemorrhage occurs in 6.7 per thousand deliveries. An averaged sized unit delivering 3500 women per year would therefore expect to manage 24 cases every year, or two per month. **Therefore, this is not a rare condition.**

- Fewer than 1% of parturients are admitted to ICU, but major haemorrhage accounts for the majority of these.
- From a global perspective, the World Health Organization (WHO) calculates that in the year 2000 worldwide there were **132 000** maternal deaths from haemorrhage—mostly in sub-Saharan Africa and Asia.

Effective management of obstetric haemorrhage can be subdivided into

- Organizational aspects.
  - Prevention.
  - Preparation.
  - Planning.
  - Processes.
  - Protocols.
- Clinical aspects.
  - Education.
  - Teamwork.
  - Practice.
  - Communication.
  - Expertise.
  - Leadership.

Organizational aspects

Prevention

- Identify the patient at risk and ensure appropriate delivery occurs in the appropriate place.
- Multidisciplinary antenatal care should include a referral pathway to a Consultant-led anaesthetic assessment clinic at an early stage for any parturient considered 'high risk' for delivery.
- Identify known risk factors for haemorrhage, including:
  - Increasing maternal age (becoming more common).
  - Multiple pregnancy (increasing due to assisted conception).
  - More women with complex medical problems.
  - Increasing CS rates are leading to an increased incidence of placenta praevia/accreta.
- Beware the previous CS with placenta praevia. These are the most 'high risk' patients for massive haemorrhage and may involve placenta accreta.
- Ideally, delivery is best performed at a unit that can provide all the necessary standard and innovative interventions, i.e. interventional radiology, cell salvage, recombinant factor VIIa, obstetricians familiar with B-Lynch sutures and tamponade (Rusch) balloons, specialist obstetric anaesthetists, on site ITU and blood bank provision.
- If these criteria cannot be met, careful consideration should be given to electively transferring the patient to a unit where such services are available.
- The unpredictable nature of obstetrics can make this simple rule more complex in practice; high risk patients booked for delivery at a specialist centre can go into labour or bleed near the local unit. Thus, even the smallest units can be involved in the initial management prior to transfer.

Preparation

- A team approach is essential. CEMACH repeatedly emphasizes the need for robust, multidisciplinary systems for communication and effective action. These must be clearly understood and regularly rehearsed by every member of the labour ward team. Without these being in place, the patient may still die despite individual clinical skill and effort.
- The understanding of this essential team approach has led to the development of multidisciplinary 'scenario-based' joint training courses for anaesthetists, obstetricians and midwives, overseen by the Advanced Life Support Group (ALSG).
- Staff of the unit should be encouraged and facilitated to attend and regularly update their skills on courses such as MOET (Managing Obstetric Emergencies and Trauma) and ALSO (Advanced Life Support in Obstetrics).
- Teams require leadership, and the Lead Consultants in Obstetrics and Anaesthetics should work together with midwives to develop the necessary team skills in every unit.

Planning, protocols, practice and audit

- Senior midwives, obstetricians and anaesthetists should meet regularly to develop local protocols dealing with the clinical management and the organization/processes needed to cope with a major haemorrhage on their own unit.
- The issues will differ in each hospital, and the following questions should be addressed:
  - How are blood samples physically sent to the laboratories and blood bank?
  - How is portering organized to transport blood?
  - Where is the blood fridge and who has the key?
  - Do switchboard and blood bank understand the level of urgency of the requests made to them?
- There should be a clearly agreed 'code' via the hospital bleep system to alert the whole team to a major haemorrhage on the delivery suite.
- Problems and systems failures are often only identified during an emergency, so 'fire drills' and simulations are essential.
- Such exercises should also be run 'out-of-hours' when realistic assessment of responses can be made.
- Planning should involve haematologists, laboratory staff, porters, ward clerks, healthcare support workers, etc. as necessary.
- Early analysis of the SaFE (Simulation and Fire drill Evaluation) study from the South West England region has now provided evidence that after appropriate training and drills, improvement is seen in both knowledge (as evaluated by MCQ scores) and communication skills (as evaluated by patient-actor perspective scores). This study has demonstrated that this can be achieved with in-house training just as effectively as at simulation centres.
- Necessary equipment, e.g. blood warmers, pressure infusors and monitoring devices, should be identified, obtained and maintained.
- Copies of the local protocols should be issued to all relevant staff and be prominently displayed on the labour ward.
- Compliance with the local protocols should be the subject of regular multidisciplinary audit, with identified failings being promptly addressed.

Clinical management overview

Overview

The aim is to restore circulating volume and prevent tissue hypoxia. Initial resuscitation will be the same whatever the cause of the haemorrhage.

Subsequent obstetric management will depend on whether the baby is delivered and/or viable. In most cases, the patient will require an anaesthetic for exploration of the uterus and surgical haemostasis.

- Senior anaesthetic and obstetric help should be sought immediately.
- Initiate the 'major haemorrhage emergency phone call'.
- The initial management is often started, of necessity, by junior staff.
- CEMACH emphasizes that major haemorrhage requires Consultant anaesthetist(s), Consultant obstetrician(s) and senior midwifery staff to be involved.
- The blood bank and the Consultant haematologist will need to be alerted, and in complex cases a vascular surgeon/interventional radiologist may be required.
- The operating obstetrician should be confident that she/he can perform a caesarean hysterectomy—not all obstetricians have this experience, and the involvement of more than one operating surgeon is often appropriate.

Role of the anaesthetist

The anaesthetist will need to initiate and lead

- Resuscitation and stabilization.
- Estimation of blood loss and appropriate ordering of blood and blood products, including liasing with haematologists and blood bank.
- Optimization for theatre and administration of appropriate anaesthesia to permit surgical exploration.
- Administration of drugs to control haemorrhage.
- Accurate and appropriate fluid replacement.
- Invasive monitoring.
- Organization of subsequent critical care, e.g. intensive or high dependency care.

Initial resuscitation and stabilization

Any resuscitation should follow the obstetric ABC principle as follows:

- Tilt.
- 100% oxygen.
- ABC with rapid initial assessment and correction as found.
- Diagnosis and definitive treatment.

Tilt

- Avoid supine aorto-caval compression by either placing the patient in the left lateral position or providing 15° left lateral tilt with a wedge under the right hip.
- If the patient is supine, the gravid uterus will compress the vena cava and prevent adequate VR to the heart. CO can be reduced by up to 30%, exacerbating hypotension due to blood loss and preventing effective resuscitation.
- If neither manoeuvre is possible, the uterus must be manually displaced to the left.

Oxygen

- **Administer 15L/min oxygen** via a tight-fitting face mask with a reservoir bag.
- Turn the wall oxygen flowmeter to maximum—this will achieve optimal oxygen saturation of the blood remaining in the circulation and help to prevent tissue hypoxia.
- In addition, nitrogen in the FRC of the lung will be washed out and replaced by oxygen—this provides a valuable reservoir for continuing oxygenation of pulmonary blood should respiratory compromise occur.

Airway

- A severely shocked patient may lose consciousness due to hypotension and require tracheal intubation to protect the airway from gastric acid aspiration and to maintain adequate oxygenation/ventilation.

Breathing

- This may become inadequate and the patient may require ventilation as consciousness is lost, and severe tissue hypoxia and metabolic acidosis supervene.

Circulation

- Rapid assessment of the estimated blood volume lost should be done while simultaneously:
  - Establishing IV access with two large-bore cannulae (14G).
  - Establishing basic monitoring: pulse oximeter, non-invasive BP, ECG as soon as practicable; but **do not delay fluid resuscitation**—HR and capillary refill are reliable clinical indicators of hypovolaemia.

Common pitfall: normal BP does not exclude major blood loss in the pregnant patient

The physiologically increased plasma volume and red cell mass of pregnancy means total blood volume can be increased up to 40%. Up to 40% blood volume can be lost (1500–2000mL) before hypotension appears, because blood is shunted away from the fetoplacental unit (750mL/min) to maintain flow to vital organs.

Early signs of impending decompensation occur with a normal blood pressure

- Tachycardia >100bpm.
- Fetal distress.

- Skin pallor with increased capillary refill time (>2s, or the time it takes to say 'capillary refill').
- Decreased/absent urine output (this is not usually known in the acute situation).

Signs of life-threatening hypovolaemia, i.e. >50% blood volume loss include

- Hypotension.
- Tachypnoea.
- Mental clouding, progressing to unconsciousness.

- **Take 20mL blood for Hb, coagulation screen, and cross-match 6 units of blood** (include baseline biochemistry).
  - A venous blood gas analyser for acid–base status and lactate is available in most delivery units and can aid the management of ongoing bleeding.
  - Ensure that all blood samples are correctly labelled, and inform blood bank of the degree of urgency.
  - It is often useful to delegate a team member to this task, and also to assign someone to record all events, with timings, at this point.
- **Infuse 2L of crystalloid** (Hartmanns/normal saline) rapidly and set up blood warmers and pressure infusors as soon as available.
  - The patient may need to be transferred to theatre at the same time, and the obstetricians should be establishing the diagnosis and deciding on treatment to stop the bleeding.
  - A second anaesthetist should be ensuring theatre drugs and equipment are ready, including haemostatic drugs and inotropes.

Assess the response to initial volume replacement

- 15–30% blood loss (750–1500mL) will respond to crystalloids alone; tachycardia will improve and remain improved.
- 30–40% blood loss (1500–2000mL) will have a transitory response to crystalloids and will require colloid infusion while waiting for cross-matched or group-specific blood.
- >40% blood loss (>2000mL) is life-threatening and requires immediate transfusion; use O-negative blood if group-specific is not available.

Assess the need for invasive monitoring

- Invasive monitoring can be a very helpful adjunct to the management of the mother with a major haemorrhage but fluid resuscitation **MUST NOT** be delayed during attempts to place CVP and arterial lines. **Wait until a second anaesthetist can aid insertion**.
- An arterial line is required for most cases where blood loss is >2000mL or rapid enough for the mother to be haemodynamically unstable, both for accurate real-time invasive BP monitoring and sequential blood gas analysis to monitor the degree of metabolic acidosis.
- A CVP line gives some useful extra information on volume status, and enables central administration of vasoactive drugs.

- CVP placement can be complicated by carotid arterial puncture, haematoma and pneumothorax, and the risks/benefits should be carefully considered, especially in the presence of a coagulopathy.
- If considered necessary, an internal jugular line should be placed under ultrasound guidance whenever possible.
- Right-sided heart pressures may become less accurate indicators of volume status if pulmonary oedema or myocardial failure supervene, in which case specialist advice from the Intensive Care Team is then appropriate to review the need for further CO monitoring, e.g. PiCCO, or echocardiography.
- A urinary catheter is mandatory with any blood loss >1500mL as urine output is an important indicator of the adequacy of volume replacement.

Early assessment of the need for additional assistance, equipment and blood products will save time, e.g.

- Haemocue® measurement of Hb.
- Platelets, FFP and cryoprecipitate, which may be on site or need to be urgently obtained from the blood transfusion centre some distance away.

Directed therapy

Diagnosis

Establishing the diagnosis may require:

- Examination of lower genital tract for tears or lacerations.
- Exploration of the uterus and pelvis if suspect:
  - Unresponsive uterine atony.
  - Retained products.
  - Uterine rupture.
  - Uncontrolled surgical bleeding.
- Assessment of coagulation status in the event of:
  - DIC.
  - Dilutional coagulopathy.

Definitive treatment

- Surgery.
- Additional oxytocic drugs.
- Drugs to reduce bleeding, e.g. tranexamic acid, aprotonin.
- Uterine tamponade techniques.
- Interventional radiology and arterial embolization.

Continuing resuscitation, appropriate fluid replacement and targeted correction of haematological abnormalities must occur simultaneously with definitive treatment to stop the bleeding.

Causes of obstetric haemorrhage

Antepartum

- Ectopic pregnancy (10 deaths in CEMACH 2003–2005 report).
- Placenta praevia (3 deaths).
- Placental abruption (2 deaths).
- Vasa praevia.
- Uterine rupture.

Postpartum

- Uterine atony.
- Retained products.
- Uterine inversion.
- Lacerations.
- Placenta accreta.

4Ts: definitive treatment/directed therapy

A more practical, working classification of major obstetric haemorrhage is to think: is the problem with Tone, Tissue, Trauma or Thrombin?

- Tone, e.g. uterine atony.
- Tissue, e.g. retained placental fragments, clots or membranes.
- Trauma, e.g. tears, lacerations, uterine rupture or inversion.
- Thrombin, e.g. DIC, dilutional coagulopathy or thrombocytopenia.

Tone

Prevention and initial treatment of uterine atony

- Mechanical.
  - The simple 'rubbing-up' of a contraction is an effective midwifery skill which should be used early.
  - Bimanual compression can be used at vaginal or operative delivery and can be a life-saving initial measure.
- Drugs.
  - ***Syntocinon***® is a synthetic analogue of the posterior pituitary hormone oxytocin. It causes uterine contraction via oxytocin receptors in the myometrium, and is the first-line drug to prevent and treat uterine atony.
  - At CS, it is given as a slow bolus IV injection of 5IU.
  - This can be repeated, but more rapid administration or larger bolus doses can cause hypotension, ECG abnormalities and pulmonary oedema, particularly in the parturient with pre-existing cardiac problems or with major haemodynamic instability.
  - Due to its short half-life, a bolus of oxytocin should be routinely followed by an IV infusion of 40IU over 4h in cases where PPH is anticipated or occurring.

Secondary treatment of uterine atony

- ***Ergometrine*** 0.5mg IM or IV causes uterine and vascular smooth muscle contraction through 5-hydroxytryptamine (5-HT) receptor stimulation. It has a slower onset but longer duration of action than oxytocin and its effect lasts for up to 3h after im injection. It should be considered if atony fails to respond to oxytocin. It can cause hypertension, headache, nausea and vomiting due to its generalized vascular vasoconstrictor effects, and should be used cautiously in pre-eclampsia and heart disease.
- ***Prostaglandins*** PGE_2 ***and*** PGF_2 stimulate myometrial contraction, and have variable effects on the cardiovascular system depending on the dose, and mode of administration. These agents should be considered if oxytocics fail to achieve adequate myometrial contraction.
  - ***Carboprost*** (Haemabate: 15-methyl PGF_2) is a potent synthetic analogue of $PGF_{2\alpha}$ which is given IM (or intramyometrially) in doses of 250 micrograms. It can be repeated every 15min to a maximum total dose of 2mg. Carboprost can cause hypoxia due to intrapulmonary shunting caused by pulmonary vascular smooth muscle constriction. It should NOT be given IV and should be used with caution in pre-eclampsia or cardiac disease. In practice, a drug that can only be given every 15min has limited applicability in rapid, massive haemorrhage.
  - ***Misoprostol*** is a synthetic PGE_1 analogue that increases uterine tone. It is administered rectally in a dose of 600–1000 micrograms and is reported to be very effective and cheap. Its use in PPH remains unlicensed, and this is the subject of current controversy, especially as regards its use in poorer countries.

Tissue

- The uterus must be emptied for effective contraction to occur. Remaining fragments of placenta, blood clot or membranes must be removed.
- This can sometimes be done gently after a vaginal delivery without anaesthesia, but frequently requires more detailed examination and adequate anaesthesia.
- Abnormally adherent or invasive placenta (accreta, percreta) can pose particular problems necessitating hysterectomy, but in extreme cases the placenta may invade outside the uterus and have to be left *in situ*.
- If haemorrhage is not ongoing, methotrexate has been described to aid reabsorption.

Trauma

- Lacerations and tears to the uterus or lower genital tract are a common and frequently underestimated cause of haemorrhage, and must be carefully explored and repaired.
- Surgical procedures will require adequate anaesthesia, which in most major haemorrhage with ongoing bleeding and haemodynamic instability requires a GA.
- Regional anaesthesia should only be considered if the patient is fully resuscitated, haemodynamically stable and has satisfactory clotting.
- The standard rapid sequence obstetric GA technique may have to be modified in the patient who has suffered a massive haemorrhage, where a bolus of thiopental/suxamethonium could cause significant hypotension.
- Alternatives include induction with ketamine 1–5mg/kg, opiate–benzodiazepine mixtures, etomidate or volatile agents; this will be a decision for a senior anaesthetist, with the risk of acid aspiration balanced against the risk of haemodynamic decompensation.

Thrombin

- Initial fluid resuscitation is based on volume replacement and clinical assessment, and Hb is not a good indicator of blood loss in acute bleeding.
- It has been shown in clinical reconstruction scenarios that blood loss is underestimated by up to 35% by all clinical groups except anaesthetists, who overestimate by up to 4% but are the most accurate.
- Results from initial samples can take up to 45min to be available. Consider the use of near-patient testing:
  - Haemocue® is a very useful near-patient testing device that gives an accurate baseline Hb reading in 30s using 1 drop of blood.
  - Many blood gas analysers have a Hb as part of their multianalysis functions.

Although neither will give information on platelet numbers and coagulation tests, and therefore are not a substitute for laboratory tests, they are a very useful initial estimate of the magnitude of the problem after clear fluid resuscitation.

Blood transfusion and coagulation factors

Red cell transfusion

The blood bank provides red cells in additive solution, and there is a hierarchy of transfusion choices depending on urgency. Transfusion should aim for a Hb of 8.0g/dL; overtransfusion is unnecessary. The use of a rapid infusor device is strongly encouraged in massive haemorrhage.

- O-negative blood for emergency use should be available on labour ward or within 5min distance.
- Uncross-matched group-specific blood can be issued 5–10min after the sample is received at the laboratory.
- Fully cross-matched blood (order 6–8 units) will take 30–50min.
- 'Electronic issue'—if the patient has had two recent 'group and screen' samples processed through the same laboratory, the electronic issue system allows the release of an unlimited number of units of blood immediately. Many units are now setting up this system for elective CS and other high risk mothers. Some units are making this routine for all mothers.
    - It saves blood and laboratory time because there is no need to perform unnecessary cross-matching.
    - Fully cross-matched blood can be issued within 10min to a patient.
- Cell salvage can provide a useful source of red cells to reduce the patient's exposure to allogeneic blood and conserve the supply in massive bleeding. It is now being used widely in the UK, and initial fears about possible contamination with amniotic fluid have not been borne out in practice. Its use in obstetrics requires the use of a leucocyte depletion filter (Pall RS filter) to ensure effective removal of all elements of amniotic fluid. If the mother is Rhesus negative there is a potential for fetal red cell exposure, and a Kleihauer test should be performed within 72h and an appropriate calculated dose of anti-D given.

Platelets

- Platelets are stored in the transfusion centre, not necessarily at your hospital blood bank—anticipate the need for platelets early and liaise with the haematologist.
- Maintain platelet count above 50×10^9. A fall to this level is typical of a two blood volume replacement, or sooner if there is DIC.
- Start with 1 adult therapeutic dose = 4 units, for every 4 units of transfused red cells.
- Very low platelet counts are associated with abruption, and early recognition and aggressive treatment is required.

FFP and cryoprecipitate

- In the event of massive, uncontrolled haemorrhage, blood products should be given on clinical grounds rather than awaiting laboratory results.
- Give 4 units of FFP for every 4 units of red cells transfused if ongoing bleeding.
- Check coagulation screen frequently depending on the clinical situation and after each intervention.
- Keep APTT and PT <1.5 × normal (indicates <25% activity and usually seen after 200% blood volume replacement).
- Conventional FFP dose is 15–20mL/kg, i.e. average adult dose is 4–6 units; 2 unit doses are ineffective. Recent studies suggest that 30mL/kg is needed to increase coagulation factors reliably above 30%.
- Aim to keep the fibrinogen level >1g/L (a fall to this level is typical at 150% blood volume replacement). FFP is fibrinogen deplete, and cryoprecipitate (5 unit pools) may be required as an adjunct to FFP.
- Normothermia is essential for haemostasis, therefore IV fluid warmers and surface warming devices, e.g. Bair Hugger®, are essential.

Fibrinogen concentrate

- Is an ultrapurified concentrate of fibrinogen made from pooled blood donation.
- It can be useful when given with the other coagulation factors in FFP to raise rapidly a low fibrinogen <0.5g/L seen typically in DIC and abruption.

Recombinant factor VIIa

- New models of coagulation emphasize the interaction of tissue factor and factor VIIa in initiation, amplification, propagation and localization of fibrin clot.
- This reaction bypasses all the other 'classical' coagulation cascade elements and generates thrombin on the platelets at the site of bleeding.
- Recombinant factor VIIa is genetically engineered from hamster kidney cells using human factor 7 gene.
- Given by bolus IV injection over 5–10min, 2h half-life, dose 90 micrograms/kg. It costs £4000 for each dose in a 70kg adult, repeated every 2–3h. Individual hospitals will usually have guidelines for authorization.
- It is currently only licensed for use in patients with haemophilia, but there is much interest currently in off-licence use for many forms of haemorrhage, including obstetric, with many anecdotal reports of impressive and rapid reduction in bleeding.
- More information from trials or registers is awaited.
- It is ineffective if the patient is acidotic or if insufficient coagulation products have been given. It is recommended that the fibrinogen level is corrected to >1g/L prior to administration.

Antifibrinolytics: drugs to inhibit clot lysis

Tranexamic acid

- Is an antifibrinolytic agent and can be given by slow IV injection at a dose of 0.5–1.0g.
- It competitively inhibits the conversion of plasminogen to plasmin, thereby preventing fibrin degradation and stabilizing clot formation.
- This agent has a place in arresting haemorrhage which is unresponsive to the above interventions.

Aprotonin

- Is a polypeptide proteolytic enzyme inhibitor extracted from cow lung.
- It acts on plasmin and kallikrein and slows fibrinolysis; however, it has a high incidence of anaphylaxis (1 in 200) and has been the subject of a recent (October 2006) FDA warning about significant renal and cardiovascular toxicity.
- Although found in most textbooks, aprotonin has limited application in practice.

If the equipment and expertise is available, there is a role for global tests of coagulation, e.g. thromboelastography (TEG). This can be near-patient testing or laboratory based.

New innovations

If the uterus remains atonic and bleeding continues after initial measures, specialist techniques and innovative therapies are now appropriate. The early use of physical methods to control ongoing bleeding, especially if only partially or unresponsive to uterotonics, is changing the management of major obstetric haemorrhage and reduces the side effects associated with the overuse of uterotonics. In the past, hysterectomy would be the definitive life-saving treatment and, whilst this may still be appropriate in some cases, effective alternatives are now available with which the anaesthetist needs to be familiar.

Balloon tamponade of uterus

- Hydrostatic balloons can be used within the uterine cavity to control haemorrhage, for both atony and placenta accreta.
- The Rusch balloon can be inflated with 600mL of saline and left in situ for 48h, then gradually deflated over several hours.
- A Senstaken balloon for oesophageal varices and even a condom have been used with success in this situation.
- The uterus can also be packed with gauze, but this requires a more traumatic removal. A Penrose drain may facilitate easy removal without the need for re-opening the abdomen.

B-Lynch brace suture

- This is a surgical technique of 'folding' the atonic uterus down on itself to provide compression haemostasis. In the CEMACH 2000–2002 report, there were no deaths in patients in whom this had been used, and obstetricians should familiarize themselves with the technique and be prepared to ask for help if they are unfamiliar with its use.
- The use of the B-Lynch suture can avoid the need for hysterectomy, and there are reports of successful pregnancies after its use.

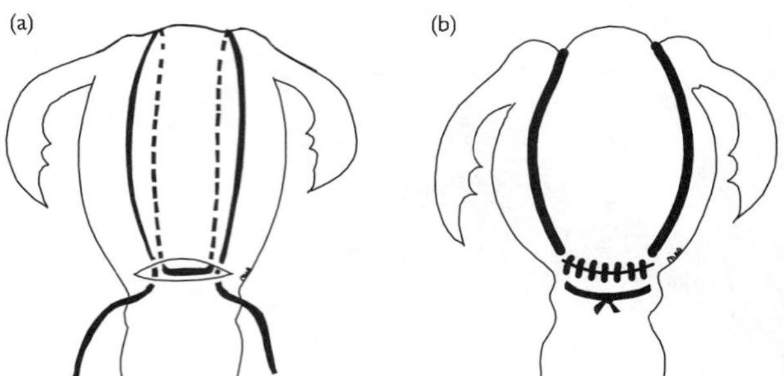

Fig. 16.1 B-Lynch suture. (a) A single suture is inserted as shown. (b) As it is drawn tight, the fundus of the uterus is compressed against the lower segment. The uterus is now physically unable to relax.

Other surgical techniques

Bilateral internal iliac artery ligation

- This is reported as successful in 50% of cases of atony and placenta accreta. The complications include ligation of external iliac artery, trauma to iliac veins, ureteric injury and retroperitoneal haematoma.

Bilateral uterine artery ligation

- This is reported as successful in 95% of cases. Various stepwise uterine devascularizations have also been described.

Temporary aortic compression/clamping

- This may be useful as a temporary measure while awaiting specialized help.

Interventional radiology

- If the bleeding is coming from one or more discrete vascular sites, the feeder artery can be catheterized (access usually being obtained via the femoral artery) and embolized with absorbable gelatin foam. The bleeding point is identified by prior contrast injection, and the foam is reabsorbed within 10 days.
- As with the B-Lynch suture, there were no deaths in the CEMACH 2000–2002 report in those major haemorrhage patients treated with this new technique.
- The problem lies with setting up the equipment. During a massive haemorrhage, the patient will be too unstable to move to the radiology suite, and there are technical difficulties with performing the procedure in theatre with the X-ray C-arm.
- At present, few units have the technology or expertise to perform this life-saving procedure, and consideration could be given to electively transferring very high risk cases to a unit that has such facilities.
- In such elective cases where haemorrhage is anticipated, the embolization catheters can be sited preoperatively.

Anaesthesia

The choice of anaesthesia must be left to the individual skill and experience of the anaesthetist.

General rules include

- If the mother does not already have a regional anaesthetic consider a GA if:
  - Haemorrhage is severe.
  - There is ongoing haemodynamic instability.
  - Diagnosis is uncertain.
- If there is a spinal or epidural *in situ* then it may safely be continued as automatically giving a GA may make haemodynamic instability worse.
- There are many case reports of caesarean hysterectomies performed solely under regional techniques.

Indications for converting a regional to a general anaesthetic are

- Maternal unconsciousness due to hypotension.
- Severe maternal anxiety.
- Inadequate anaesthesia, especially during prolonged surgery.

Continuing care

The mother who has suffered a major haemorrhage must be cared for afterwards in an appropriate environment. Once haemostasis is achieved, the patient should be transferred to an appropriate ITU/HDU setting for further management. Maternal deaths have been attributed to substandard care in the postpartum period.

- All mothers where the bleeding has been estimated >1500mL should be admitted to an HDU environment, even if apparently stable.
- The length of time on HDU will depend on haemodynamic stability over the first 6h after delivery.
- Observations should be made on an HDU chart with frequent measurments of BP and pulse, urine output, respiratory rate and fluid balance.
- In all settings, there must be close ongoing liaison between obstetricians, obstetric anaesthetist and ICU/HDU staff.
- Regular Hb and coagulation studies will need to be performed every 4–6h if received transfusion >8 units of packed RBCs.

Indications for transfer for ventilation in an ICU

- Ongoing bleeding—especially if associated with coagulopathy.
- Hypothermia.
- Severe oliguria/anuria.
- Evidence of pulmonary oedema or increased oxygen requirements.
- Poorly corrected metabolic acidosis with an increased lactate.

Review

- Cases of major haemorrhage should be reported to the local hospital critical incident reporting system.
- All staff involved should ideally conduct a 'rapid review' of the case within 48h to examine the effectiveness of the systems involved, to define lessons learned and to organize/provide counselling as necessary in the event of a bad outcome.
- A review of the causes and management of the haemorrhage should be made at the local critical incident meeting.
- Maternal deaths should be reported to the National Patient Safety Agency and CEMACH in due course.

Further reading

Lancet Maternal Survival Series Steering Group. Maternal mortality: who, when, where, and why (Review). *Lancet* 2006; **368**: 1189–1200.

Waterstome M *et al*. Incidence and predictors of severe obstetric morbidity: case–control study. *British Medical Journal* 2001; **322**: 1089–1093.

O'Rourke N *et al*. Cesarean delivery in the interventional radiology suite: a novel approach to obstetric hemostasis. *Anesthesia and Analgesia* 2007; **104**: 1193–1194.

Haynes J *et al*. Use of recombinant activated factor VII in massive obstetric haemorrhage. *International Journal of Obstetric Anesthesia* 2007; **16**: 40–49.

Allam MS, B-Lynch C. The B-Lynch and other uterine compression suture techniques. *International Journal of Gynecol and Obstet* 2005; **89**: 236–241.

Catling S, Joels L. Cell salvage in obstetrics: the time has come. *British Journal of Obstetrics and Gynaecology* 2005; **112**: 131–132.

Add SC reference July IJOA.

Catling S. Blood conservation techniques in obstetrics: a UK perspective. *International Journal of Obstetric Anaesthetic* 2007; **16**:241–249.

Chapter 17

Pre-eclampsia

Stuart Davies and Hywel Roberts

Introduction

- Overall, pre-eclampsia is the second most common cause of maternal deaths in developed countries, causing 7.5 deaths per million maternities.
- Deaths from severe pre-eclampsia are most commonly caused by cerebral haemorrhage and pulmonary oedema/respiratory failure. The incidence of cerebral haemorrhage seems to have fallen with improved BP control in recent years. Hepatic rupture/haematoma, HELLP syndrome and eclampsia also cause deaths. ARF is a serious complication, but in itself does not cause death.
- Substandard care has been identified as a contributing factor in many of these deaths. It is hoped that increased emphasis on screening, early diagnosis, early involvement of senior clinical staff and increasing use of management protocols will reduce the number of deaths still further.
- Pre-eclampsia in the developing world is rarely diagnosed early, and as many as 50 000 deaths a year are attributable to eclampsia alone.
- Placental abruption/haemorrhage, fetal IUGR and risk of early delivery cause increased perinatal morbidity and mortality.

Classification and diagnosis of hypertensive disorders in pregnancy

Pre-eclampsia (PET) is a multisystem disorder occurring exclusively after the 20th week of pregnancy and affecting up to 8% of all pregnancies. It is one diagnosis that forms part of the spectrum of hypertensive disorders of pregnancy. It can be separate from other hypertensive disorders or overlap with them, as some women with other causes of hypertension are much more likely to develop pre-eclampsia.

Hypertension in pregnancy is defined as a manual BP reading >140mmHg systolic and/or 90mmHg diastolic (using Korotkoff phase V) on two consecutive occasions >4h apart or one BP reading of ≥110mmHg diastolic. Most automated BP monitors underestimate BP, and a high index of suspicion should lead to manual checking with an appropriate size cuff.

Classification of hypertensive disorders of pregnancy

Pre-existing/chronic hypertension
Occurs in 5% of pregnancies.

Hypertension diagnosed before pregnancy or before 20 weeks gestation.
- ***Essential***—no underlying cause.
- ***Secondary***—associated with disease.

Chronic hypertension is associated with an increased risk of PET (25%).

Pre-eclampsia/pregnancy-associated hypertension
Occurs in 12% of pregnancies.
Hypertension diagnosed after 20 weeks gestation with a normal booking BP.
- Gestational hypertension/PIH—no proteinuria or other features of PET.
- Pre-eclampsia—hypertension with at least 300mg proteinuria in 24h (or at least 2+ on urine dipstick testing).

Risk factors for PET

- First pregnancy or >10yrs since previous pregnancy: 10 × increase.
- New paternity multigravida pregnancy: 10 × increase.
- Previous PET requiring early delivery: 20% chance.
- Family history of PET (1st-degree female relatives): 4–8 × increase.
- Partner previously fathered an affected pregnancy: 2 × increase.
- Age >40 years.
- BMI >35 at 'booking': 4 × increase.
- An increase in BMI between pregnancies.
- Chronic hypertension (BP >140 systolic at 'booking'): 20% chance.

- Multiple pregnancy: 2 × increase.
- Hydropic fetus.
- Associated medical conditions.
  - Diabetes mellitus.
  - Renal disease.
  - Antiphospholipid syndrome and other connective tissue disorders.

Doppler assessment

- Early identification of the high risk pregnancy can be performed using Doppler assessment of the uteroplacental circulation.
- By 20 weeks gestation a normal pregnancy should develop a low resistance Doppler wave form.
- In a low risk population at 20 weeks gestation, 20% of pregnancies will go on to develop pre-eclampsia if a low resistance circulation has not developed.

Diagnosis

- The three features of pre-eclampsia, increased BP, proteinuria and oedema, are important in the diagnosis.
- Hypertension or proteinuria may be mild but the disease severe.
- Pre-eclampsia may manifest itself almost entirely as severe IUGR.
- The diagnosis of HELLP (haemolytic anaemia, elevated liver enzymes and low platelets), which is thought to be part of the spectrum of pre-eclampsia, can be associated with no proteinuria and normal blood pressure.
- Many cases of eclampsia occur with no previous recordings of raised BP.
- Other surrogate markers of pre-eclampsia such as a raised uric acid and haematocrit rarely help other than to confirm the diagnosis if hypertension and proteinuria are already present.
- Uric acid can be normal in severe pre-eclampsia.

Pathophysiology of pre-eclampsia

- The exact cause of pre-eclampsia is unknown, but it appears to be a multisystem disorder mediated by widespread endothelial cell dysfunction. Inadequate placentation seems to trigger reduced placental blood flow. Sometimes there is overt placental insufficiency and fetal growth retardation.
- In younger women, there may be abnormal development of the placental vascular bed with failure of the normal invasion of the trophoblast by the spiral arteries.
- In older women, atherosclerotic vascular disease may be the cause of reduced placental blood flow, and a diagnosis of PET may indicate a higher risk of future cardiovascular events.
- Generally, the circulation is in a state of vasoconstriction, with intravascular hypovolaemia and abnormal capillary permeability.
- In addition, there may be activation of the coagulation cascade, platelet aggregation and fibrin deposition in blood vessels.

Cardiovascular changes

- Generalized vasoconstriction leads to increased SVR and hypertension (especially diastolic).
- Capillary permeability leads to redistribution of plasma into the interstitial space.
- Intravascular depletion and hypovolaemia occur as a consequence of the above.
- Peripheral oedema is seen due to:
  - Increased capillary permeability.
  - Hypoalbuminaemia, therefore reducing colloid oncotic pressure (COP).
  - Increased capillary hydrostatic pressure due to increased SVR and the effects of the gravid uterus.
- Pulmonary and cerebral oedema may occur in severe cases and can be life-threatening. Excessive administration of IV fluids, fluid shifts at delivery and LV dysfunction may contribute to their severity.

Respiratory changes

- Pulmonary oedema—seen more frequently postpartum.
- Increased lung water causes reduced lung compliance and increased work of breathing.
- Upper airway oedema—face, neck, tongue and larynx. Voice changes and difficult intubation are early changes, with stridor occurring late. The cricoid cartilage may be difficult to palpate.

Renal changes

- Endothelial damage leads to protein loss and decreased albumin/COP.
- Decreased glomerular filtration leads to increased serum uric acid, which is an indicator of disease severity.
- Tubular ischaemia secondary to vasoconstriction and hypovolaemia.
- ARF requiring dialysis is rare but is a serious prognostic indicator due to its association with severe disease.

Hepatic changes

- Oedema, haemorrhage and ischaemic necrosis of the liver.
- Raised aspartate aminotransferase (AST), alanine aminotransferase (ALT) and γ-glutamyltransferase (GGT)—rapidly rising titres are a poor prognostic sign (see HELLP syndrome, page 464).
- Liver capsule distension—may present with epigastric pain. This may cause a subcapsular hepatic haematoma or even hepatic rupture—both are life threatening.

CNS changes

- Cerebral oedema and raised ICP.
- Cerebral vasoconstriction.
- Cerebral ischaemia due to combination of the above factors—may precipitate eclamptic seizures.
- Cerebral haemorrhage secondary to hypertension.
- Variable neurological symptoms and signs—headache, vomiting, visual disturbance, confusion, decreased Glasgow Coma Score (GCS), hyper-reflexia and clonus.

Haematological changes

- Thromobocytopaenia.
- Haemolysis and anaemia.
- Coagulopathy—usually in severe disease with hepatic dysfunction.
- DIC is rare—usually in association with haemorrhage or placental abruption.

Fetoplacental unit

- IUGR is often seen.
- There is a significant risk of placental abruption.

Antenatal management of pre-eclampsia

Primary prevention

Several strategies show promise for reducing the incidence of PET:

- ***Low dose aspirin*** seems to reduce the risk of PET by ~19% overall. The NNT (number needed to treat) varies depending on the baseline risk from 69 (in low risk women) to 18 (in those 'at high risk' of PET). There also seems to be an associated reduction in fetal mortality.
- ***1g calcium per day*** as a dietary supplementation may reduce the incidence of PET—the benefit being greatest in those women with low dietary calcium.
- ***Antioxidants (vitamins C and E)*** have showed some promise, but may be associated with increased rates of preterm delivery.

Secondary prevention/preatment

- Oral antihypertensive drugs are used in the management of mild/moderate PET. There is good evidence that oral antihypertensives reduce the incidence of severe hypertension by up to 50%. Evidence that they improve any other outcome measures, e.g. hospital admission, progression of PET, CVA (cerebrovascular accident) or fetal outcomes, is unproven. There is no evidence that the commonly used antihypertensives worsen IUGR.
- Methyldopa is often used for the treatment of mild/moderate hypertension and has a long safety record. Drowsiness is a common side effect.
- Oral labetalol or calcium channel antagonists, e.g. nifedipine, are alternatives. There is no current evidence to suggest that any of these agents is superior to any other, but labetalol should be avoided in asthmatics and the babies once delivered are at increased risk of hypoglycaemia.
- Other β-blockers are not used in pregnancy due to concerns regarding IUGR.
- Diuretics are not recommended because of the associated intravascular depletion and risk of renal impairment.
- Angiotensin-converting enzyme (ACE) inhibitors and ACE receptor antagonists are contraindicated in pregnancy due to teratogenicity demonstrated in animal studies.
- Mother and fetus require frequent monitoring to assess disease progression.
- Early management of BP may extend the pregnancy to allow better fetal maturity.

Severe pre-eclampsia

Definitions vary, but ~5 per 1000 maternities have 'severe' PET in developed countries. It should be noted that no criterion detects all women with severe PET, as some women present with eclampsia and no prodromal symptoms. It is also possible to have severe PET with normal BP measurements. In these cases, the diagnosis should be made on grounds of clinical suspicion and probability.

Definition

- BP >170 systolic and/or >110 diastolic (confirmed on repeat measurement 4–6h later), associated with proteinuria >1g/L.
- Moderate PET (BP >140 systolic and/or >90 diastolic confirmed on repeat measurement and proteinuria >300mg in 24h) with ≥2 of the signs below:
  - Severe headache.
  - Visual disturbance.
  - Clonus (three or more beats).
  - Papilloedema.
  - Epigastric pain and/or vomiting.
  - Liver tenderness.
  - Platelet count $<100\times10^9$/L.
  - Abnormal LFTs (ALT/AST >70IU/L).
  - Features of HELLP syndrome (see below).

Eclampsia

- Eclampsia is defined as one or more convulsions superimposed on any degree of pre-eclampsia.
- It affects 5 per 10 000 maternities in the UK and is associated with ~2% mortality.

HELLP syndrome

This is a rare, severe form of PET characterized by rapid deterioration and the following features:

- **H**aemolysis.
- **E**levated **L**iver enzymes.
- **L**ow **P**latelets.

Management

General supportive measures

- Multidisciplinary management—senior obstetric, anaesthetic, midwifery and critical care staff, either managed in a high dependency area of delivery suite or in the Critical Care Unit.
- Maintain patent IV access at all times.
- Administer oral ranitidine 150mg 6hly if delivery imminent or there is risk of eclampsia.
- BP should be measured every 15–30min (or continuously by invasive arterial monitoring).

- Hourly oxygen saturations, HR and respiratory rate, and 4hly temperature should be documented.
- Accurate fluid balance recording is essential. Catheterization for accurate hourly urine measurement.
- Daily blood tests should include U&E, LFTs, serum calcium, phosphate and magnesium, serum uric acid, FBC and coagulation profile. Blood bank should hold a 'group and save' sample if delivery is imminent.
- More severe cases may require monitoring of blood tests more frequently than daily and may also require regular analysis of arterial blood samples. Placement of an arterial cannula should be considered to facilitate this sampling.
- Regular assessment of fetal well-being should be according to local protocols (CTG, Doppler, etc).

Control of blood pressure

- Acute antihypertensive treatment should be started in all women with BP >160 systolic, >125 mean or >110 diastolic to reduce the incidence of cerebral haemorrhage.
- Treatment may also be considered for women with lesser degrees of hypertension if there are other markers of 'severe' PET.
- BP should be measured by manual sphygmomanometry every 15min until stabilized and then every 30min. Non-invasive automatic BP monitoring should be compared periodically with manual sphygmomanometer measurement to assess its accuracy.

Oral treatment regimens

- Oral labetalol 200mg, repeat every 1–2h until BP controlled then 200mg TID to 300mg QDS maintenance.
- Nifedipine slow release preparation 10mg orally (NOT sublingually)—maintenance varying from 10mg BD to max 60mg/day in divided doses.
- Oral labetalol and nifedipine combined regimen.
- Methyldopa 250mg TID increased up to a maximum of 3g per day.

Intravenous treatment regimens

- Treatment should be overseen by senior anaesthetic and obstetric staff.
- IV antihypertensive treatment may be more appropriate than oral if the BP is very high (e.g. >180 systolic, 125 mean, 110 diastolic) or the patient is unable to take oral medication (unconscious, vomiting).
- CTG monitoring is mandatory predelivery.
- Consideration should be given to a bolus of 250mL colloid before initiation of IV antihypertensive therapy (depending on the patient's fluid status). There is some evidence that a fluid bolus may sometimes actually lower BP and good evidence that it reduces the incidence of hypotension on initiation of vasodilator therapy.
- The aim should be to lower MAP to <125mmHg.
- In general, IV treatment should be continued until the patient's condition improves after delivery.
- Continuous intra-arterial BP measurement is advisable.

In general, labetalol is the drug of choice. Hydralazine is an alternative if β-blockade is contraindicated or ineffective, but may cause FHR abnormalities.

- Labetalol—50mg slow IV bolus then infusion (500mg in 50mL)—60mg/h initially (6mL/h) doubled every 15min until control is reached or on 480mg/h (48mL/h) maximum.
- Hydralazine—give 250mL colloid bolus over 20min, then administer IV hydralazine 5mg over 20min. Wait at least 20min before repeating the dose as the drug has a relatively slow onset of action. Maximum of 4 bolus doses may be given. Once control is achieved, start infusion 50mg in 50mL, 1–5mL/h, titrated according to response.
- Oral nifedipine may be added (dose as above) as a second-line drug if required. Nifedipine's action may be synergistic with magnesium and so caution is advised with this combination.

Other antihypertensive drugs which may be added for resistant cases include GTN and sodium nitroprusside (SNP). The decision to commence additional treatment should be made by a senior anaesthetist or critical care specialist.

Magnesium sulphate

- May be beneficial to prevent eclampsia in the most severe cases of pre-eclampsia.
- The incidence of eclampsia is 1% without magnesium.
- Magnesium sulphate has been shown to reduce this by 50%.
- Its use is generally restricted to the most severe cases, with evidence of cerebral irritation and clonus.
- Care is required with its administration in the face of renal impairment.
- Magnesium sulphate should be used as first-line management if an eclamptic fit occurs.

Timing and mode of delivery

In all but the most urgent cases, the timing and mode of delivery should be carefully considered. The woman should be stable, fluid status should be optimized, high BP and seizures should be treated. The most senior staff available should be present in unstable cases, and special care provision should be available for the baby. Delivery during normal 'working' hours is preferred.

Before 34 weeks gestation

- Women should receive corticosteroids to aid fetal lung maturity if delivery is anticipated before 34 weeks gestation. Where possible, delivery should be delayed for 24–48h after administration of corticosteroids. It may be necessary to re-assess the risks/benefits of delivering the baby after this period.
- Before 24 weeks gestation, survival of the baby is unlikely, and delivery is considered only if necessary to save the mother's life.
- Between 24 and 34 weeks, the chances of survival increase steadily, although there is a significant risk of disability before 28 weeks.
- The evidence currently does not exist to support either an 'Expectant' or 'Interventionist' strategy before 34 weeks, and so a clinical decision based on individual risks vs benefit will have to be made.
- Delivery before 34 weeks would usually be by CS.

After 34 weeks gestation

- Survival of the baby approaches 100% and delivery is curative for the pre-eclampsia (although it may take a few days to resolve and symptoms often worsen immediately after delivery).
- Most women with severe PET after 34 weeks gestation should therefore be delivered as soon as their clinical condition allows.
- A trial of labour may be warranted if the condition of the cervix is such that induction of labour could be successful and the fetal condition and presentation are satisfactory.
- A CS will be required otherwise.

Fluid balance

General principles

- Excessive fluid administration is harmful in severe pre-eclampsia, and causes worsening pulmonary and cerebral oedema.
- Fluid restriction has been shown to be safe in severe pre-eclampsia, and fluid intake should generally be limited to 1mL/kg/h—administered through an infusion pump to avoid accidental overinfusion.
- Fluid restriction should be continued until resolution of the illness causes a spontaneous diuresis.
- Fluid intake and output must be carefully recorded and, for this purpose, an indwelling urinary catheter is required. In general, a urine output of >0.5mL/kg/h is satisfactory.
- Oxygen saturations should be monitored regularly for the onset of pulmonary oedema (<94% on air is a worrying sign), and any changes in neurological state should raise the suspicion of cerebral oedema.
- ARF requiring renal replacement therapy (RRT) is an uncommon complication of pre-eclampsia alone but confers a high mortality due to its association with severe disease and haemorrhage. Most cases of ARF in pre-eclampsia are associated with haemorrhage.
- The risk of ARF is higher if there is pre-existing chronic renal impairment or if NSAIDs are used.
- Fluid balance is particularly difficult in a patient who has concurrent blood loss.
- Volume replacement without excess should be aimed for, but this is often easier said than done—particularly if the haemorrhage is severe.
- Good clinical judgement by an experienced team, possibly supplemented by invasive monitoring, is important.

CVP measurements

- Can aid fluid balance management in severe disease associated with oliguria.
- Is most helpful when pre-eclampsia is complicated by haemorrhage.
- May be unreliable, and pre-eclamptic patients can develop pulmonary oedema with a normal or low CVP measurement.
- Changes in CVP readings, rather than absolute values, are more important.

Diuretic administration

- Does not alter the outcome or progression of the disease.
- Many pre-eclamptic patients will produce a diuresis after IV furosemide 20mg.
- Diuretics can therefore be useful in the overall management of fluid balance.
- A progressively positive fluid balance is associated with pulmonary oedema, and diuretic administration when the mother is in 1500–2000mL positive balance can prevent this complication.

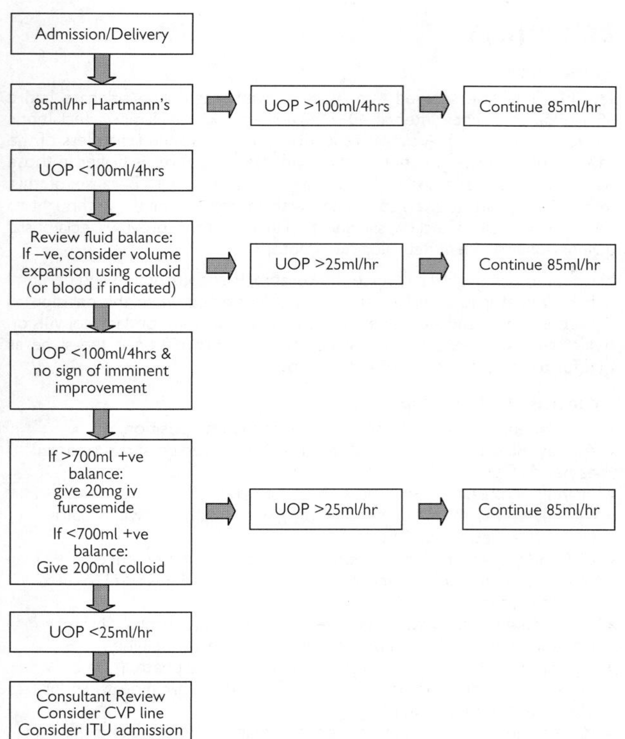

Fig. 17.1 Fluid balance in severe pre-eclampsia/eclampsia. UOP = urinary output.

Eclampsia

Prevention

The MAGPIE trial showed that women given magnesium sulphate had a 58% (95% conficence interval 40–71%) lower risk of eclampsia (eclamptic convulsions/seizures). A similar reduction in risk was seen regardless of the severity of pre-eclampsia but, as the incidence of seizures is higher in those with severe pre-eclampsia, the number NNT is lower. Because of this, magnesium is usually given to women with severe PET or those thought to be at higher risk of eclampsia due to family history, previous eclampsia/epilepsy or prominent neurological symptoms.

Magnesium is thought to reverse the cerebral vasoconstriction and cerebral ischaemia that lead to eclampsia. It is usually started when the decision to deliver is made and continued for 24h after delivery or last convulsion (whichever is the later). The regimen used for prevention is the same as that for treatment of eclampsia (see below).

Treatment of eclampsia

- The patient should be turned into the left lateral position.
- Airway, Breathing and Circulation should be assessed and supported as per ALS protocol.
- High flow oxygen by face mask should be given.
- Venous access should be secured (any size initially but will require large bore if going for CS).
- ECG/oxygen saturation/BP monitoring should be commenced.
- Blood sugar should be checked by finger prick and 25–50mL of 50% dextrose given if <5mmol/L.
- Fetal well-being should be assessed as soon as practical as this may influence the decision on proceeding to immediate delivery.
- The drug of choice for eclampsia is magnesium sulphate. (Use of IV diazepam has been associated with increased maternal death and is less effective than magnesium).
- Most eclamptic fits are short lived, and magnesium therapy is given to prevent a second fit.
- Contraindications to magnesium include
  - Hypersensitivity to magnesium.
  - Hepatic coma.
  - Severe renal failure.
  - Myasthaenia gravis.
  - Respiratory rate <14/min.
  - Absent/diminished tendon reflexes.
  - Caution with concurrent use of nifedipine or muscle relaxants.

Magnesium therapy

The usual doses of Mg^{2+} should be reduced (typically halved) in the presence of significant renal dysfunction, e.g. urinary output <100mL/4h or abnormal urea/creatinine.

Magnesium loading dose

For those women not on magnesium already.

- Give 4g IV over 5min.
- Draw up 10mL of 50% magnesium sulphate (5g) with 40mL of normal saline to give a total volume of 50mL. Give 40mL over 5–10min.

For those already on magnesium infusion.

- Take blood for urgent Mg^{2+} level then give extra 2g IV (20mL of above mixture) over 10min.

Signs of magnesium toxicity include

- Muscle weakness/respiratory depression.
- Absent tendon reflexes.

Severe toxicity may cause

- Muscle paralysis/respiratory arrest.
- Heart block/cardiac arrest.

- Regular checking of respiratory rate and maternal reflexes reliably detects toxicity in the majority of cases.
- Routine checking of serum magnesium level is no longer considered necessary, but serum magnesium should be checked if there are concerns regarding toxicity, in the presence of renal disease or if there are recurrent convulsions (when it may be subtherapeutic).

Absent tendon reflexes and respiratory rate <14/min are indications to stop the infusion and check serum magnesium level.

Treatment of suspected magnesium toxicity

- Support respiratory/cardiovascular systems as per ALS algorithm.
- Calcium gluconate 1g (10mL) over 10min should be given for signs of significant toxicity.
- The infusion should be restarted at half the previous rate once respiratory depression has resolved.

Other side effects of magnesium

- May potentiate the effects of depolarizing muscle relaxants.
- May prevent the appearance of fasciculation with suxamethonium (but no effect on subsequent myalgia).
- Magnesium may lower BP by vasodilation. Although sometimes useful, it is not routinely given for this purpose.
- Inhibition of uterine contraction.

Complications of eclampsia

- Failure to recover consciousness rapidly, recurrent convulsions, evidence of significant aspiration or the need for immediate CS are indications for intubation.
- Rapid sequence induction with thiopental and suxamethonium should be performed. Long-acting muscle relaxants may make diagnosis of recurrent seizures more difficult and should be used sparingly.
- Immediate delivery of the fetus should be considered if there are recurrent convulsions or fetal compromise.
- If convulsions are not recurrent and there is no fetal distress, it is usually best to control the seizures with magnesium and achieve cardiovascular stability before proceeding to delivery of the baby.

Intensive care management of severe pre-eclampsia

Admission to an ICU environment may be required for some women with severe pre-eclampsia. In all cases, delivery of the baby and control of haemorrhage/surgical complications take priority, and admission to the ICU should be for management of ongoing problems postdelivery.

- Indications for ICU admission postdelivery include:
  - Need for prolonged intubation/airway protection.
  - Decreased level of consciousness/cerebral oedema.
  - Need for ventilatory support, e.g. pulmonary oedema.
  - Difficult to control hypertension/cardiovascular instability.
  - Recurrent seizures.
  - ARF requiring RRT.
- Minimal haemodynamic monitoring in an ICU would include an arterial line (to facilitate regular blood sampling/arterial blood gas analysis) and a CVP line.
- A CVP $<$4mmHg may indicate need for fluid, whilst $>$6mmHg is associated with an increased risk of pulmonary oedema.
- More advanced monitoring in an ICU environment might include invasive haemodynamic monitoring, e.g. PAFC, PICCO, LIDCO or oesophageal Doppler.
- Pulmonary oedema, if severe, may require intubation and ventilation. High FiO_2 and positive end-expiratory pressure (PEEP) may be required initially.
- ARF may require RRT, but subsequent chronic renal failure is very rare. Indications for RRT include hyperkalaemia, acidosis and fluid overload. It may be necessary to perform RRT without anticoagulation, depending on the clinical situation.
- Treatment of cerebral oedema is essentially supportive—intubation to protect the airway and standard neurointensive care measures to control raised ICP whilst fluid overload is treated.

Anaesthetic management of patients with pre-eclampsia

Labour

Women may present in labour and subsequently be found to have signs of pre-eclampsia—usually proteinuria and mild hypertension. Alternatively, some women diagnosed with pre-eclampsia may be assessed as suitable for induction of labour. In these women, treatment of hypertension and anaesthetic review should be undertaken prior to attempted induction of labour as their risk of CS is higher.

- All women with pre-eclampsia in labour should have antacid prophylaxis.
- Continuous CTG monitoring is recommended during labour.

Epidural analgesia

- Early epidural analgesia is recommended for most women with pre-eclampsia during labour to control surges in BP due to pain.
- Prior to insertion of epidural analgesia, coagulopathy should be excluded.
- A recent (<6h) platelet count should be available. If this is >100, there is no need to carry out further coagulation studies unless there is some other indication, e.g. cholestasis of pregnancy.
- A platelet count <70 is an absolute contraindication to regional blockade, and alternative analgesia should be provided, e.g. Entonox or IV PCA opioids.
- A platelet count between 70 and 100 should involve a 'risk/benefit' assessment for each individual patient by the most senior anaesthetist available. Formal coagulation tests should be checked as part of this assessment.
- Technique of insertion should be as usual, but excess fluid preloading should be avoided. It may be wise for the epidural to be sited by the most experienced person available.
- A poorly functioning epidural should not be accepted. The epidural should be working well enough such that the anaesthetist is confident to use it for either instrumental delivery or CS.
- ***Postdelivery***, before removing the epidural catheter:
  - Re-check the platelet count if a significant period of time has elapsed since the last count. This is especially important if the platelet count was low, or if it was falling rapidly preinsertion.
  - The same acceptable platelet counts should be applied to catheter removal as to epidural insertion.
  - If the platelet count is too low for safe removal, options are either to wait until recovery of the platelet count or give platelet transfusion if removal is urgent.

Caesarean section

- Ideally the patient should be fully preassessed, fasted and have received antacid prophylaxis.
- The BP should be controlled, and up to date blood tests should be available.
- Magnesium prophylaxis should be started if necessary.
- Blood bank should have a recent blood sample. Cross-match may be indicated.
- In the urgent situation, some or all of this preparation may not be possible.
- Large-bore venous access is mandatory, but excess fluid administration should be carefully avoided. Use of colloid solutions may limit the amount of fluid required intraoperatively.
- Need for invasive haemodynamic monitoring should be assessed on a 'case by case' basis, but an arterial line can be very useful and there should be a low threshold for its insertion.
- NSAIDs for postoperative analgesia should be avoided in moderate/ severe PET as it tends to cause oliguria and may increase the risk of ARF.
- Standard DVT prophylaxis should be provided postoperatively unless contraindicated, e.g. bleeding, platelet count <100.

Regional anaesthesia

- Regional anaesthesia is preferable to GA if it can be safely performed.
- Regional anaesthesia is NOT contraindicated after an eclamptic fit if the mother has regained consciousness.
- As well as the usual contraindications, a recent platelet count should be available. If this is >100 then there is no need to carry out further coagulation studies unless there is some other indication, e.g. cholestasis of pregnancy.
- A platelet count <70 is a contraindication to regional blockade and a GA will usually be required. A platelet count between 70 and 100 should involve a 'risk/benefit' assessment for each individual patient by the most senior anaesthetist available. Formal coagulation tests should be checked as part of this assessment if time allows.
- Fluid preloading should be minimized—consider use of colloid.
- 'Prophylactic' vasopressors should either not be used or used with extreme caution.

Spinal anaesthesia

- Spinal anaesthesia has the advantage of simplicity, familiarity and usually gives a better quality of block than epidural anaesthesia.
- There has been concern that a sudden vasodilation due to spinal anaesthesia might cause significant hypotension in some patients. In practice this is rarely seen, and most patients with pre-eclampsia tend to have less hypotension than other patients. Where seen, hypotension must be carefully treated—restoring similar BP to prespinal levels while avoiding hypertension.
- Response to vasopressors may be exaggerated in patients with pre-eclampsia so they should be used sparingly.
- The usual doses of LAs/opiates should be used for spinal anaesthesia in pre-eclampsia.

Epidural anaesthesia

- Epidural anaesthesia has been the traditional, preferred technique for CS in pre-eclampsia. However, spinal anaesthesia or a CSE technique have proven to be safe.
- Any BP changes are likely to be more gradual than with spinal anaesthesia.
- The catheter may already be *in situ* if the patient has been labouring, and the block can be extended if the operation becomes prolonged.
- 'Top-ups' should be with the usual agents with which the user is familiar, but they should be given cautiously with full monitoring (including CTG) in theatre.
- Continuation of epidural analgesia into the postoperative period may aid analgesia and BP control.
- Drawbacks of epidural anaesthesia include greater technical difficulty, slower onset of block and sometimes a less satisfactory block. Poor blocks are associated with severe peripheral oedema.

Combined spinal–epidural

- The CSE technique uses a low dose spinal anaesthetic 'topped-up' with subsequent epidural injections.
- It potentially combines a relatively rapid, predictable block with minimal cardiovascular derangement and the ability to extend the block if required, including use for postoperative analgesia.
- Its main disadvantage is its greater technical difficulty, and it should not be attempted unless the operator is familiar with the technique.

General anaesthesia

GA for CS in pre-eclampsia may be required if:

- Immediate delivery is required—life of mother or fetus at risk.
- There is thrombocytopenia/abnormal coagulation (or need for urgent CS before blood test results available).
- Poorly controlled convulsions.
- Severe haemorrhage/high risk of haemorrhage.
- Patient refuses regional anaesthesia.
- Technical failure of regional anaesthesia.
- Other contraindication, e.g. aortic stenosis, sepsis.

Management of general anaesthesia

- A senior anaesthetist should be available.
- BP and convulsions should be as well controlled as time allows.
- Large-bore venous access is mandatory and invasive monitoring may be required.
- Careful airway assessment is mandatory—voice changes/hoarseness/stridor should alert to the possibility of laryngeal oedema.
- If present, stridor should be treated with 0.2mg/kg dexamethasone IV and 5mg nebulized adrenaline prior to intubation. Fibreoptic intubation should be considered.

- A smaller tracheal tube than usual may be necessary. It may be wise to keep the patient intubated at the end of the procedure until the swelling subsides and there is a 'leak' around the endotracheal tube.
- Lesser degrees of pharyngeal oedema may still increase the risks of failed intubation.
- Careful preoxygenation followed by a modified rapid sequence induction is the most common technique.
- A short-acting opiate (e.g. alfentanil 10–20 micrograms/kg) is recommended before induction to reduce the hypertensive response or tachycardia related to laryngoscopy and intubation. If opiates are used prior to delivery of the baby, the neonatal team should be informed.
- Other agents that have been used to control BP during induction are labetalol and magnesium sulphate.
- Induction with thiopental 3–5mg/kg—a slightly lower dose than usual being required due to the concurrent administration of opiates. Muscle relaxation is achieved with suxamethonium 1–1.5mg/kg.
- It should be noted that muscle fasciculation may not be seen following suxamethonium, especially if the patient is on magnesium. Magnesium may also prolong the effects of non-depolarizing muscle relaxants.
- Anaesthesia is maintained with the usual agents in usual doses. Cardiovascular system stability should be maintained and paO_2 and $paCO_2$ kept within the normal range.
- Intraoperative control of BP may be achieved with volatile anaesthetics and/or IV labetalol/hydralazine.
- Any concurrent pulmonary oedema may make ventilation/oxygenation more difficult. PEEP/high FiO_2 may be required.
- Control of convulsions, level of consciousness, condition of the airway, FiO_2 requirement and concurrent factors, e.g. haemorrhage, will dictate whether the patient is extubated at the end of the procedure or transferred to ITU.
- Where possible, the patient should be extubated at the end of surgery.

Further reading

Dyer RA *et al.* The role of the anaesthetist in the management of the pre-eclamptic patient. *Current Opinion in Anaesthesiology* 2007; **20**: 168–174.

Dyer RA *et al.* Prospective, randomized trial comparing general with spinal anesthesia for cesarean delivery in preeclamptic patients with a nonreassuring fetal heart trace. *Anesthesiology* 2003; **99**: 561–569.

Altman D *et al.* Do women with pre-eclampsia, and their babies, benefit from magnesium sulphate? The Magpie Trial: a randomised placebo-controlled trial. *Lancet* 2002; **359**: 1877–1890.

CLASP (Collaborative Low-dose Aspirin Study in Pregnancy) Collaborative Group. CLASP: a randomised trial of low-dose aspirin for the prevention and treatment of pre-eclampsia among 9364 pregnant women. *Lancet* 1994; **343**: 619–629.

Poston L *et al.* Vitamin C and vitamin E in pregnant women at risk for pre-eclampsia (VIP trial): randomised placebo-controlled trial. *Lancet* 2006; **367**: 1145–1154.

Aya AG *et al.* Spinal anesthesia-induced hypotension: a risk comparison between patients with severe preeclampsia and healthy women undergoing preterm cesarean delivery. *Anesthesia and Analgesia* 2005; **101**: 869–875.

Visalyaputra S *et al.* Spinal versus epidural anesthesia for cesarean delivery in severe preeclampsia: a prospective randomized, multicenter study. *Anesthesia and Analgesia* 2005; **101**: 862–868.

Embolic disease

Stuart Davies, Kath Eggers, Karthikeyan Chelliah and Stephen Stamatakis

Venous thromboembolism

Pregnancy is a prothrombotic state, therefore the incidence of DVT and pulmonary embolism (PE) is increased during both the antenatal and postnatal periods.

- The CEMACH 2003–2005 report confirms that PE is the leading cause of direct maternal deaths.
- There were 41 deaths reported in 2003–2005, giving a calculated incidence of 1.94 per 100 000 maternities.
- PE can occur during the antenatal, peripartum or postpartum period.
- There is a higher incidence of PE and consequently death following an untreated DVT than a treated DVT.

Risk factors

In the 19th century Virchow identified a triad of risk factors for venous thromboembolism:

- Venous stasis.
- Injury to the blood vessel intima.
- Changes in the coagulation properties of blood.

Many of the important risk factors related to pregnancy are based on the above triad:

- Pregnancy itself increases the risk 5-fold.
- Mothers aged >40yrs are at very high risk.
- Increasing parity.
- Caesarean section.
- Family history.
- Obesity.
- Hypertensive disease of pregnancy.
- Immobility.
- Dehydration.
- Haematological conditions, e.g. antithrombin deficiency, protein C and S deficiency.
- Long-distance travel.

Clinical presentation

- Presentation varies from progressive dyspnoea to sudden cardiovascular collapse.
- The symptoms can be non-specific, so a high index of suspicion is required, particularly when a patient has risk factors.

Symptoms

- The most common symptoms are dyspnoea, pleuritic chest pain and haemoptysis.
- Patients can be asymptomatic or have an atypical presentation.
- Other symptoms are cough, leg pain and back pain.
- In massive PE, central chest pain, convulsions and cardiac arrest can occur.

Signs

- Tachycardia and crepitations on chest auscultation may be the only findings.
- Look for signs of a DVT (more commonly in the right leg).
- In a massive PE, evidence of right heart failure can occur. Look for features such as jugular venous distension, an enlarged liver and parasternal heave.

Differential diagnosis

- Differential diagnoses are extensive.
- Consider all the causes for chest pain and dyspnoea, including myocardial infarction, myocarditis, pericarditis, pneumonia, pleuritis and musculoskeletal pain.

Investigations

- Investigations in PE are crucial, because clinical assessment alone is unreliable.
- Failure to diagnose PE is associated with high mortality, but incorrect diagnosis of the condition unnecessarily exposes the patient to the risks of anticoagulant therapy.
- There is no single test which has a high sensitivity and specificity to diagnose PE.
- A combination of tests according to the clinical features will increase the sensitivity and specificity.

Blood tests

- D-dimer is formed when cross-linked fibrin within the thrombus is lysed by plasmin. Elevated levels usually occur with PE.
- However, because elevations of D-dimer can occur in other conditions, e.g. liver disease, infection, postoperative period, it has a low positive predictive value.
- A negative result can help to exclude PE.

Arterial blood gas

- Hypoxaemia with normal or low $PaCO_2$ may occur.
- Normal blood gases do not exclude even a major PE.

ECG

- May be normal, but sinus tachycardia and non-specific ST segment and T wave changes are the most common findings.
- Right axis deviation, RBBB, S1 Q3 T3 pattern are rare.

Chest X-ray

- Findings are often non-specific.
- Atelectasis, collapse, consolidation, focal infiltrates and raised hemidiaphragm may occur. Wedge-shaped infarction is rare.
- The radiation risk to the fetus is minimal.

Bilateral duplex Doppler ultrasonography of legs

- Should be done in all suspected cases of DVT, including calf, thigh and groin regions.

Ventilation/perfusion (V/Q) scan

- This is a useful test with minimal radiation exposure risk.
- V/Q scans detect areas of lung that are ventilated but not perfused, as occurs in PE.
- The results are reported as normal, low, intermediate or high probability of PE based on patterns of V/Q mismatch. A completely normal scan can essentially exclude PE, but a high probability scan provides enough evidence of PE in those patients with a high clinical suspicion.
- Perfusion deficits may occur in many other lung conditions such as pleural effusion, chest mass, pulmonary hypertension, pneumonia, and COPD (chronic obstructive pulmonary disease).

Echocardiogram

- Echocardiogram is a very useful non-invasive bedside test, which may reveal a large PE demonstrated by RV dysfunction.

Pulmonary angiography

- This is the gold standard test, but it is an invasive test with high radiation exposure and can be difficult to interpret. An arteriogram with intraluminal filling defects or abrupt cut-off to flow is a positive result.
- It is useful in intermediate or low probability V/Q scans in patients with a high clinical suspicion.
- The use of non-invasive spiral CT and MRI has superseded the use of pulmonary angiography.

Spiral/helical CT

- Traditional CT is not suitable for evaluating PE, because it is difficult to opacify the pulmonary arteries with contrast for the time required to complete imaging (~3min). A spiral CT image can be completed within a single breath hold (~20s).
- Other advantages are: it is non-invasive, readily available and easy to perform.

CT pulmonary angiography (CTPA)

- CT with radiocontrast is effectively a pulmonary angiogram imaged by CT. It is increasingly used as the mainstay in diagnosis.
- Whereas the V/Q scan displays the secondary effect of the PE on the pulmonary vasculature, CTPA actually visualizes the clot.
- Other advantages include better availability, cost-effectiveness, identification of alternative diagnoses, and the ability to image pelvic and lower extremity veins in the same study.
- The disadvantages are a large contrast load and a high radiation dose.

MRI

- A useful tool to evaluate the pulmonary arteries and diagnose PE.
- It avoids exposure to radiation and radiographic contrast.
- It is also useful in identifying an alternative diagnosis.

Management

Supportive therapy

- Ensure adequate Airway (100% oxygen), Breathing, Circulation.

Anticoagulation

- Anticoagulation should not be delayed while awaiting investigations in highly suggestive cases.
- Heparin is the drug of choice.
  - IV UFH, e.g. commence infusion at 1000U/h.
  - Aim for dose to ensure APTT 1.5–2.5 times the normal for the early treatment period and change to LMWH later.
  - Fractionated heparin or LMWH: has advantages over UFH. It has a high bioavailability, is longer acting, needs less monitoring and has fewer side effects.
  - DO NOT START LMWH if there is a possibility of early delivery as the effects of an anticoagulant dose is long lasting (24h) and difficult to reverse.

The Royal College of Obstetricians has published the following guidelines for antenatal prophylactic and therapeutic doses of LMWH.

Table 18.1 Prophylactic doses for venous thromboembolism

	Enoxaparin (100U/mg)	**Dalteparin**	**Tinzaparin**
Normal body weight	40mg daily	5000U daily	4500U daily
Body weight <50kg	20mg daily	2500U daily	3500U daily
Body weight >90kg*	40mg 12hly	5000U 12hly	4500U 12hly

* These doses apply to a woman who has a BMI of >30 kg/m^2 in early pregnancy.

Table 18.2 Therapeutic doses for venous thromboembolism

	Enoxaparin (100U/mg)	**Dalteparin**	**Tinzaparin**
Therapeutic dose	1mg/kg 12hly	90U/kg 12hly	90U/kg 12h*

* The manufacturer recommends 175U/kg once a day.

Therapeutic dosing should be monitoring against regularly anti-factor Xa assays to ensure the correct treatment dose.

WARFARIN is not preferred antenatally for venous thromboembolism because of unacceptable side effects for mother and fetus. It is useful in the postpartum period after initial heparin therapy.

For information on placement of regional techniques for women on anticoagulants, see p 180.

Other specific treatment options

- Thrombolysis.
- Pulmonary embolectomy.
- Vena cava filters for recurrent PE despite adequate anticoagulation.

These treatment options are indicated for the management of a major PE causing significant cardiovascular compromise. The decision to use such options will depend on individual patient assessment and multidisciplinary team discussion.

Thrombolysis therapy

- Has been described in pregnancy.
- Is not recommended except in extreme life-threatening collapse.
- Is associated with a very high risk of antepartum and postpartum haemorrhage, which can cause fetal demise and may significantly complicate the management of the collapsed parturient.

Pulmonary embolectomy

- Has been described as an open and percutanious procedure.
- May be life saving in the severely compromised parturient.
- Open procedures, especially associated with cardiac bypass, are associated with a very high incidence of fetal demise.

Further reading

Kher A *et al.* The management of thrombosis in pregnancy: role of low-molecular-weight heparin. *Thrombosis and Haemostasis* 2007; **97**: 505–513 (Review).

Scarsbrook AF, Gleeson FV. Investigating suspected pulmonary embolism in pregnancy. *British Medical Journal* 2007; **334**: 418–419 (Review).

Royal College of Obstetricians and Gynaecologists. Thromboembolic disease in pregnancy and the puerperium: acute management. Green top RCOG guidelines: www.rcog.org.uk.

Amniotic fluid embolus

Description

- AFE is a rare but devastating condition responsible for 17 maternal deaths in the CEMACH 2003–2005 report.
- Entry of amniotic fluid into the maternal pulmonary circulation causes profound effects upon gas exchange and haemodynamic status, frequently leading to cardiorespiratory arrest.
- Coagulopathy occurs within 30min, if the patient survives that long.
- The incidence is reported as between 1 in 8000 and 1 in 80 000 deliveries.
- Deterioration is rapid, with up to half of deaths within 1h of presentation.
- Early recognition is associated with improved survival.
- Mortality may be as high as 80%.

Aetiology

- May occur at any time during pregnancy, and has been described after termination of pregnancy, amniocentesis and immediately postdelivery.
- Risk factors include advanced maternal age, multiparity, trauma, precipitant labour or delivery of a large baby, obstructed labour, placental abruption and CS.
- The role of uterine stimulation as a cause or effect of AFE is uncertain; however, they appear to be associated with one another.

Pathophysiology

- An underlying mechanism of anaphylaxis has been proposed since fetal tissue can be found in the maternal circulation in asymptomatic individuals.
- Right heart failure occurs due to intense pulmonary vasoconstriction.
- LVF ensues, with pulmonary oedema, hypoxia and cardiorespiratory arrest.

Clinical features

- Presentation may be subtle in the first instance with premonitory symptoms, e.g. restlessness or altered behaviour followed by:
  - dyspnoea.
  - seizures.
  - cardiovascular collapse.
  - coagulopathy.
- Coagulopathy is severe with marked features of DIC. Severe haemorrhage is associated with the condition, and frequently is a major factor in maternal collapse and death.

Diagnosis

- Clinical: usually by exclusion.
- High index of suspicion with:
  - Severe hypoxia.
  - Collapse.
  - Coagulopathy (DIC).

- Laboratory: fetal squames may be aspirated from the pulmonary vasculature using a pulmonary artery flotation catheter, but this is not diagnostic of AFE.
- At postmortem: fetal elements (squames and lanugo hair) should be looked for in the pulmonary vasculature.

Differential diagnosis

Other causes of cardiorespiratory arrest
- Major haemorrhage.
- Pulmonary thromboembolism.
- Air embolus.
- Acute anaphylaxis.

Other causes of cardiac failure
- Acute coronary syndrome.
- Cardiomyopathy.

Other causes of altered neurological status
- Eclampsia.
- Local anaesthetic toxicity.
- Intracranial haemorrhage.

Management

- No specific therapy exists, with supportive care being the mainstay of treatment.
- Multidisciplinary involvement (senior obstetrician, anaesthetist, intensivist, haematologist).
- Supportive treatment: **A**irway, **B**reathing, **C**irculation.
- Cardiopulmonary resuscitation if required.
- Expedite delivery of the baby if appropriate.
- Invasive cardiovascular monitoring (arterial line, CVP monitoring).
- Treatment of cardiac failure.
- Treat haemorrhage and correct coagulopathy.
- Transfer to ITU for ongoing critical care.

Long-term sequelae

If the patient survives the insult of emboli and coagulopathy, long-term recovery may be complicated by neurological deficits.

AFE register

UK Obstetric Surveillance System (http://www.npeu.ox.ac.uk/UKOSS/) has established a voluntary database for all cases of suspected AFE. It aims to gather more information on the epidemiology of the disease. By comparing outcomes of different cases, it is hoped advances in management can be achieved.

Intraoperative blood cell salvage

Specific concerns regarding AFE have meant that blood cell salvage has traditionally not been routinely used in obstetric practice. The decision to employ the technique must be balanced against the risks associated with donor transfusion. From the clinical trials to date, it appears the risk remains theoretical since no cases of AFE or DIC have been associated with cell salvage when used with the appropriate filter.

Further reading

Tuffnell DJ. United kingdom amniotic fluid embolism register. *British Journal of Obstetrics and Gynaecology* 2005; **112**: 1625–1629.

NHS National Institute for Health and Clinical Excellence. Intraoperative cell salvage in obstetrics. November 2005. http://www.nice.org.uk/guidance/IPG144.

Moore J, Baldisseri MR. Amniotic fluid embolism (Review). *Critical Care Medicine* 2005; **33** (10 Suppl): S279–S285.

Venous air embolism

Description

- Massive air embolus is a rare phenomenon in obstetrics, but is potentially lethal.
- Has been described during CS, manual removal of placenta and termination of pregnancy.
- Air may be entrained into the uteroplacental veins, which form an open plexus during removal of the placenta.
- Minor air embolus is probably very common during CS, and showers of small bubbles can be seen using Doppler ultrasound in the vena cava during routine surgery.
- This observation is a possible explanation for the frequent maternal complaint of heaviness or tightness in the chest around the time of placental removal.
- Fluid administration sets also provide a route for air to enter the circulation.
- Symptoms may manifest after 0.5mL/kg/min of air has entered the circulation.

Pathophysiology

- A large bolus of air enters the RV and obstructs outflow into the pulmonary circulation.
- Smaller amounts of air can enter the pulmonary vasculature, with the development of pulmonary hypertension and subsequent RVF.

Clinical features

- Presentation will vary according to the rate and volume of air that enters the circulation.
- Clinical signs are a late indication of air embolism.
- Fluctuating symptoms of restlessness and dyspnoea are frequently seen as a prequel to a major collapse.
- In the awake patient, air embolism may present as severe chest pain, dyspnoea, haemoptysis or altered mental status.
- Clinical signs include cyanosis, tachypnoea, tachycardia, raised jugular venous pressure (JVP), hypotension, a 'millwheel' murmur on auscultation of the heart.
- If the patient is under a GA, consider the diagnosis if there is a sudden fall in end-tidal CO_2, accompanied by hypoxia and ECG abnormalities (e.g. tachydysrhythmias, AV block, acute ischaemic changes).
- Massive air embolism can present with cardiorespiratory arrest, usually in pulseless electrical activity (PEA).
- Paradoxical emboli can occur in patients with a PFO, causing neurological signs and cardiac symptoms.

Differential diagnosis

Respiratory distress

- Bronchospasm.
- Pneumothorax.
- Pulmonary oedema.

Other embolic phenomena

- Thromboebolism.
- AFE.

Primary cardiac event

- Acute coronary syndrome.
- Cardiomyopathy.

Other causes of PEA

- Consider the 4 Hs (Hypoxia, Hypovolaemia, Hyper/hypokalaemia, Hyperthermia) and 4Ts (Tension pneumothorax, Tamponade—cardiac, Toxins, Thrombosis—coronary or pulmonary)

Diagnosis

- Initially difficult as it is a rare cause of collapse in obstetrics. A high index of suspicion is required.
- Special monitoring to detect venous air embolism, e.g. transoesophageal echo, precordial Doppler, oesophageal stethoscope, is not routinely used in obstetric anaesthesia.
- If GA is employed, capnography will detect most clinically significant emboli.
- The final diagnosis is usually one of exclusion after the other two causes of embolic collapse have been investigated:
  - High right-sided pressures on echo and CVP.
  - Cardiovascular collapse.
  - No evidence of coagulopathy.
  - No evidence of thrombolic event from duplex Doppler scans, V/Q and CTPA.

Management (ABC approach)

- Airway: check for a patent airway.
- Breathing:
  - Stop nitrous oxide if administered (as this will expand intravascular gas) and administer 100% oxygen.
  - If the capnograph trace has suddenly changed, check for leaks or disconnection.
  - CPAP or PEEP has been proposed since the rise in mean intra-thoracic pressure will elevate CVP, in turn limiting the extent and progression of an air embolus.
- Circulation:
  - Flood the wound with saline and compress the open veins of the uterus.
  - Check all lines for the presence of air.
  - Give an IV fluid bolus and use vasopressor agents to raise the CVP.
  - Classical description is to aspirate air from the right ventricle using a CVP line with the patient in the left lateral position in a head-down tilt.
  - Cardiopulmonary resuscitation if there is cardiopulmonary arrest. The act of chest compression may help break up the bubbles of air, dispersing them into the pulmonary vasculature where they are absorbed.

Prevention

- Exteriorization of the uterus while suturing during CS is associated with an increased incidence.
- Avoid all air in IV lines and syringes. This is essential if patients are known to have a PFO.

Further reading

Webber S *et al.* Gas embolism in anaesthesia. *BJA CEPD Reviews* 2002: **2**: 53–57.

Lowenwirt IP *et al.* Nonfatal venous air embolism during cesarean section: a case report and review of the literature (Review). *Obstetrical and Gynecological Surveys* 1994; **49**: 72–76.

Fomg J *et al.* Precordial Doppler diagnosis of haemodynamically compromising air embolism during caesarean section. *Canadian Journal of Anaesthesia* 1990; **37**: 262–264.

Chapter 19

The collapsed and compromised parturient

Rachel Collis and Stuart Davies

Assessment of the critically ill mother

The critically ill obstetric patient poses many problems during clinical assessment and management:

- The physiological changes of pregnancy and the large physiological reserve in younger mothers can complicate clinical assessment. A high index of suspicion is required.
- Medical conditions might present differently during pregnancy and, not only may they complicate pregnancy, but also pregnancy may alter the disease state.
- Obstetric critical care involves simultaneous assessment and management of both mother and fetus, who have differing physiological profiles.
- The treatment of the mother will have an impact on the fetus in both the ante- and postnatal periods, but the treatment of the mother takes priority.
- Good communication and multidisciplinary management involving senior obstetricians, anaesthetists and intensive care specialists is essential.

The assessment of the critically ill mother should be similar to an assessment of any critical ill patient, with the following considerations regarding the differential diagnosis:

- **Specific pregnancy-related problems** e.g. haemorrhage, eclampsia, PE, AFE.
- **Non-pregnancy-related problems**, e.g. trauma, sepsis, and their ongoing effect and risks to the mother and fetus.

The **ABCDE** approach will help systematic assessment. Early warning scores should be used more often on obstetric wards, with modifications for the altered physiology of pregnancy.

- *A*: *Airway assessment*—the airway may pose difficulties due to anatomical, physiological or pathological changes, e.g. airway oedema due to pre-eclampsia.
- *B*: *Breathing*—100% oxygen should be administered, as there is decreased vital capacity and an increased oxygen requirement in pregnancy. Adequacy of ventilation should be assessed. Tachypnoea is an early sign of an underlying medical problem. Auscultate the chest for any added sounds, e.g. crepitations in pulmonary oedema secondary to pre-eclampsia.
- *C*: *Circulation*—assess capillary refill (normally <2s and usually shorter in pregnancy), colour, conscious level, JVP, urine output and also any evidence of concealed or overt haemorrhage. Check pulse and BP. Avoid aorto-caval compression. Establish large-bore IV access.
- *D*: *Disabilty*—dapid assessment of neurological status includes AVPU system (A alert, V response to vocal stimuli, P response to pain, U unresponsiveness), GCS and pupillary assessment.

Recommendations of CEMACH

Intensive care should start as soon as it is needed and does not need to wait for admission to an ICU. It is possible to provide the majority of immediate intensive care treatment in an obstetric theatre.

FBC, electrolyte measurement and coagulation should be tested on a regular basis.

- An arterial line should be inserted early. Blood gas analysis should be performed early, and a metabolic acidosis should always be investigated further. There is a normal increase in metabolic acidosis in pregnancy and labour, but this is not associated with a lactic acidosis. An acidotic pH with a metabolic acidosis is usually abnormal. Where indicated, fluids and inotropes should be started without delay.
- Consideration should be given to improved stabilization and elective intubation prior to transfer.

Transfer of the critically ill mother

The principles of transfer to intensive care of the critically ill mother are the same as that of any adult critically ill patient, but with additional specific issues related to pregnancy.

- Good multidisciplinary communication and planning is essential.
- Ensure ongoing treatment, e.g. fluids, antihypertensive drugs, are all continued during transfer.
- Avoid any aorto-caval compression in the antenatal patient and ensure monitoring of both the mother and the fetus during transit.
- Essential maternal monitoring should include ECG, pulse oximetry, BP and urine output.
- Consider invasive BP and CVP monitoring in any haemodynamically unstable patient, and end-tidal capnography is recommended in all ventilated patients.
- All the monitors and the ventilator should be checked for function and battery status prior to transfer.
- Check the oxygen cylinder is full prior to the transfer. For long journeys you may require more than one oxygen cylinder.
- Resuscitation equipment and drugs should be checked and ready for the transfer.
- Appropriate personnel, who are experienced and trained in transfer procedures should accompany the patient.
- Ensure notes and investigations go with the patient.

Further reading

Clutton-Brock T. Trends in intensive care. *CEMACH Why Mothers Die 2000–2002*. RCOG Press.

Association of Anaesthetists GB and Ireland. *Recommendations for the Safe Transfer of Patients with Brain Injury*. AAGBI Press, 2006.

Cardiac arrest

Maternal cardiorespiratory arrest is an uncommon event, occurring in ~1 in 30 000 pregnancies that are near term. Cardiorespiratory arrest or collapse in a parturient can be due to any cause that affects non-pregnant patients along with those specific to pregnancy. The initial diagnosis may be unclear and there may be a number of differential causes to consider.

Immediate resuscitative measures

- Position the patient in full left lateral, if patient has a CO.
- Administer 100% oxygen, using a tight-fitting mask.
- Establish IV access and administer a fluid bolus.
- Ascertain if there are any pre-existing medical conditions, e.g. cardiac disease.

Exclude all reversible causes

- 4Hs; hypoxaemia, hypovolaemia, hypo/hyperkalaemia, hypothermia.
- 4Ts; tension pneumothorax, tamponade, thromboembolism, toxic/ therapeutic disturbances.

Causes specific to or more common in pregnancy

- **Haemorrhage**
  - Obstetric haemorrhage can often be concealed, and usually young, fit parturients can appear cardiovascularly stable despite excessive ongoing bleeding. Always communicate your concerns to the obstetrician and ensure a senior obstetrician examines the patient.
  - Commence fluid resuscitation, using blood (O-negative or group-specific if necessary) and blood products early to prevent a significant coagulopathy.
  - For further management of obstetric haemorrhage, see p 433.
- **Thromboembolic disease**, including PE is more common in pregnancy due to the hypercoaguable pregnancy state.
  - Anticoagulate if history and examination suggestive of diagnosis.
  - CTPA is the diagnostic test of choice.
- **Amniotic fluid embolism**
  - Presents with acute hypotension proceeding to circulatory collapse, hypoxia, convulsions and coagulopathy, either during labour or at time of delivery.
  - Usually a diagnosis after all others have been excluded and often not confirmed until the postmortem.
- **Eclampsia**—for further management, see p 470.
- **Magnesium toxicity** should be considered in patients receiving magnesium therapy. It may be secondary to overdosage or reduced excretion resulting from renal impairment.
  - Treatment: stop magnesium infusion, give 10mL IV calcium gluconate 10% or 10mL IV calcium chloride 10%.

- **Anaesthetic related**:
  - Oesophageal intubation causing hypoxaemia. Always confirm endotracheal tube placement with end-tidal CO_2 monitoring. If in doubt, replace the endotracheal tube
  - Failed intubation and failed ventilation—commence failed intubation drill. See p 324.
  - Total or high spinal anaesthesia—high sensory block, profound hypotension, bradycardia may lead to reduced conscious level.
- **Systemic local anaesthetic toxicity**
  - Prodromal symptoms, e.g. perioral tingling, dizziness, tinnitus, followed by convulsions ± cardiovascular collapse.
  - IV lipid treatment for bupivacaine toxicity, 100mL of 20% Intralipid® is recommended.
- **Cardiac disease**
  - Patients with adult congenital heart disease, ischaemic heart disease or peripartum cardiomyopathy can decompensate rapidly.
  - Consider any past medical history, older mothers, smoker or presence of chest scars.
  - An echocardiogram should be considered an early investigation, e.g. to confirm a cardiac cause for pulmonary oedema.

Factors impeding resuscitation in pregnancy

- **A**irway—more difficult in pregnancy due to airway oedema, breasts impeding attempts at intubation.
- **B**reathing—ventilation more difficult due to reduced chest compliance. Mothers are less tolerant of apnoea, due to decreased FRC and increased metabolic demands, leading to rapid desaturation, with the risk of hypoxic brain damage.
- **C**irculation—aorto-caval compression dramatically reduces VR and CO. Positioning the mother in full left lateral is essential in the presence of some CO. However, in its absence effective chest compression is impossible in this position and therefore a compromise of 15–30° (see below) is used. There should be early consideration of emergency CS if early resuscitative measures are unsuccessful, as it is difficult to perform effective cardiopulmonary resuscitation (CPR) if the patient is not supine.

Management

- Be prepared to be the team leader.
- Call for senior help early including: obstetric, anaesthetic, paediatric and midwifery staff.

A systematic approach to the collapsed patient is required:

- **A**irway—assess and maintain patency.
- **B**reathing—ensure adequate ventilation with 100% oxygen.
- **C**irculation—establish large-bore IV access.
- **D**isability—assess neurological status, e.g. in head injury.
- Assess fetus—may need immediate CS delivery.

Institute appropriate treatment at each step.

Follow current Resuscitation Council UK Adult ALS guidelines (Fig. 19.1) with the following modifications for the parturient:

- **Reduce aorto-caval compression** by tilting the mother left lateral (>15° but <30° to allow effective chest compressions).
  - This can be done using a purpose-made wedge, e.g. a Cardiff wedge, pillows or rolled up blanket under the right hip and lumbar region.
  - Alternatively, a human wedge is made by someone kneeling on the floor and pulling the mother's pelvis on to their knees to maintain lateral tilt, or ask an assistant to displace the uterus manually by pushing it to the left and towards the mother's head.
  - In the case of the trauma patient, the whole spinal board can be tilted.
  - Elevation of the legs will help VR to the heart if appropriate.
- **Early application of cricoid pressure (until airway secured), intubation and ventilation** because of the increased risk of regurgitation and aspiration in pregnancy.
  - Ventilate with 100% oxygen using a self-inflating bag, with a reservoir bag, and mask with cricoid pressure applied until the airway is secured with a cuffed endotracheal tube.
  - Be aware that difficult tracheal intubation is more common in pregnancy, often necessitating other laryngoscope blades, etc., and a smaller endotracheal tube may be needed if there is airway oedema.
- **Perform chest compressions higher on the sternum**, i.e. slightly above the centre of the sternum.
- **Remove fetal/uterine monitors** before defibrillating the patient.
- **Emergency (perimortum) CS** should be undertaken within 4min and delivery accomplished by 5min from the time of cardiac arrest, if resuscitation is not successful. This improves the chance of maternal, and therefore fetal, survival (see p 518).
  - Continue CPR throughout and afterwards.
  - Transabdominal open cardiac massage may be necessary. This is possible at laparotomy.

Further management

- If the mother responds quickly to resuscitation measures, the viability of the fetus needs to be assessed by an ultrasound scan, and a management plan for delivery made in conjunction with the ongoing investigation and treatment of the mother.
- Transfer the mother to an appropriate place depending on the cause of the collapse, e.g. theatre or intensive care for ongoing management (see p 510).

Investigations

These will depend on the cause of arrest and stability of the patient:

- FBC, U&E, blood glucose, LFTs, clotting studies.
- Blood group and save ± cross-match blood.
- Arterial blood gas.
- Chest X-ray.

- ECG.
- Echocardiogram.
- V/Q scan, spiral CT scan, or CTPA if a PE is suspected.
- CT head.

Summary

- CPR should be started promptly once indicated.
- Be aware of the physiological changes in pregnancy that affect resuscitation.
- Emergency CS aiming to deliver baby within 5min of maternal cardiopulmonary arrest is indicated if ALS is not successful.
- Good multidisciplinary communication and care is essential.
- The parturient's family must be cared for and kept informed of events.
- Assign someone to document the events, time and management accurately.
- Regular 'fire drills' are good practice, as maternal cardiac arrest is a rare occurrence.

Further reading

American Heart Association. American Heart Association Guidelines for Cardiopulmonary Resuscitation and Emergency Cardiovascular Care. Part 10.8 Cardiac arrest associated with pregnancy. *Circulation* 2005; **112**: 150–153.

Morris S *et al.* Resuscitation in pregnancy. *British Medical Journal* 2003; **327**: 1277–1229.

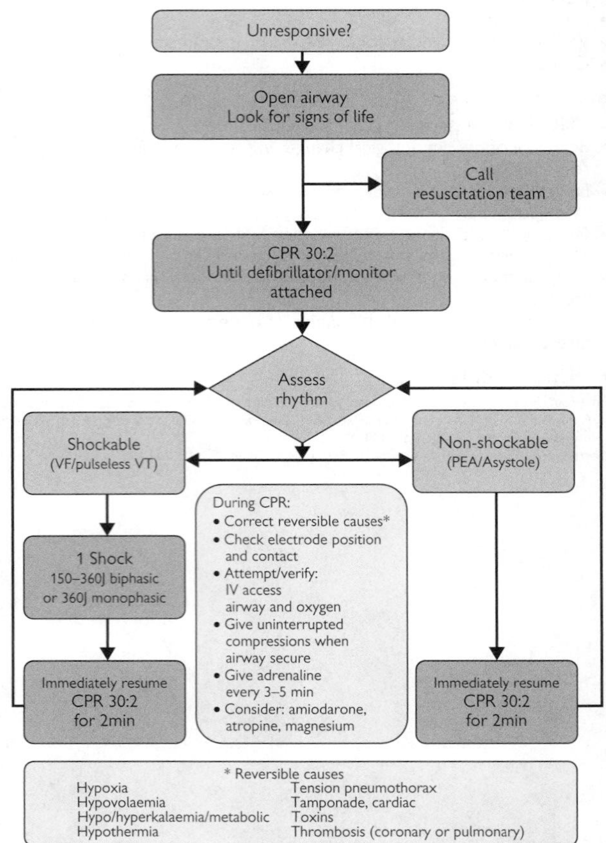

Fig. 19.1 Adult Advanced Life Support Algorithm.

Perimortem caesarean section

An emergency CS needs to be considered as soon as a pregnant mother has a cardiopulmonary arrest. It should be performed if resuscitation is not successful at 4min and delivery completed by 5min to improve the chance of both maternal and fetal survival and outcome.

- Emptying the uterus significantly improves maternal outcome with relief of aorto-caval compression, therefore permitting performance of CPR in the supine position. This leads to:
  - More effective chest compressions and ventilation.
  - Reduced oxygen consumption and circulatory demands.
  - Increased VR.
- Case reports have shown a dramatic return of maternal pulse and BP once the uterus is emptied.
- A gestational age ≥20 weeks has been given as a cut-off for emergency CS because below this a gravid uterus is unlikely to compromise maternal CO significantly.
- Precious minutes should not be wasted moving the mother to theatre or preparing a sterile field. This may mean performing the CS in a less than ideal environment, e.g. in the Accident and Emergency (A&E) department or antenatal clinic. In reality, minimal equipment is likely to be needed, e.g. a scalpel and a pair of artery forceps, as the surgical field is likely to be bloodless if there is no CO.
- A classical uterine incision may allow quickest delivery of the infant.
- Continue CPR throughout and afterwards.
- Consider transabdominal open cardiac massage.
- Fetal prognosis is poor, becoming worse with prolonged time to delivery. Remember to call for the paediatricians early.
- Transfer the mother and baby to the appropriate place, e.g. theatre or ICU once stable, for ongoing treatment.
- Unfortunately, even under ideal circumstances, death is the usual outcome for both the pregnant woman who suffers a cardiac arrest, and her baby.
- Training in maternal CPR for those looking after pregnant women is essential, with regular updates. Practise fire drills, e.g. in the A&E department, are useful.

Further reading

American Heart Association. American Heart Association Guidelines for Cardiopulmonary Resuscitation and Emergency Cardiovascular Care. Part 10.8 Cardiac arrest associated with pregnancy. *Circulation* 2005; **112**: 150–153.

Katz VL *et al.* Perimortem cearean delivery. *Obstetrics and Gynecology* 1986; **68**: 571–576.

Peters CW *et al.* Cardiac arrest during pregnancy. *Journal of Clinical Anesthesia* 2005; **17**: 229–234.

High regional blocks: causes

This is a term used to describe a central neuroaxial block that rises to upper thoracic level and above with associated cardiorespiratory symptoms.

Can be divided into

- High block that extends to the upper thoracic or lower cervical dermatomes which can cause some cardiorespiratory compromise and maternal anxiety; but does not cause diaphragmatic paralysis.
- Total spinal where the block extends to the upper cervical dermatomes and brainstem, which leads to complete paralysis, respiratory failure followed rapidly by desaturation, airway compromise and cardiac arrest if not dealt with appropriately.

It is important to recognize the two situations, because the management, although overlapping, is different.

Mechanism of high blocks/total spinal

- Spinal.
  - Excessive dose.
  - Patient position.
- Spinal injection after an epidural.
- Epidural.
  - As a result of excessive dosage (high epidural block).
  - Unintentional injection of LA into the subarachnoid space.
- Subdural.
- CSE.
- Epidural top-up after a recent spinal injection.

Spinal anaesthetic

- Only likely to cause a high block.

Excessive dosage: it is common in non-obstetric practice to use 3–4mL of 0.5% heavy bupivacaine for lower limb orthopaedic and lower abdominal surgery. These doses may lead to excessive blocks in the pregnant woman who can have an acceptable intra-abdominal block with doses from 1.5 to 2.5mL of bupivacaine 0.5%.

- Experience with the 'usual' non-obstetric spinal doses of LA in pregnant women has shown that there can be significant variability in the extent of block achieved.
- Increased intra-abdominal pressure from the pregnancy causing epidural venous engorgement and a reduction of both epidural and subarachnoid space is thought to be a major factor.
- The reduced LA requirements are seen as early as 8–12 weeks pregnancy, well before the mechanical effects of gravid uterus are present. The explanation is that either pregnant nerve fibres are more sensitive to LAs or there is enhanced diffusion of LA across the nerve membrane.
- High progesterone levels in CSF and/or blood during pregnancy may be the cause of the different response to subarachnoid injection of LA during late pregnancy.

- The dose of LA during pregnancy should be reduced by at least 25% compared with similar non-pregnant patients and tailored to the individual parturient depending on gestation (smallest dose in the full-term parturient).

Position: may also play a part in the aetiology. High intra-abdominal pressure and engorged epidural veins may make the pregnant woman more vulnerable to developing an excessive block, in a flat or slightly head-down position, compared with a non-pregnant patient.

Spinal anaesthesia after an epidural

- May cause either a high block or a total spinal.
- The subarachnoid space is squeezed by the volume of LA already in the epidural space, facilitating cephalad spread of subarachnoid LA.
  - If a spinal block is performed within 45min of an epidural top-up the dose should be reduced by 25%.
- Drug flux is movement of drug from the epidural space to the subarachnoid space via the dural hole made by the spinal needle. Some of the LA from the epidural space can pass through the dural hole and enter the subarachnoid space, further extending the block.

Excessive epidural doses

- Only likely to cause a high block.
- Large doses of epidural LA can give rise to a high block associated with cardiorespiratory features.
- This is usually seen when one is faced with a block, which after top-up for operative delivery, is unequal. When the final block height is achieved, it may lead to a high block especially on one side.
- This is more likely to happen after a single bolus volume >20mL or divided boluses >30L total volume.
- An early presentation is unilateral Horner's syndrome.

Subdural block

- Causes a high block or modified type of total spinal.
- Incidence is quoted to be 0.82%.
- Results from unintentional catheterization of the subdural space at insertion, as well as delayed migration of the epidural catheter.
- The block behaves more like an epidural than a subarachnoid block.
- Time to maximal block ranges from 20 to 30min but the extent produced by a given volume of LA is greater.
- Subdural block is often patchy, asymmetric, with minimal motor block and hypotension.
- Retention of sacral sensation distinguishes it from spinal block.
- As it extends intracranially, a subdural block can involve the cranial nerves and can cause unconsciousness.
- A subdural block can unexpectedly lead to a sudden subarachnoid block.
  - A sudden increase in pressure generated in the subdural space by the injection of LA may rupture the arachnoid.
  - The onset of a subarachnoid block in the absence of CSF during placement of the catheter, inability to aspirate fluid through the catheter before injection and free flow of CSF after injection confirms this.

Unintentional subarachnoid block

Accidental dural puncture during epidural placement

- May cause a high block or a total spinal.
- 65% of the time this is recognized at the time by the free flow of CSF through the epidural needle.
- 35% of the time it is due to the catheter puncture. It may not be as obvious, and a negative aspiration of CSF via the catheter does not guarantee that it is not placed in the subarachnoid space.
- Administration of a test dose should help identify subarachnoid placement of a catheter.
- If unrecognized, injection of a large volume of LA may rapidly lead to a high/total spinal.
- A high block may result from an epidural injection of LA given into the intervertebral space adjacent to an inadvertent dural perforation with a 16 or 18G Tuohy needle.
- It is suggested that the frequent uterine contractions of labour can result in some of the LA solution being forced through the puncture hole into the subarachnoid space.
- If an epidural catheter is resited after an inadvertent dural puncture this should be performed above and well away from the original interspace to minimize this risk.
- A multiholed catheter may be placed partly in the epidural and partly in the subarachnoid space.
  - With initial slow injection, the LA emerges from the proximal holes.
  - With a subsequent rapid injection, LA will emerge from the distal holes, resulting in a subarachnoid block.
  - The block may have features of an epidural, subdural and subarachnoid block.

Catheter migration from the epidural into the subarachnoid space

- May cause a high block or a total spinal.
- High blocks occurring on second or subsequent top-ups may be due to migration, of an originally correctly placed epidural catheter, into the subarachnoid space.
- However, a postmortem study has shown that the epidural catheter is unable to puncture the dura.
- It is likely that the epidural catheter in this circumstance was originally in the subdural space and, because it provided some analgesia, was not recognized.
- Sudden disruption of arachnoid mater results in a sudden, late, high block.

Combined–spinal epidural

- Only likely to cause a high block.
- This may result when an epidural top-up is used to augment the initial spinal injection.
- The volume effect is the mechanical compression of the dural sac by the epidural fluid displacing the CSF in the cephalad direction. This is supported by the studies demonstrating the increase in LA block even when saline is injected epidurally.

  - To minimize this risk there should be a 10min time gap between the spinal injection and the first epidural top-up.
  - The epidural top-up volume should not exceed 5mL (saline or LA solution).
- Drug flux is movement of drug from the epidural space to the subarachnoid space via the dural hole made by the spinal needle. The clinical effect of such drug flux is thought to be affected by the size of the dural hole. It is probably minimal with the conventional use of 24–27G spinal needles during this technique.
- The epidural catheter may be accidentally placed in the subarachnoid space and, because of the initial intended spinal block, a test dose through the epidural catheter can be difficult to interpret.
  - It is therefore suggested that a low concentration of LA be used.
  - Each bolus should be treated as a test dose.

High regional blocks: presentation

High block

- **Nausea and vomiting** is usually seen and may be due to hypotension or cerebral hypoxia.
- **Hypotension**
  - Although common in obstetric spinal anaesthesia, the rapidity and severity with which it occurs during high blocks can put the patients' life and the fetus at risk if treatment is delayed.
  - The major factor in the development of hypotension is the height of the block. The sympathetic outflow from the spinal cord is between T1 and L2. A block below that level has little effect on the BP. The sympathetic supply to the adrenal medulla is from T8 to L1, and a block to T8 will affect the BP by inhibition of systemic release of catecholamines in addition to venous pooling of blood in the lower half of the body secondary to vasodilatation. All these effects are compounded by any degree of aorto-caval compression, resulting in a severe fall in BP and CO.
- **Bradycardia** is usually secondary to blockade of T1–T4 cardioaccelera-tory fibres. Decreased right atrial filling from aorto-caval compression may be a contributing factor (the Bezold–Jarisch reflex), where the onset of bradycardia can be very sudden and severe (HR <20/min).
- **Respiratory difficulty**
  - Experienced due to paralysis of the intercostal muscles.
  - During pregnancy the intercostal muscles contribute more than normal during quiet respiration due to diaphragmatic splinting.
  - Patients may complain of difficulty especially in taking a deep breath or coughing, but will be able to speak normally.
- **Tingling in the hands and fingers** indicates a sensory block at T1 (beware of the anxious hyperventilating patient).
- **Somnolence**
  - Can be a difficult sign to interpret as excessive fatigue and the effect of opioids can have a similar effect.
  - When associated with a high block it is caused by the sensory component spreading several dermatomes above the motor block to the brainstem.
  - Motor function may be surprisingly unaffected; however, beware, as the patient may not complain of any difficulties before a respiratory arrest occurs.

Total spinal

- **Loss of consciousness**
  - Due to spread of LA into the brainstem.
  - Loss of airway reflexes due to involvement of cranial nerves.
- **Respiratory arrest**
  - May occur without warning.
  - Due to phrenic nerve paralysis, which may be preceded by difficulty in coughing and phonation.
  - Medullary repiratory centres may also be affected.

- **Cardiovascular collapse**
  - Profound hypotension and severe bradycardia due to total block of sympathetic nervous system.
  - Cardiac arrest may occur.

High regional blocks: assessment and management

High block

The mainstay of treatment includes prompt recognition and early treatment aimed at providing adequate oxygenation and correcting hypotension and bradycardia. Senior anaesthetic and ODP help should be sought early if simple measures are unsuccessful in stabilizing the mother.

- It is common for a mother with a block required for a CS to complain of some breathing difficulty. This is caused by the paralysis of intercostal muscles and the supine position required for surgery.
- The extent of the block should be quickly ascertained. It is common for the mother to complain of some numbness to cold in the high thoracic T1 and lower cervical C8 dermatones, i.e. inner border of arm and little finger.
- If the numbness involves the whole hand, this indicates an abnormally high block.
- The sensory block extends above the motor block and, even if there is a significant sensory block, the ability to squeeze her hand closed is a reassuring sign for the mother and anaesthetist.
- Place a firm additional pillow or wedge under the mid thoracic curve to prevent a block that has reached the lower cervical dermatomes from rising further.
- This manoeuvre will in addition allow the descent of the diaphragm and improve respiratory function. This will make the mother feel less breathless and reduce her associated anxiety.
- Administer high flow oxygen via a face mask.
- If there is doubt about respiratory effort, tidal volume can easily be assessed through most modern anaesthetic machines using a tight-fitting anaesthetic face mask.
    - The additional value of this approach is that 100% oxygen can be administered.
    - The anaesthetist stays in close contact with the mother both to reassure her and to assess her respiratory status.
    - Preoxygenation has taken place if intubation is required.
- Ensure adequate lateral tilt to prevent aorto-caval compression. (If possible, a full lateral position may be more effective).
- Lifting the legs above the level of the heart increases the VR. The patient must not be placed in a head-down position as this may extend the block and increase respiratory difficulty because of reduced pulmonary volume. Raising the knees flattens the lumbar curve and raises intra-abdominal pressure; both manoeuvres may also extend the block further.
- Atropine boluses of 300–600 micrograms are useful to treat bradycardia.

- Boluses of ephedrine 6–9mg or phenylephrine 25 micrograms as required, to restore and maintain the systolic BP. Phenylephrine may be a more useful drug (although there is frequent anxiety about its use in a patient who is bradycardic). It is a more potent drug than ephedrine, has a more direct α action, is therefore effective against an excessive sympathetic block and improves VR.
- IV fluids should be administered rapidly (e.g. 1000mL crystalloid and/or 500mL colloid) and repeat as necessary. Fluid therapy should not be used alone and, if it is not rapidly effective, the early use of other manoeuvres (change of position and vasopressors) should be adopted.
- Reassurance is extremely useful to calm the anxious mother.
- Sometimes it is not possible to achieve good haemodynamic stability with a high block even if the mother remains conscious. Delivery of the baby will improve this and may be indicated. Further anaesthesia is not usually necessary unless the block progresses and respiratory function declines.
- Depending on the circumstances, the block may progress (to a total spinal), and preparation should be made to protect and secure the airway as appropriate. The operating theatre on a maternity unit is usually the safest place.

Total spinal

The complaining agitated patient may have a high block BUT beware of the silent non-complaining somnolent patient.

- The hypotension can be of sudden onset if it is secondary to an extensive subarachnoid block, when it presents as sudden loss of consciousness and collapse. However, it can be of slower onset if due to subdural or extensive epidural block. Hypotension may be severe enough to impair cerebral perfusion and cause loss of consciousness.
- The associated loss of airway reflexes as the cranial nerves are affected may lead to aspiration of gastric contents.
- Weakness of arm and hand indicates blockade of cervicothoracic nerves.
- Once the phrenic nerve fibres (C3, 4, 5) start to be affected, difficulty in coughing and phonation develops. Respiratory arrest ensues as a result of complete respiratory muscle paralysis.
- LA action on the medullary respiratory centre will cause a direct cessation of respiration, and its effect on other brainstem functions will directly cause unconsciousness.
- Finally fixed and dilated pupils are seen.
- Early recognition and treatment is of utmost importance for successful outcome, and every anaesthetist working on the maternity ward should be able to recognize this complication and treat appropriately.
- Treatment is aimed at protecting and securing the airway with restoration of ventilation and circulation.
- Endotracheal intubation is required in almost all the cases. A small dose of an anaesthetic, sedative agent and an intubating dose of a muscle relaxant may need to be used to facilitate intubation.

- Controlled ventilation of the lungs with 100% oxygen should be instituted.
- Ensure adequate uterine displacement to prevent aorto-caval compression.
- Further management involves administration of fluids, atropine and vasopressors to support the BP. An adrenaline infusion may be required to maintain a satisfactory level of BP and HR.
- The duration of the block depends on the type and dose of the LA injected into the subarachnoid space and usually starts to recede after 1–2h.
- The patient will not require further anaesthetic/sedative agents initially as her unconsciousness is caused by the LA action on the brainstem. Additional agents will only impair the anaesthetist's ability to assess the level of consciousness and cause unnecessary additional cardiovascular compromise. Additional sedation may be needed later if she is able to respond and open her eyes before the return of adequate respiratory function.

If the cardiovascular and respiratory features are recognized early and treated effectively, the outcome of a total spinal for mother and baby is good.

Further reading

Evans TI. Total spinal anaesthesia. *Anaesthesia and Intensive Care* 1972; **2**: 158–163.

Crawford JS. Some maternal complications of epidural analgesia for labour. *Anaesthesia* 1985; **40**: 1219–1225.

Morgan B. Unexpected extensive conduction blocks in obstetric epidural analgesia. *Anaesthesia* 1990; **45**: 148–152.

Yentis SM, Dob DP. High regional block—the failed intubation of the new millenium? *International Journal of Obstetrics and Anesthesia* 2001; **10**: 159–161.

McCrae AF, Wildsmith JAW. Prevention and treatment of hypotension during central neural block. *British Journal of Anaesthesia* 1993; **70**: 672–680.

Local anaesthetic toxicity

Modern obstetric anaesthetic practice frequently involves the use of regional techniques, using large amounts of LA agents to establish effective analgesia and anaesthesia. Consequently, obstetric patients are at risk of developing systemic toxicity of LA drugs.

Systemic LA toxicity depends on a number of factors

- Site of injection (e.g. epidural space, pudendal block infiltration).
- Total dose (in mg)—see below.
- Intravascular injection—this is the most common reason for systemic toxicity and is often unrecognized. The epidural veins in the obstetric patient are congested, and cannulation with the epidural catheter is common. Aspiration may not reveal blood as epidural veins are thin walled and may collapse.
- Speed of injection—slow injection of the LA drug will allow detection of toxicity earlier and is an important safety measure.
- The degree of protein binding and the presence of acidosis.
- The agent being used—levo-bupivicaine is recognized for its enhanced cardiovascular safety profile.

The British National Formulary guidelines recommend a total maximum dose (in mg) of bupivacaine or levobupivacaine of 150mg over a 4h period.

- Although a guide, the clinical manifestation of LA toxicity will depend on all the factors above, and in particular accidental intravascular injection.
- In the event of IV injection, a much smaller total dose of LA would be required to cause life-threatening complications.

Presentation

The manifestation of systemic toxicity may present acutely, as is the case of accidental IV administration, or insidiously through systemic absorption. LAs act as membrane stabilizers within the heart and brain, leading to the following symptoms:

CNS complications

Early excitation followed by CNS depression.

- Anxiety, light headed or drowsy.
- Facial paraesthesia especially around the lips and tongue because of increased blood flow.
- Tinnitus.
- Loss of consciousness.
- Convulsions.
- Coma and apnoea.

Cardiovascular system complications

- Arrythmias including VF/VT.
- Bradycardia and eventually asystole.
- Hypotension.
- Cardiac arrest.

Prevention

- Careful aspiration and observation of epidural catheters.
- Slow administration of increased concentration doses.
- If the patient has the first signs of LA toxicity (usually perioral tingling), stop injection and reaspirate via the catheter.

The use of adrenaline in LA administration is well known as a mechanism for the detection of inadvertent IV injection. Its use in obstetric patients is controversial as many patients are tachycardic and hypertensive, therefore the sensitivity and specificity are both low.

Management

- **A and B.** Maintain airway and give 100% O_2. Intubate and ventilate if indicated, e.g. patient obtunded/cardiovascular system collapse. Treat convulsions with diazepam.
- **C.** Left lateral tilt or wedge to reduce aorto-caval compression. Treat bradycardia with atropine and hypotension with appropriate vasopressors, e.g. ephedrine, phenylephrine or adrenaline. Continue until clinical improvement. Consider IV vasopressor infusion for inotropic support. In event of cardiac arrest—Resuscitation Council ALS algorithm applies with emphasis on early delivery and avoidance of aorto-caval compression.
- CPR may have to be sustained for a considerable time, as cardiac arrest secondary to LA toxicity is very resistant to normal resuscitation practices (see below).
- IV bretylium may be used in the event of ventricular arrythmias.

The use of Intralipid for LA-associated cardiac arrest

- Strong evidence now suggests that the use of a lipid emulsion (Intralipid® 20%) markedly improves outcome in cardiac arrest secondary to bupivacaine systemic toxicity (its use with other LA has been implied but not as yet tested).
- The impressive animal trials are now supported by human case reports.
- A suggested protocol for human use is as follows. As yet it is not the first-line choice of treatment for ventricular arrhythmias associated with LA, but may become so in the future.

Cardiac arrest secondary to LA toxicity

- Give 1.5mL/kg Intralipid® (20%) over 1min.
- Then immediately start infusion of Intralipid® at 0.25mL/kg/min.
- Repeat the bolus dose at 3–5min intervals until 3mL/kg total dose given.
- Continue the infusion until cardiovascular system stability is restored. Increase the infusion rate to 5mL/kg/min if BP decreases again.
- Maximum recommended dose is 8mL/kg.

Further reading

Morris S, Stacey M. Resuscitation in pregnancy. *British Medical Journal* 2003; **327**: 1277–1279.

Hazinski MF *et al.* Major changes in the 2005 AHA Guidelines for CPR and ECC: reaching the tipping point for change. *Circulation* 2005; **112**: IV206–IV211.

Picard J *et al.* Editorial: Lipid emulsion to treat overdose of local anaesthetic: the gift of the blob. *Anaesthesia* 2006; **61**: 107–109.

www.lipidrescue.org

Other drug toxicity

The variety and number of drugs used in obstetric anaesthetic practice is considerable. Many have no licence in pregnancy but are used on a background of considerable clinical experience. As well as the uncommon complications such as anaphylaxis, many have side effects that can cause considerable problems to the patient, especially if they remain unrecognized by the anaesthetist.

Magnesium

Magnesium is used in the treatment of severe pre-eclampsia and the prevention and treatment of eclampsia.

Side effects are

- Flushing: if given too rapidly.
- Hypotension.
- Shortness of breath.
- Muscle weakness/paralysis, if given in an excessive dose especially in the presence of renal impairment. The patient on a magnesium infusion should have regular assessment of reflexes, and a serum magnesium level measured 4h after establishing the treatment.

Special consideration for the obstetric anaesthetist

- Suxamethonium neuromuscular blockade is not affected by magnesium but the muscle fasiculations are suppressed, making the timing of intubation difficult. A standard dose of suxamethonium 1–1.5mg/kg should be used. Its duration of action is unchanged.
- Magnesium will prolong and enhance non-deporalizing neuromuscular blockade. The dose of non-depolarizing muscle relaxant should be reduced, and attempts at reversal and extubation made only after assessment with a peripheral nerve stimulator.
- Care must be taken well into the postoperative period as recurarization has been described, which may lead to aspiration in the high risk obstetric patient and respiratory failure. The mother must have her respiratory rate and oxygen saturation monitored in a well-lit room.
- IV calcium gluconate or chloride (10mL of 10% solution as a bolus) may be used if severe magnesium toxicity is present. Further management may include additional IV calcium and supportive care, often requiring critical care input.

Spinal/epidural opioids

Opioids in spinal and epidural blocks are commonly used, and their side effect profile is similar by both routes. Fentanyl, morphine and diamorphine are shown to improve block quality, and the longer-acting opioids contribute to better postoperative analgesia and maternal satisfaction.

Side effects are

- **Pruritus (trigeminal nucleus)**
  - A troublesome and very common side effect.
  - Although commonly prescribed, chlorpheniramine does not have a direct effect as the itch is not due to histamine release, but the mother may find this drug beneficial because of its sedative properties.

- A reduction in itch intensity has been described in some patients given ondansetron, and it may be worthwhile giving this drug to a mother who is also nauseous.
- Subanaesthetic doses of propofol may be beneficial but should not be given without full and immediate anaesthetic support.
- Naloxone will reverse the pruritus associated with opioids but may also reverse the analgesic effect. An initial dose of 50 micrograms is recommended.
- Reassurance that the 'itch' is not an 'allergic' reaction is the most important strategy, as it is a relatively short-lived problem (<24h).

- **Delayed gastric emptying**
  - This is well described after all epidural opioids and is dose related.
  - Mothers receiving epidural fentanyl in labour will be at risk.
- **Nausea and vomiting**
  - Should be treated with conventional antiemetic therapy.
- **Urinary retention**
  - Uncommon in obstetric practice, BUT bladder emptying must be carefully monitored and enquired after.
- **Maternal respiratory depression**
  - Uncommon in obstetric practice at the spinal doses often used.
  - May be increased risk if given with systemic IV opioids.
  - Respiratory rate and sedation scores should be compulsory for a period of 12–24h in a well-managed clinical area after long-acting opioids (morphine or diamorphine) in the intrathecal and epidural space.
- **Neonatal respiratory depression**
  - Major respiratory depression in the neonate is rare after conventional epidural or spinal doses in obstetric practice.
  - Epidural opioids have been implicated in poor establishment of breastfeeding.

Vasoconstrictors

Ephedrine, phenylephrine and metaraminol are all used in obstetric anaesthesia to counteract the hypotension associated with neuraxial blockade.

Ephedrine

- An indirect α- and β-agonist, ephedrine has a long history of clinical use in obstetric anaesthesia.
- It gained popularity because placental blood flow was not impaired in experimental animal models compared with other agents.
- β effect predominates and is therefore ineffective if the mother is already tachycardic.
- Should not be used if maternal or fetal tachycardia is to be avoided.
- Current evidence shows that fetal acidosis is more common with ephedrine probably secondary to fetal β-adrenoceptor activity.
- Ephedrine remains popular because of its ease of use and its long history of obstetric anaesthetic experience.
- Standard dose is as a 3–6mg bolus, rather than as an infusion.
- Tachyphylaxis rapidly occurs due to depleted stores of presynaptic noradrenaline, and will become clinically ineffective.

- If the mother remains hypotensive after 30mg total dose, she should be repositioned with increased tilt or full left lateral and/or a different vasopressor used.

Metaraminol and phenylephrine

- α-Agonists that are now gaining popularity as adverse effects with ephedrine use have been noted.
- More experimental work has been carried out on phenylephrine in obstetric practice, and its use has therefore been popularized although data suggesting that it is superior to metaraminol are lacking.
- Infusions have been shown to be more efficacious in preventing episodes of hypotension but the risk of drug toxicity may be higher as the total dose of drug given by infusion will be greater and there is more potential for human or equipment error.
- These potent agents may of course be more likely to cause severe hypertension and maternal bradycardia if used inappropriately and without experience.
- If used in excessive doses, their α agonist effects will cause vasoconstriction in the placental bed and fetal acidosis.
- Pre-eclamptic patients may be very sensitive to these agents, and additional care should be taken to avoid adverse effects in this group of women.

Antiemetics

Many women require antiemetics throughout pregnancy and during labour as nausea and vomiting occur frequently. All classes of these drugs are commonly used and are generally considered to be safe and effective; however, their use is unlicensed.

Prochlorperazine

- Is an antidopaminergic drug and occasionally may cause extrapyramidal side effects.
- Extrapyramidal effects have been reported in the neonate.

Ondansetron

- The HT_3 antagonists have few safety data in pregnancy and so should be avoided as a first-line agent.
- Is effective and safe in labour and postdelivery.

Dexamethasone

- Effective and safe antiemetic, although prolonged use of corticosteroids in pregnancy is contraindicated because of an association with fetal growth restriction.

Non-steroidal anti-inflammatory drugs

- Diclofenac is the most commonly used NSAID.
- May be teratogenic and should be avoided in the first trimester.
- Should be avoided in the third trimester due to the risk of premature closure of the ductus arteriosus, leading to fetal pulmonary hypertension.

Caution in prescribing postdelivery in the following setting

- In patients where bleeding has been problematic.
- Low platelet counts <100.

- Oliguria due to hypovolaemia or renal impairment.
- Pre-eclampsia/eclampsia because of the renal component of the disease. NSAIDs can be introduced after assessment of renal function and a normal platelet count has been established.

Uterotonics

Oxytocin

- Oxytocin is normally produced by the posterior pituitary and is structurally very similar to vasopressin.
- May cause hyperstimulation of the uterus, uterine dysfunction and fetal distress when used to promote or induce labour.
- It has some antidiuretic activity and can contribute to oliguria and fluid overload.
- This is especially likely in the context of PPH where a large amount of fluid/blood will be required in conjunction with an oxytocin infusion.
- Rapid bolus causes flushing, peripheral vasodilatation and hypotension.
- Maximum single bolus of 5U IV given slowly, followed by an infusion postdelivery to avoid complications.

Ergot alkaloids

- Ergometrine is the classic example of this group; however, Syntometrine® (a combination of ergometrine and oxytocin) is also frequently used. It is used clinically postpartum IM to promote tetanic uterine contraction and decrease blood losses.
- May be given IV, IM or intramyometrially to treat large blood losses.
- The IV route is associated with marked hypertension.
- Nausea and vomiting.
- A slow IV injection (dilute in 100mL of normal saline) will decrease the incidence and magnitude of these side effects.
- Avoid in pre-eclampsia/severe essential hypertension.

Prostaglandins

- Synthetic prostaglandins (analogues of E_2 and $F_{2\alpha}$) are used for the induction of labour and in the treatment of PPH.
- Haemabate® is an example of this group used in the treatment of PPH.
- Most frequently given by the IM and intramyometrial route.
- May cause severe:
  - Bronchospasm (contraindicated in asthmatics).
  - Cyanosis.
  - Systemic hypertension.
  - Diarrhoea (20–30%).
  - Pulmonary hypertension.
  - Pulmonary oedema.
  - Arrhythmias (including VF).
  - Anaphylaxis.
- It is important to realize that these drugs may convert one life- threatening situation, e.g. uterine atony and PPH, to another!
- β-Agonist treatment may be required to treat bronchospasm and may increase uterine atony.

Anaphylaxis

- IgE-mediated type B (not dose-related) hypersensitivity reaction. The causative antigen combines with IgE on mast cells and basophils, leading to the mass release of histamine and seretonin.
- Presentation includes facial swelling, airway obstruction, bronchospasm rash, oedema, erythema, profound hypotension and shock. This condition is of major concern in the parturient and is associated with poor fetal outcome.
- Presentation may be within seconds of drug administration or over minutes.
- Common triggers in anaesthetic practice include muscle relaxants, latex, antibiotics, NSAIDs, hypnotics, colloids and opioids (in decreasing order of frequency).
- A history of prior exposure is not required as cross-sensitivity is possible.

Immediate management

- **Call for help (remember obstetric team).**
- **Remove suspected trigger.**

A and B

- Maintain airway and give 100% O_2.
- Intubate and ventilate if significant upper airway obstruction.

C

- Left lateral tilt or wedge to minimize aorto-caval compression.
- Adrenaline 50 micrograms IV increments (0.5mL 1:10 000 solution) or 0.5–1mg. IM. Repeat as necessary to support BP and continue until clinical improvement.
- Elevate legs and commence rapid IV fluid resuscitation.
- Expedite early delivery and paediatric support if situation not rapidly improving.

Further management

- Chlorphenamine 10–20mg by slow IV injection for less severe reactions.
- Hydrocortisone 100–300mg IV.
- Consider continued inotropic support with adrenaline (0.05–0.1 micrograms/kg/min) or noradrenaline (0.05–0.1 micrograms/kg/min), and critical care transfer. *Noradrenaline can be especially useful if the hypotension pressure is resistant to treatment with adrenaline.*
- Consider nebulized bronchodilators (salbutamol 2.5–5mg) if continuing bronchospasm.
- Leak test endotracheal tube before extubation to exclude possible airway oedema.

Differential diagnosis

- AFE (very similar presentation) but profound DIC is common with an AFE.
- Latex sensitivity. Risk factors include healthcare workers, spina bifida, need for recurrent bladder catheterization and some fruit allergies (including banana, kiwi and tomato).
- Cardiac disease of pregnancy, which is the most common indirect cause of maternal death. Can present with cardiogenic shock and wheeze secondary to cardiac failure.

Investigation/follow-up

- ***Plasma tryptase***. Take 10mL blood after resuscitation and up to 1h following the reaction. Store at –20°C and inform biochemistry. Note down time of sample on form and in the patient notes. A further sample should be taken at 6–24h post reaction.
- Arrange anaesthetic follow-up and immunology referral for further investigation.
- Suspected drug reactions require CSM reporting (yellow card). Information on allergy investigation centres and a national anaesthetic reaction database can be found on the AAGBI website (www.aagbi.org/allergies).
- A clear record of the allergy must be made in the notes, a full explanation given to the patient and a Medic alert bracelet issued.

Further reading

Association of Anaesthetists of Great Britain and Ireland and the British Society of Allergy and Clinical immunology. *Suspected Anaphylatic Reactions Associated with Anaesthesia*. 2003.

Soar J *et al.* European Resuscitation Council Guidelines for Resuscitation. Section 7. Cardiac arrest in special circumstances. *Resuscitation* 2005; **67S1**: S135–S170.

Aspiration

This is rare in modern practice, but Curtis Mendleson (1913–2002) first highlighted the serious consequences of pulmonary aspiration in 1946. This leads initially to a chemical pneumonitis and atelectasis of varying degree. Later the condition can be complicated by the development of ARDS and/or polymicrobial pneumonia. In Mendleson's original description, deaths were caused by asphyxiation due to solid matter. The chemical pneumonitis associated with the aspiration of gastric acid, although serious, recovered without specific treatment in all cases.

Aspiration continues to be a small but important cause of anaesthetic-related maternal deaths. Failure to manage the airway appropriately and secure rapid endotracheal intubation exposes the mother to the risk of aspiration.

Relevant gastrointestinal physiology

- Gastro-oesophageal reflux is common in pregnancy.
- pH studies show increased gastric acidity.
- Increased intragastric pressure due to the pregnancy.
- Decreased lower oesophageal tone.
- In labour, there is decreased gastric emptying associated with pain and opioid drugs.

Additional risk factors

- Poor cricoid application (due to left lateral tilt).
- Failed intubation (reported to be up to 1 in 250 pregnant women).
- Peripartum opioids, either systemic or regional.
- Obesity.
- Diabetes mellitus (gastroparesis) increasingly common in pregnancy.
- Non-fasted women—this is a controversial area, but aspiration, however rare, may be used as an argument against feeding in labour, especially as it is the aspiration of solid material that is most life-threatening.

Prevention

The following changes in clinical practice have significantly decreased the incidence of aspiration:

- Increased use of regional techniques.
- Antacid prophylaxis in labour and prior to operative delivery.
- Fasting or light diet only in labour.
- Improved training in obstetric anaesthesia.

Presentation

- Presents initially as tachypnoea, tachycardia and raised airway pressures, decreased O_2 saturations and localized wheeze/crepitations. The extent of the symptoms and signs depends on the acidity and volume of the aspirate.
- ARDS is possible within 24–72h, presenting with increasingly high airway pressures and respiratory rate, low paO_2 and high $paCO_2$. A prolonged period of ventilation may be necessary.

Management

Acute management

- Call for help. Inform obstetricians.
- Maintain airway and give 100% O_2.
- Check endotracheal and cuff. Re-intubate if required.
- Suction airway until aspirates clear.
- Avoid excessive IPPV until suctioned.
- Consider bronchodilators if there is marked bronchospasm.
- Consider bronchoscopy/lavage if clinically no improvement.
- Pass nasogastral tube and empty stomach.

Further management

- Liaise with critical care and plan for transfer.
- Evidence of high oxygen requirement may indicate that postoperative ventilatory support may be required.
- If there is evidence of atelectasis, consider physiotherapy and CPAP.
- Prophylactic antibiotics are not required.
- Corticosteroids do not affect outcome.

Investigations

- Chest X-ray—early changes include diffuse infiltrative shadowing in the right lower lobe, classically with a variable degree of atelectasis, which may be profound if bronchial occlusion has occurred. The left lateral tilt used in obstetric patients can change this pattern, and infiltrates are seen more commonly on the left.
- Arterial blood gases.
- Bronchoscopy—consider if aspiration of solids is possible, severe atelectasis or little clinical improvement.

Trauma in the obstetric patient

The principles of trauma resuscitation are the same for pregnant and non-pregnant patients. Pregnancy causes major physiological changes and altered anatomical relationships involving almost every organ system. These changes may alter the response to injury. Trauma is the major cause of death in young people, and the pattern of death demonstrates a trimodal distribution:

- Instantaneous—within seconds to minutes of the injury.
- Early—from a few minutes to a few hours.
- Late—hours to weeks.

When attending a pregnant trauma victim, it must be remembered that there are two patients; successful outcome for the fetus relies on prompt resuscitation of the mother and early consultation with other specialties. A systematic approach to resuscitation with the appropriate team can prevent deaths especially during 'the golden hour'.

Anatomical alterations of pregnancy relating to trauma

First trimester

- The uterus lies within the pelvis and it and the fetus are therefore well protected from traumatic damage.

Second trimester

- The uterus expands into the abdomen but the fetus remains somewhat protected, now by the proportionally large volume of amniotic fluid.

Third trimester

- The uterus is now large and increasingly thin walled, which makes the fetus more vulnerable; the fetal head lying within the pelvis is at danger in the case of maternal pelvic fracture.
- The lack of elasticity of the placenta when compared with that of the uterus exposes it to shearing forces, thus causing placental abruption.
- The bowel is pushed to the upper part of the abdomen posteriorly and is therefore relatively protected.

Physiological changes of pregnancy relating to trauma

- There is often initial haemodynamic stability despite blood loss of up to 1500mL (Grade 3–4 shock), due to the expansion of plasma volume of 50% normally seen in late pregnancy.
- The CO is increased and SVR decreased, resulting in an overall decrease in BP during second trimester. The BP returns nearly to normal values at term.
- The supine position can reduce CO by 30% from the second trimester because of aorto-caval obstruction.
- The haematocrit is reduced.
- Vasoconstriction in placental vasculature occurs easily in response to hypotension and circulating catecholamines during trauma causing increased vascular resistance, reduced blood flow and fetal hypoxaemia.
- Increased oxygen consumption and lowered arterial carbon dioxide can make interpretation of arterial blood gases difficult.

Assessment and treatment

- Ideally any injured pregnant woman needs to be seen and treated as early as possible after injury by a multidisciplinary team including anaesthetist, surgeon, obstetrician, paediatrician and midwife.
- During the primary survey, life-threatening injuries are identified and treated using the A B C D E sequence of resuscitation.
- During the secondary survey, other important injuries which might not be life threatening are identified and treated during a head to toe, back to front examination.

Special measures for mother and fetus are required

- Injured mother must be resuscitated in a position that minimizes aorto-caval obstruction.
- If a spinal injury is suspected, a lateral tilt on a spinal board or lateral displacement of the uterus may be needed.
- Fetal monitoring is required for at least 4h, even after trivial trauma, using a CTG.

Maternal monitoring should continue for 24h with specific attention to

- Uterus—fundal height, position of fetus, contractions, irritability.
- Vagina—evidence of blood, amniotic fluid.
- Cervix—effacement suggesting preterm labour.

If a patient has been multiply injured

- X-rays of chest and pelvis are mandatory at some stage when the patient is stable. This MUST NOT be deferred because of the pregnancy.
- Cervical spine X-ray including the C7/T1 junction can be difficult to achieve and time should not be wasted; if there is any doubt in a critical situation, assume the neck is unstable and treat other life-threatening injuries.
- Nominate a team leader to ensure a systematic approach to resuscitation and reassessment of the multiply injured patient.

Airway

Acute airway obstruction may result from:

- Anatomical distortion from trauma.
- Debris such as blood or vomit.
- Oedema from inhalation injury and head injury.

Immediate recognition and resolution is vital

- Basic and advanced airway manoeuvres with cervical spine control and oxygenation.
- Immobilization of the neck is achieved with a correct sized stiff collar, tapes and sand bag.

If considering endotracheal intubation, expect a difficult airway

- Term pregnancy and laryngeal oedema.
- Head not in the 'sniffing the morning air' position.
- Increased risk of regurgitation.
- Collar impedes movement of jaw and mouth.

- A rapid sequence induction is required using thiopental and suxamethonium.
- Nasogastric and nasotracheal tubes are contraindicated if a base of skull fracture suspected.

Breathing

- Inspection—respiratory rate, depth, symmetry, bleeding, wounds.
- Palpation—tenderness, asymmetry, crepitus, midline trachea.
- Percussion—hyper-resonance or dullness.
- Auscultation—loss of air entry.

Clinical examination should identify these life-threatening injuries

- Tension pneumothorax—treated with needle thoracocentesis in the second intercostal space, mid-clavicular line with a 16G needle.
- Open pneumothorax—three-sided occlusive dressing.
- Flail chest—consider lung contusion and need for ventilation.
- Massive haemothorax—chest drain losses of 1500mL of blood or continued loss of 200mL in 1h needs a thoracotomy.
- Cardiac tamponade—difficult to diagnose, Becks triad of muffled heart sounds, raised JVP, reduced arterial pressure, aspiration required with ECG monitoring.

Circulation

- Site two 14/16G cannulae in the antecubital fossae.
- Blood should be sent for FBC, cross-match, U&E and glucose.
- Rapidly infuse 2L of warmed Hartmann's solution and check response.
- Apply compression to any external source of bleeding, e.g. open femoral fracture and obvious vascular injuries.
- Avoid aorto-caval obstruction in any shocked pregnant patient.

During fluid therapy, patients may be classified as

- Stable.
- Responding to fluid therapy.
- Transient responders.
- Non-responders.

Fetal compromise demonstrated with the CTG may the first sign of maternal haemorrhage. Further monitoring, fluid and surgery may be required.

Any suspected source of bleeding must be identified

- Chest.
- Abdomen—diagnostic peritoneal lavage, if abdominal injury suspected.
- Retroperitoneal space—large engorged pelvic vessels that surround the gravid uterus can contribute to massive retroperitoneal bleeding after blunt trauma.
- Pelvis—sacroiliac joints and symphysis pubis widen in pregnancy.
- Extensive placental separation or AFE can cause DIC with depletion of fibrinogen, clotting factors and platelets. If this occurs, appropriate therapy should be given in liaison with the Consultant Haematologist.

- As little as 0.01mL of fetal blood can cause isoimmunization of Rhesus-negative mothers. Ig therapy should be considered in all Rhesus-negative mothers, irrespective of the extent and site of trauma, within 72h.
- A Kleihauer–Betke test to assess isoimmunization should be performed. A maternal blood smear allows detection of fetal RBSs in the maternal circulation. A positive test is also an accurate predictor of premature labour.
- Diagnostic peritoneal lavage has been used to detect free blood in the abdominal cavity. However this may be technically difficult, and ultrasound [especially focused abdominal sonography for trauma (FAST)] may be preferred to detect haemorrhage.

Disability

Non-pregnant and pregnant patients are assessed alike with the AVPU score:

- A—awake and orientated.
- V—responds to voice.
- P—responds to pain.
- U—unresponsive.

Eclampsia is a complication of pregnancy that may mimic head injury. The diagnosis needs to be considered if a patient has a head injury. Look for evidence of hyper-reflexia, peripheral oedema and proteinuria.

Environment

The patient needs to be completely exposed to assess for injury. The ambient temperature needs to be increased to prevent hypothermia and further clotting abnormalities.

Domestic violence is rapidly becoming a major cause of injury to women during cohabitation, marriage and pregnancy—17% of injured patients experience trauma as a result of another person. This needs to be considered.

Some indicators include

- If the partner insists on being present for interview and examination and monopolizes discussion.
- Diminishing self-image, depression, history of suicide attempts.
- Self-blame.

Secondary survey

This does not begin until the primary survey has been completed and the immediate life-threatening injuries identified and treated.

Other important potential injuries include:

- Simple pneumothorax.
- Haemothorax.
- Aortic disruption.
- Diaphragmatic injury.
- Blunt cardiac injury.

Fetal survival is completely dependent on adequate resuscitation of mother. Fetal survival does not necessarily equate with the injury severity score, and fetal demise can occur with trivial maternal trauma and at any gestational age.

Vigilant monitoring of mother and fetus is needed.

Specific maternal and fetal injury

Blunt injury

- The abdominal wall, uterine myometrium and amniotic fluid act as buffers to direct fetal injury from blunt trauma.
- Direct injuries to fetus and uterus causing rupture can occur during motor vehicle accidents and indirect ones from shearing forces resulting in abruptio placentae.

Penetrating Injury

- As the gravid uterus increases in size, the remainder of the viscera are relatively protected from penetrating injury, while the risk of uterine injury increases.
- Energy is absorbed by the uterus from any penetrating injury, resulting in good maternal survival and poor fetal survival.
- Maternal volume status should be monitored with early placement of CVP.
- An abnormality of fetal heart baseline, repetitive decelerations, absence of acceleration or beat-to-beat variability may indicate fetal compromise.
- A vaginal examination is mandatory to assess cervical effacement and dilatation, fetal presentation and relationship of fetal presenting part to ischial spines.

Uterine rupture

If this has occurred, peritoneal signs may be difficult as usual peritoneal signs are attenuated.

- Abdominal guarding and tenderness may be present.
- Odd lie of uterus with an inability to feel fundus.
- Suspicion of uterine rupture requires surgical exploration.
- Placental abruption is a leading cause of death after blunt trauma and occurs after relatively minor trauma in late pregnancy.
- Vaginal bleeding can be occult (30%).
- Uterine tenderness, premature contractions, irritability, tetany may occur.
- The fundal height may increase.
- Maternal shock is very likely.

Amniotic fluid embolism

- If fluid is identified at the vagina after rupture of membranes with a pH of 7–7.5, there is a possibility of a life-threatening AFE and a consumptive coagulopathy.

Outcome

- Pregnancy is likely to end unsuccessfully with placental, uterine or direct fetal injury.
- Fetal death occurs in 80% of cases where there has been maternal haemorrhagic shock.
- Maternal survival may depend on surgical evacuation of uterus and fetus.
- Postmortem CS is advised in the event of fatal maternal trauma since it may result in fetal salvage despite prolonged hypoxaemia.

Sepsis

Sepsis remains a common direct cause of maternal mortality in the CEMACH reports. During pregnancy, the susceptibility to endotoxins is increased, with diabetic mothers and women on steroid therapy being at higher risk of systemic sepsis following infection. Severe sepsis in pregnancy has a high mortality (30–50%).

Definitions

- Bacteraemia: bacteria in the bloodstream.
- Systemic inflammatory response syndrome (SIRS), has been defined as a combination of two or more of the following features:
  - Temperature >38°C OR <36°C.
  - HR >90bpm.
  - Respiratory rate >20/min or $PaCO_2$ <4.3kPa.
  - WCC >12 000/mm^3 or <4000/mm^3 or >10% immature forms.
- Sepsis is SIRS in the presence of a proven or suspected infection.
- Septic shock is defined as sepsis plus hypotension, despite adequate fluid resuscitation, plus organ perfusion abnormalities.

WCCs are normally elevated in pregnancy (10 000–18 000/mm^3), making diagnosis of early infection difficult. However, bacteraemia is common in the fit and healthy obstetric population, but only 0–4% of these women develop septic shock following infection.

Pathophysiology of sepsis

In a septic patient, the severity of illness is determined by the extent of the inflammatory response rather than by the infection itself. The initial response to sepsis is the release of primary mediators; tumour necrotic factor, interleukin-1 and other cytokines. These mediators are produced from activated macrophages. These primary mediators then stimulate production of secondary mediators, such as prostaglandins, leukotrienes, coagulation and complement cascades, platelet-activating factor and nitric oxide (NO). At the cellular level, the effects caused by these mediators include vasodilatation, increased capillary permeability, impaired tissue oxygenation and myocardial depression. This promotes anaerobic metabolism in tissues and lactic acidosis.

Causes of sepsis in obstetric patients

- Chorioamnionitis.
- Pyelonepheritis.
- Wound infection.
- Pneumonia.
- Acute appendicitis.
- Acute cholecystitis.
- Pancreatitis.
- Postpartum endometritis.
- Necrotizing fascitis.

Common microbes responsible for sepsis in the developed world include *Streptococcus* group A and B, *Escherichia coli*, and some anaerobes such as *Listeria monocytogenes*, *Gardnerella vaginalis* and *Staphylococcus aureus*. The infective organisms ascend the genital tract and colonize the uterine cavity. Once established, spread may occur via the bloodstream, leading to pelvic sepsis and abscess formation. If not treated, septic thrombus of the pelvic veins, septicaemia and septic shock may occur.

Predisposing factors include

- Prolonged rupture of membranes.
- Prolonged labour.
- Operative delivery.
- Perineal trauma/episiotomy.
- Retained products of conception.
- History of pelvic sepsis.

Clinical manifestation

- Pyrexia or hypothermia.
- Offensive lochia.
- Pelvic pain.
- Tachycardia.
- Tachypnoea.
- Altered mental state.
- Hypotension.
- Neutrophilia or neutropenia.
- Isolated thrombocytopenia.
- Other complications, e.g. DIC, ARDS, renal failure or hepatic failure.

Not all febrile episodes are infection related. Conversely about one-third of septic patients have no fever or are hypothermic, which is associated with increased mortality. Pyrexia increases uterine activity and induces preterm labour.

Differential diagnosis

Other causes of fever, which may not be associated with infection, are other inflammatory responses;

- Fever associated with prostaglandin administration and normal labour.
- Epidural analgesia is associated with a progressive rise in temperature.
- Endocrine (e.g. hyperthyroidism, malignant hyperthermia, hypoadrenalism).
- Central causes (e.g. intracranial haemorrhage).
- Drug related (including drug withdrawal).
- Following transfusion of blood or blood products.

Management

In the management of patients with sepsis, the anaesthetist has a major role in maintaining tissue oxygenation.

- Maintain a patent **A**irway with adequate **B**reathing and oxygenation.
- Fluid resuscitation to maintain **C**irculation—almost all septic patients are vasodilated.
- Transfer to critical care for continuing support.

Monitoring in early stages should include

- Temperature.
- Pulse.
- Respiratory rate.
- BP.
- Arterial saturation (SpO_2).
- Hourly urine output.

Assess baseline investigations

- FBC.
- U&E.
- Blood cultures.
- Coagulation profile.
- LFTs.

- If the patient remains hypotensive despite adequate fluid resuscitation, vasopressors should be commenced to normalize CO or increase CO to above normal parameters.
- The pregnant woman is susceptible to pulmonary oedema even with minimal or modest fluid overload.
- Noradrenaline is the appropriate vasopressor in septic shock.
- Start appropriate broad-spectrum antibiotics and seek microbiology advice at an early stage.
- Urgent blood, urine, high vaginal, endocervical and other appropriate cultures should be taken, ideally before starting antibiotics.
- Consider surgical intervention if needed to evacuate the uterus or drain an abscess.
- Exclude other sources of infection, e.g. chest, urine and blood.
- Tight control of blood glucose in septic patients using insulin infusion improves outcome.
- In septic shock, low dose steroids, hydrocortisone 5mg 6hly for 7 days has been proven to be useful.
- Consider activated Protein C within 24–48h of onset of infection if no contraindications are present.
- ***Surgical intervention*** is required for:
  - Evacuation of retained products of conception.
  - Evacuation of retained placenta.
  - Myometrial necrosis.
  - Myometrial abscess.
  - Necrotizing fasciitis.
  - Any other closed space infections.

Chapter 20

The fetus

Christine Conner

Fetal circulation *in utero*

Oxygen and nutrients are brought to the placenta by the maternal uteroplacental circulation, with delivery to the fetus by the separate fetoplacental circulation.

Uteroplacental circulation

- Maternal CO together with the spiral arteries within the uterine myometrium and decidua determine blood flow to the intervillous space and fetus.
- Physiological adaptations in pregnancy increase the maternal CO by 40%.
- Oxygen-carrying capacity is increased up to 28% by an increase in the red cell mass.
- Spiral arteries become more tortuous and lose elasticity through placental trophoblast invasion to adapt to the increasing demand of blood supply to the placenta.
- Trophoblast erosion of the spiral arteries occurs in two phases to produce a low pressure, high blood flow system within the placenta.

  - Phase 1 occurs in the first trimester and involves trophoblast erosion of the decidual portions of the spiral arteries.
  - Phase 2 in the second trimester involves trophoblast erosion into the myometrial portion of the spiral arteries.

- The loss of elasticity within the spiral arteries removes vasoregulation. Therefore, blood flow to the placenta is directly proportional to the maternal CO.
- Oxygenated blood enters the intervillous space from the spiral arteries as jets of blood directed towards the chorionic plate of the placenta.
- Transplacental gas exchange occurs by simple diffusion.
- Blood then flows towards the basal placental plate, aided by uterine contractions and movement of the chorionic villi.
- Deoxygenated blood drains into the uterine veins.

Umbilical circulation

- In the fetus, the placenta performs the functions of the lungs and kidneys.
- Two umbilical arteries (UAs) carry 50% of the fetal CO to the placenta.
- One UA arises from each fetal internal iliac artery and leaves the fetus through the umbilical cord to the placenta.
- In the placenta, the arteries divide into small branches, which enter the chorionic villi where further subdivision into arterioles and capillaries and transplacental gas exchange occur.
- Fetal blood then flows through corresponding venous systems, which drain into a single umbilical vein carrying oxygenated blood back to the fetus through the umbilical cord.
- Approximately 50% of the blood from the umbilical vein passes into the ductus venosus, which enters the IVC, bypassing the fetal liver.

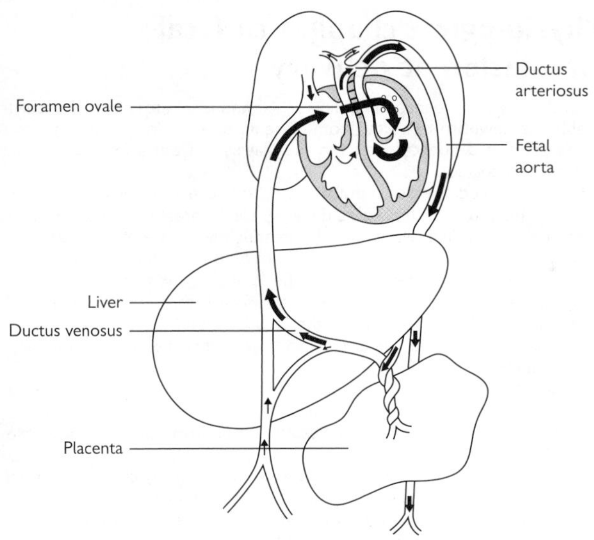

Fig. 20.1 Fetal circulation.

- On reaching the heart, a large proportion of blood within the IVC is directed by the crista dividens through the foramen ovale into the left atrium, avoiding entry into the right heart channel.
- This oxygenated blood passes into the left ventricle from where it is pumped into the aorta.
- From the aorta, two large carotid arteries distribute a large share of the oxygenated blood to the cerebral circulation.
- The smaller portion of blood in the IVC that does not pass through the foramen ovale mixes in the right atrium with deoxygenated blood carried by the superior vena cava (SVC) and the coronary sinus.
- This blood passes to the right ventricle from where it is pumped into the pulmonary circulation.
- Pressure within the pulmonary circulation is much higher than in the aorta, resulting in most of the blood being diverted along the ductus arteriosus, which joins the aorta below the origins of the carotid arteries.
- Less than 10% of the fetal CO enters the pulmonary circulation.
- The blood which passes down the fetal aorta to supply the viscera contains mainly blood that has circulated through the head and arms together with a lesser amount from the LV.
- Two-thirds of the blood from the aorta is pumped along the umbilical arteries to the placenta, with a small amount entering the femoral arteries to the legs.

Physiological changes to fetal circulation at delivery

At birth, a rapid sequence of cardiovascular and respiratory events occur to enable the newborn to switch from placenta to lungs for effective gaseous exchange. This sequence results in the transition from a fetal to an adult pattern of circulation.

- Labour-induced stresses stimulate catecholamine and steroid responses within the fetus, which prepare the lungs for air breathing by reducing the amount of lung fluid secretion and increasing the release of lung surfactant.
- Uterine contractions reduce the flow of blood into the intervillous space, resulting in deterioration in the fetal blood gas status.
- Compression of the fetal thorax as it descends through the birth canal at delivery helps expel some of the fetal lung fluid. Fluid within the alveolar spaces and tracheobronchial tree is absorbed into pulmonary lymphatics.
- Expansion of the fetal thorax as it emerges from the vagina at delivery enables the proximal airways to fill with air.
- Clamping of the umbilical cord results in a deterioration of blood gases and low arterial pO_2.
- This change is detected by the carotid and aortic body chemoreceptors and provides a very powerful stimulus to initiate breathing.
- Exposure to other sensory stimuli with delivery (temperature, pain, pressure, tactile stimuli) helps to initiate breathing.
- Entry of air into the lungs raises the interstitial pO_2, resulting in a reduction in PVR, an increase in pulmonary blood flow, a rise in the pO_2 and increased filling of the left atria.
- Clamping of the cord removes the low resistance placental circulation, with a resulting increase in SVR and reduced VR to the right atrium.
- The pressure gradient within the atrial chambers reverses with the increased pressure in the left atrium, resulting in a functional closure of the foramen ovale.
- This separates the circulatory system into two halves—the right and left.
- The fall in the PVR causes a reversal of blood flow within the ductus arteriosus shunt.
- The perfusion of the ductus arteriosus with oxygen-rich blood together with locally produced vasoactive substances results in its closure.

Physiological remnants of the fetal circulation

- The foramen ovale becomes the adult fosse ovalis.
- The ductus arteriosus becomes the adult ligamentum arteriosum.
- The extrahepatic portion of the umbilical vein becomes the adult ligamentum teres hepatis.
- The ductus venosus becomes the adult ligamentum venosum.
- The proximal portions of the fetal right and left umbilical arteries become the adult umbilical branches of the internal iliac arteries.
- The distal portions of the umbilical arteries become the adult medial umbilical ligaments.

Fetal haemoglobin

The partial pressure of oxygen within the umbilical vein at term is between 30 and 40mmHg. To meet its tissue oxygen requirements at this relatively low pO_2, the fetus has made adaptations to hypoxia.

- At term, the fetal haemoglobin concentration is high, between 16 and 18g/dL, which increases the oxygen-carrying capacity of the blood.
- Fetal haemoglobin is predominantly (60–80%) HbF, which has a higher affinity for O_2 than adult haemoglobin (HbA).
- This enables fetal blood to take up oxygen more readily from maternal blood.
- The O_2 dissociation curve for HbF is steeper than that for HbA over the range of pO_2 found in fetal tissues, allowing better delivery of oxygen to these tissues.
- The anatomy of the fetal circulation ensures that the pO_2 within the ascending aorta is 30% higher than in the descending portion, providing more oxygenated blood to the developing brain and heart muscle than to the other fetal organs.

Assessment of fetal well-being during pregnancy

Obstetric patients are risk stratified at booking into two main groups:

- Low risk: no identifiable risk factors. They will have the majority of their care in community-based midwifery-led antenatal clinics.
- High risk: identified by either their past obstetric or medical history. Their care in pregnancy will be co-ordinated through hospital obstetrician-run antenatal clinics.
- All obstetric patients require antenatal fetal assessment, but the frequency and forms of assessment will vary according to risk.
- Patients who initially start as low risk may, during the course of either their pregnancy or labour, develop obstetric complications necessitating additional fetal assessment.

Fetal growth

- Normal fetal growth is dependent on an adequate supply of oxygen and nutrients to and across the placenta with sufficient fetal uptake, together with overall regulation of the growth process.
- Any factor which interferes with these processes can result in IUGR.
- The severity of the IUGR will depend on the gestational age at onset, the magnitude of the injury and the success of adaptive mechanisms.
- Factors affecting fetal growth can be broadly subdivided into maternal, uterine, placental and fetal categories.

- ***Maternal factors*** include:
    - any chronic medical condition.
    - smoking.
    - alcohol and drug addiction.
    - maternal age <16 and >35 years.
    - low BMI.
- ***Uterine abnormalities*** include:
    - congenital uterine malformation.
    - uterine fibroids
- ***Placental factors*** include:
    - impaired trophoblast invasion as seen with pre-eclampsia.
    - placental abruption.
    - placental infarction.
    - chorioamnionitis.
    - placenta praevia.
- ***Fetal factors*** include:
    - chromosomal abnormalities.
    - structural abnormalities.
    - congenital infection.
    - inborn errors of metabolism.
    - multiple pregnancy.

- All obstetric patients require assessment of fetal growth.
- Any method employed to assess fetal growth requires an accurate knowledge of gestational age.
- Most of the tests currently used detect the small for gestational age (SFG) fetus rather than the fetus with IUGR.
- The IUGR fetus is one who has failed to reach its own growth potential. Not all SFG fetuses will be suffering from IUGR, as many will be healthy constitutionally small babies.
- Differentiating the pathological IUGR fetus from the healthy SFG fetus is clinically important as IUGR is associated with an increased risk of:
  - stillbirth.
  - prematurity.
  - intrapartum fetal distress.
  - perinatal morbidity.
- Tests used to assess fetal growth are more sensitive and specific when applied to high risk pregnancies compared to the low risk population.

Symphyseal fundal height

- A useful screening test for all obstetric patients.
- The measurement is taken from the top of the maternal symphisis pubis to the top of the uterine fundus and is measured in centimetres.
- Between 20 and 35 weeks gestation, the normal symphyseal fundal height (SFH) should approximate the number of weeks of gestation with an acceptable variation of ±2cm.
- After 35 weeks gestation, the margin of error is ±3cm.
- It does not differentiate between SFG and IUGR and is subject to significant intra- and interobserver error.
- Serial SFH measurements increase its sensitivity as a screening test.
- Sensitivity is further limited by factors including:
  - Maternal obesity.
  - Uterine fibroids.
  - Abnormal amniotic fluid volume.
  - Abnormal fetal lie.
  - Multiple pregnancies.
- Customized charts which adjust for maternal factors, including BMI, parity and ethnicity, improve the sensitivity and increase the antenatal detection of SFG babies.
- Further investigation, in the form of an ultrasound examination, is required if the SFH measurement differs by more than the expected for gestation.

Ultrasound biometry

- Ultrasound is the best available method for detecting a SFG fetus and in monitoring growth.
- Any fetus thought to be at risk of IUGR, from either the maternal obstetric or medical history, should be assessed with serial ultrasound biometry.
- The fetal biparietal diameter, head circumference (HC), abdominal circumference (AC) and femur length are the measurements obtained at ultrasound examinations.

- Growth charts are available for each of these measurements, and most are based on cross-sectional rather than longitudinal population studies.
- On most charts, the 5th, 50th and 95th centiles are plotted.
- The AC, which includes the fetal liver, the size of which is dependent on stored glycogen and hence fetal nutrition, is the best measurement for detecting IUGR.

Two patterns of growth restriction exist

- **Symmetric IUGR** where both head size and AC are simultaneously reduced, with a HC/AC within normal limits.
  - Constitutionally small babies at the lower end of the normal range.
  - Pathological due to an insult early in pregnancy at the time of general organ growth. This includes congenital abnormalities, chromosomal abnormalities and congenital infections.
- **Asymmetric IUGR** is the result of fetal adaptation to an inadequate supply of nutrition in order to protect the developing brain.
  - AC is reduced more than the head measurements, giving an increased HC/AC ratio.
  - Usually seen in conditions with a later pathological onset, e.g. pre-eclampsia, placental abruption or infarction.
- Ultrasound scanning also enables assessment of the amniotic fluid volume (AFV) and the UA Doppler status, which are both useful in distinguishing the healthy SFG fetus from the one with IUGR.

Amniotic fluid volume

- After 16 weeks gestation, the fetal kidneys produce most of the AFV.
- If the supply of oxygen and nutrients to the growing fetus is insufficient, adaptations occur, with redistribution of fetal blood away from the kidneys in favour of the brain and the myocardium.
- The reduced blood flow to the kidneys results in an overall reduction in the AFV.
- Ultrasound provides the most reliable method of assessment of AFV, which is expressed as the amniotic fluid index (AFI).
- Oligohyramnios is defined as either an AFI of <5cm or a single maximum pocket of <2cm.
- The perinatal mortality is increased in pregnancies with reduced AFV on ultrasound scanning compared with those where the AFV is normal.

Umbilical artery Doppler

- Assessment of the UA Doppler waveform is widely used in the antenatal surveillance of pregnancies with IUGR.
- The UA Doppler waveform is affected by the resistance of blood flow within the placenta and the degree of villous formation.
- Normal placental villous formation produces a low resistance system facilitating forward flow of blood within the UA throughout the fetal cardiac cycle, described as positive end-diastolic flow (EDF) (Fig. 20.2a).
- Various parameters including the resistance index can be calculated from the UA Doppler waveform and are used to assess the degree of resistance within the UA (Fig. 20.2a).

- Conditions such as IUGR and pre-eclampsia are associated with an inadequate maternal vascular response to placentation and result in increased resistance in the placental circulation.
- With increasing placental resistance, the EDF decreases (Fig. 20.2b).
- Further damage with increasing resistance will eventually lead to no forward flow, known as absent EDF (Fig. 20.2c) or, in extreme cases, to reversal of flow, known as reversed EDF (Fig. 20.2d).
- By this stage, ~60–70% of the villous vascular tree is damaged.
- Abnormal UA Doppler flow patterns indicate an increased risk of fetal hypoxia and acidaemia.
- Both perinatal mortality and morbidity rates increase with the degree of abnormality within the UA Doppler recording.

Management of IUGR

Once fetal IUGR has been confirmed by serial scanning, the subsequent management will depend on the gestation.

- With early-onset IUGR before 32 weeks gestation or symmetric IUGR, consider chromosomal abnormalities, congenital anomalies and congenital infection.

  - Detailed anomaly scan to look for structural abnormalities.
  - Consider fetal karyotyping.
  - Maternal viral screen (TORCH screen for toxoplasmosis, rubella, cytomegalovirus and herpes simplex).
  - Maternal corticosteroid administration, in case preterm delivery <36 weeks is required, to help fetal lung maturation.
  - Intensive fetal monitoring as for late-onset IUGR.

- Late-onset IUGR after 32 weeks gestation.

  - Regular fetal monitoring using ultrasound scanning assessment of the AFV, the UA Doppler status, serial biometry and CTG.
  - Consider maternal steroid administration if delivery before 36 weeks is necessary.

- If the UA Doppler waveform and other tests remain normal, continue twice-weekly fetal monitoring. Some obstetricians may consider delivery at ~36 weeks whilst others may continue monitoring until term.
- If the UA Doppler shows absent EDF but other tests are normal, consider delivery if an adequate gestation has been reached. Otherwise, careful frequent monitoring at least twice weekly.
- If the UA Doppler shows reversed EDF or the CTG or other biophysical parameters suggest hypoxia, proceed to immediate delivery.

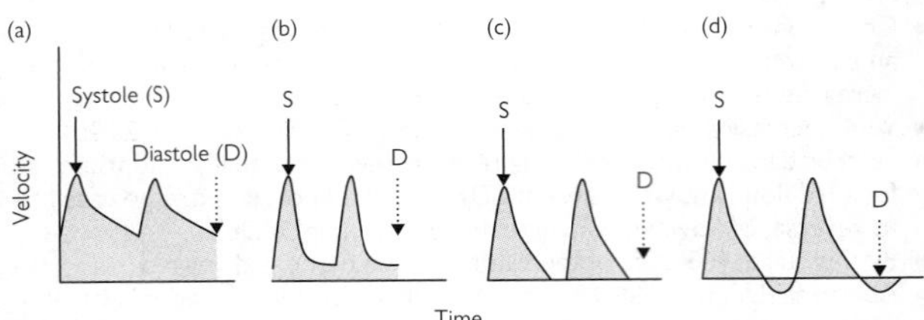

Fig. 20.2 Umbilical artery waveform patterns. (a) Normal UA Doppler with normal resistance index. (b) UA Doppler waveform showing increased resistance index. (c) UA Doppler waveform showing absent end-diastolic flow. (d) UA Doppler waveform showing reversed end-diastolic flow.

Assessment of fetal well-being during labour

Meconium

- Clear amniotic fluid drainage is a reassuring feature in labour.
- Meconium-stained liquor (MSL) is present in ~15% of all labours.
- The main factors influencing the passage of meconium are gestational age and possible fetal compromise. Therefore, the presence of MSL must be interpreted accordingly.
- Meconium is produced in the fetal gut from 10 weeks, but is rarely passed by the fetus before 34 weeks gestation. By term, MSL is present in ~30% of cases, increasing to 50% by 42 weeks.
- In preterm infants, MSL is very uncommon and is associated with infections such as listeriosis, which produce a fetal gut enteritis.
- Maternal obstetric cholestasis is associated with increased risk of MSL.
- Fresh thick meconium is frequently passed with a fetal breech. presentation in the late first and second stage due to mechanical forces on the presenting part in labour.
- Acute and subacute fetal compromise can lead to the passage of meconium.
- In very acute situations such as cord prolapse or placental abruption, this may not occur.

Grading of meconium

- Meconium is often graded according to its appearance, which will be affected by the volume of amniotic fluid around the fetus and the temporal relationship between its passage and the timing of membrane rupture.
- Meconium consistency will be determined by the diluting influence of the AFV. With decreasing amounts of amniotic fluid, the thickness of meconium will increase.
- Meconium passed several days before rupture of the membranes is often brown and described as old.
- Recently passed meconium is green and often referred to as new or fresh.

Management of meconium-stained liquor in labour

- Continuous fetal monitoring is recommended.
- If the FHR is normal, no other specific action is required in labour.
- If the FHR is abnormal, consideration should be given either to performing a fetal blood sample or immediate delivery depending on the clinical setting.

Meconium aspiration syndrome

- Aspiration of meconium into the fetal or neonatal lungs can lead to meconium aspiration syndrome (MAS).
- Meconium aspiration, defined as the presence of meconium below the vocal cords, occurs in ~35% of fetuses with MSL.
- Clinically MAS can range from a mild transitory condition to severe respiratory compromise.

- Meconium aspiration can occur *in utero*, at delivery or after birth.
- *In utero* meconium aspiration is thought to occur as a result of fetal breathing movements.
- In an infant who has not been exposed to intrauterine hypoxia, meconium aspiration usually results in mild MAS, which is asymptomatic in 90% of cases.
- In severe cases, neonatal mortality can be as high as 40%.
- Meconium causes physical airway obstruction, displaces surfactant, resulting in atelectasis, and produces a local chemical pneumonitis.

Risk factors for severe MAS

- Fetal hypoxia.
- Presence of thick meconium, more common in post-term pregnancies and with oligohydramnios.

Intrapartum prevention of MAS

- Intrapartum saline amnioinfusion is a relatively new technique shown in small studies to reduce the incidence of MAS with MSL.
- Normal saline 1L is instilled into the uterine cavity through an indwelling intrauterine pressure catheter over a 30min period, and repeated after 4–6h in prolonged labour.
- In addition to diluting the meconium concentration, it may reduce cord compression and consequently fetal hypoxia.
- The technique may not be clinically feasible in up to 50% of cases.

Management at delivery

- A paediatrician should be present for delivery in all labours where there is MSL.
- If the baby is vigorous and active following delivery, irrespective of grade of meconium, no further action should be taken.
- With a non-vigorous baby, the vocal cords should be visualized. If meconium is present on or below the cords, direct tracheal suction is required.
- Saline lavage is not recommended as it carries the risk of removing surfactant and it may facilitate further spread of meconium within the lung.
- There is no evidence to support the technique of clamping the chest to delay the first breath, nor is gastric suctioning recommended.

The cardiotocograph

The CTG is a continuous simultaneous recording of the FHR and uterine contractions, known as continuous electronic fetal monitoring (EFM).

- EFM can be performed with external transducers using Doppler ultrasound scanning to assess the FHR and a tocodynamometer, a strain gauge attached to a belt, to assess uterine contractions.
- Alternatively, internal devices such as an electrode applied directly to the presenting fetal part and a calibrated intrauterine pressure catheter can be used.
- External tocography assesses frequency and duration of contractions.
- An intrauterine pressure catheter is required to assess the intensity of contraction.

Fetal monitoring in labour

- In labour, uterine contractions restrict maternal blood supply to the placental bed, which is further compounded by the effects of pushing in the second stage.
- Each fetus has a different capacity to withstand the stress of labour.
- On admission in labour, an assessment is made to identify risk factors that may affect the fetal reserve.

Risk factors

- Maternal factors.
  - Medical problems: essential hypertension, IDDM (insulin-dependent diabetes mellitus).
  - Antenatal events: antepartum haemorrhage, pre-eclampsia.
  - Induced labour.
  - Prolonged pregnancy.
  - Past obstetric history: previous CS, previous stillbirth.
- Fetal factors.
  - Prematurity.
  - IUGR.
  - Oligohydramnios.
  - Abnormal UA Doppler studies.
  - Multiple pregnancy.
  - Breech presentation.
  - MSL.
- Intrapartum risk factors.
  - Augmentation with IV oxytocin.
  - Epidural anaesthesia.
  - Intrapartum bleeding.
  - Maternal pyrexia.
  - Development of fresh meconium in labour.
  - Abnormal FHR on intermittent auscultation.

Two options exist for fetal monitoring in labour

- For low risk cases, intermittent FHR auscultation is acceptable.
- For high risk cases, continuous EFM is recommended.

External fetal monitoring

- EFM was introduced to try and reduce perinatal mortality and cerebral palsy (CP) rates.
- Only 10% of CP cases are thought to result from intrapartum events, the remainder being due to antenatal factors.
- EFM has failed to reduce CP rates but has led to an increase in instrumental-assisted vaginal delivery.
- EFM is very sensitive in detecting fetal hypoxia but lacks specificity.
- Fetal blood sampling has helped to improve overall specificity.

CTG interpretation in labour

A systematic approach is required to ensure correct CTG interpretation.

- Any existing obstetric risk factors need to be considered.
- Assessment of uterine contractions is required to allow their effect on the FHR to be established.

Features of the FHR to be considered

Baseline rate

- The mean FHR when it is stable, over a 5–10min period with both accelerations and decelerations excluded.
- Normal baseline rate in labour is between 110 and 150bpm (Fig. 20.3).
- A tachycardia is a baseline FHR of >150bpm. Between 150 and 170bpm is termed moderate baseline tachycardia and, provided other features are reassuring, is not indicative of hypoxia.
- A bradycardia is a baseline FHR of <110bpm. Between 100 and 110bpm is termed moderate baseline bradycardia, but provided all other features are reassuring is not suggestive of hypoxia.
- A change in baseline may indicate gradually developing hypoxia.

Baseline variability

- The degree to which the baseline varies, i.e. the width of the baseline, excluding accelerations and decelerations.
- Normal variability is between 10 and 25 beats (Fig. 20.3).
- A baseline variability of 0–5bpm is classified as silent, 5–10bpm as reduced and >25bpm as saltatory.
- Normal baseline variability is an indicator of adequate oxygenation of the autonomic system.

Presence or absence of accelerations

- Acceleration is a transient increase in the FHR of ≥15bpm lasting ≥15s.
- Two or more accelerations per 20min is termed reactive and is indicative of fetal well-being (Fig. 20.3).

Presence and type of decelerations

- A deceleration is a transient decrease in the FHR of ≥15bpm lasting ≥15s.
- **Early decelerations**
  - These are due to compression of the fetal head causing stimulation of the vagus nerve producing a bradycardia.
  - Tend to appear in the late first and second stage of labour with descent of the head.
  - They are synchronous with contractions and tend to be uniform in shape (Fig 20.4).
  - If isolated and other CTG parameters normal, they are usually benign.

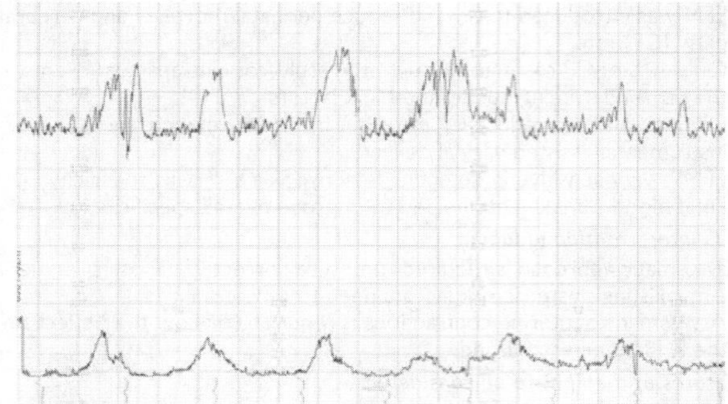

Fig. 20.3 A CTG trace showing a normal baseline and baseline variability with accelerations.

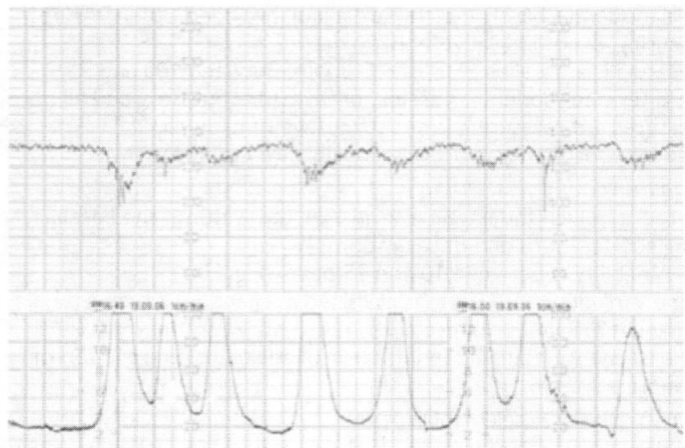

Fig. 20.4 A CTG trace showing early decelerations.

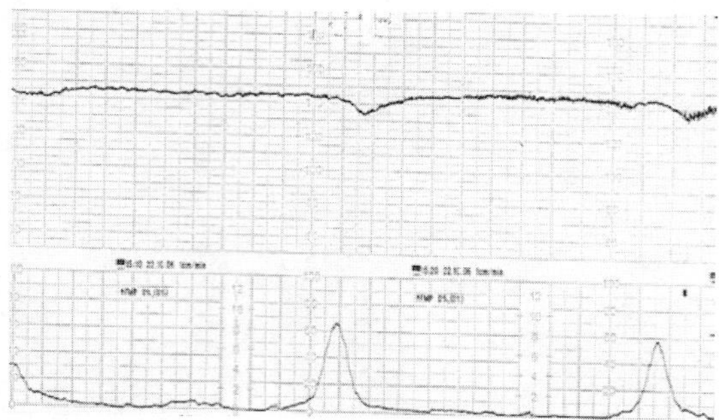

Fig. 20.5 A CTG trace showing late decelerations with reduced baseline variability.

- **Late decelerations**
  - These decelerations are late with respect to the uterine contractions and are associated with uteroplacental insufficiency.
  - The retroplacental space provides a variable-sized reservoir of oxygenated blood. In a fetus with IUGR, this reservoir will be small. At the start of a contraction, the fetus uses its reservoir of oxygen.
  - Due to restriction of uteroplacental blood supply during a contraction, a hypoxic deceleration begins and continues throughout the contraction.
  - Recovery occurs some time after the contraction when full oxygenation has been restored.
- **Variable decelerations**
  - Most common type of FHR decelerations are a consequence of umbilical cord compression with contractions.
  - As the cord can be compressed in a different way with each contraction, their appearance can vary in shape, size and timing.
  - In the cord, the umbilical vein is thinner and is compressed first before the arteries.
  - This results in loss of some of the fetal circulating volume, and autonomic responses result in an increased FHR to compensate, which is seen as an acceleration.
  - Further compression of the cord then occludes the thicker umbilical arteries with a relative restoration of the fetal circulation.
  - Stimulation of fetal baroreceptors leads to a precipitous fall in the FHR. The nadir of the deceleration occurs when both the umbilical vein and artery are compressed.
  - A normal well-grown fetus can tolerate cord compression for a considerable length of time before developing hypoxia. Small IUGR fetuses have less reserve.
  - Variable decelerations can be subclassified as typical and atypical.

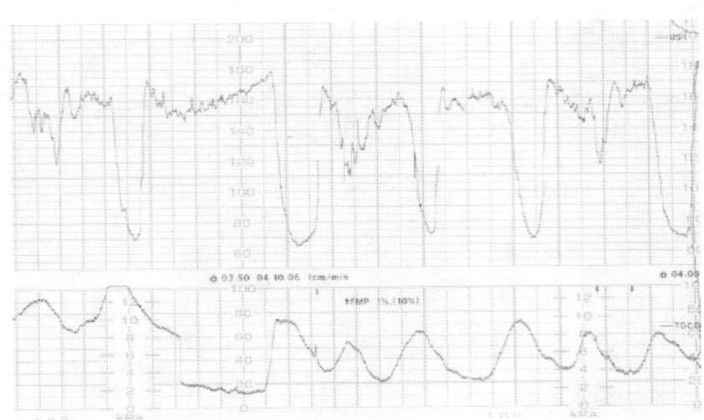

Fig. 20.6 A CTG trace showing typical variable decelerations.

- Suspicious features associated with atypical variable decelerations include reduced baseline variability, a rising baseline, late recovery, a combined variable and a late deceleration component, and a duration of >60s with a loss of >60 beats from the baseline.
- The presence of atypical variables makes progressive hypoxia more likely.

CTG classification

The CTG is classified as normal, suspicious or pathological.

- *Normal.* All four features are reassuring.
- *Suspicious.* No more than one non-reassuring feature.
- *Pathological.* Two or more non-reassuring features or one or more abnormal features.

Reassuring features on CTG

- Baseline FHR between 110 and 150bpm.
- Baseline variability between 5 and 25bpm.
- Two accelerations per 20min.
- No decelerations.

Non-reassuring or suspicious features on CTG

- Baseline FHR between 100 and 109 bpm or 151 and 170bpm.
- Baseline variability between 5 and 10bpm for >40min.
- Increased baseline variability of >25bpm.
- Variable decelerations.

Abnormal or pathological features on CTG

- Baseline FHR <100bpm or >170bpm.
- Baseline variability of <5bpm for >40min.
- Late decelerations.
- Atypical variable decelerations.
- Prolonged deceleration for >3min duration.
- Sinusoidal pattern for ≥20min.

Action with a non-reassuring CTG

When non-reassuring or pathological features appear on the CTG, a search and treatment of correctable causes should be made, e.g.

- Uterine hyperstimulation.
- Maternal hypotension from aortovenal compression or epidural top-up.
- Maternal dehydration.
- Maternal pyrexia.
- Maternal need for analgesia.

If no underlying cause is identified or the CTG does not improve despite corrective procedures, a fetal blood sample (FBS) to assess fetal acid–base balance should be considered.

- Suspicious and pathological CTG traces are not always associated with acidosis.
- Special attention should be paid to fetuses susceptible to developing acidosis more quickly, including those with IUGR, preterm, post-term, infected, where there is grade 3 meconium or minimal amniotic fluid draining.
- In addition, other factors in labour that have a significant influence on the rate of decline of the fetal pH need to be considered, e.g. use of oxytocin, difficult instrumental delivery as well as acute events such as cord prolapse, uterine scar dehiscence and placental abruption.
- With these acute events, there may not be enough time to perform an FBS and delivery should be expedited.
- FBS is only technically possible once the cervix is 3cm or more dilated.
- Occasionally, it may not be possible to obtain an adequate blood sample and, if the CTG abnormality is persistent, delivery is then necessary.

Fetal blood sample

- An explanation should be given to the mother about the indication for the procedure and the planned action following the FBS.
- Verbal consent should be obtained.
- Midwifery and anaesthetic staff should be aware that the test is taking place in case urgent delivery is necessary.

Position

- Ideally, the mother should be in either the left or right lateral position.
- The lithotomy position should be avoided because of the risk of maternal hypotension from aorto-caval compression. This can produce an iatrogenic fetal hypoxia and acidosis, leading to an unnecessary operative delivery.

Procedure

- An aseptic technique is used and an amnioscope is passed through the vagina to reach the fetal scalp.
- The fetal scalp is dried using a dental swab and then sprayed with ethyl chloride to produce a hyperaemia, which aids bleeding.
- The fetal scalp is then smeared lightly with a water-repellant gel to help the blood form into a round drop.
- Under direct vision the fetal scalp is stabbed with a 2mm blade.

- The blood droplet is allowed to form and is then drawn up by capillary action into a preheparinized thin glass tube.
- When there is a sufficiently sized sample, it is taken immediately to the blood gas analyser.

Analysis

- It is preferable to measure the pH, the base deficit, the PO_2 and PCO_2.

FBS interpretation

- It is essential to inform the anaesthetic team when an FBS is being performed as the result may necessitate immediate delivery.
- Any FBS result should be interpreted taking into account the clinical features of both the mother and baby, any previous FBS results and the progress of the labour.
- As a general guide, Table 20.1 illustrates the subsequent action required following an FBS result according to published guidelines from the Royal College of Obstetricians and Gynaecologists and NICE.

Table 20.1 Fetal blood sample

Fetal blood sample result	Action
pH ≥7.25	Repeat FBS if the FHR abnormality persists
pH 7.21–7.24	Repeat FBS within 30min or consider delivery if rapid fall since last FBS sample
pH ≤7.20	Delivery indicated

CTG plus ST analysis of the fetal ECG (STAN)

- Although the use of intrapartum EFM has been shown to reduce the incidence of neonatal seizures, it has had little impact on long-term neonatal outcome. In addition, there is concern that its use has resulted in an increase in the CS rate.
- Whilst the use of FBS can help with CTG interpretation, there are situations where this may not be technically possible, e.g. in the early stages of labour.
- In an attempt to overcome some of these issues, newer methods of intrapartum fetal monitoring have been explored. These methods include CTG in conjunction with STAN, the use of which is becoming more widespread.
- As part of the physiological response to *in utero* hypoxia, depression of the ST-segment of the fetal ECG has been observed and interpretation of such events with the CTG forms the basis of the STAN analysis.
- Application of a fetal scalp electrode (FSE) is necessary and therefore STAN can only be used in situations where this is technically possible, acceptable to the patient and where no contraindications to the use of FSE exist (e.g. risk of bleeding disorder in the fetus; maternal HIV).

- Interpretation of any ST-segment abnormalities, also know as STAN events, must be made in conjunction with the CTG findings and the overall clinical picture. In the first stage of labour, a significant STAN event will necessitate additional intervention in the form of either a FBS or delivery, depending on the overall clinical picture.
- In the second stage of labour, immediate delivery may be necessary and the anaesthetist must be kept fully informed of the situation to ensure the safest most appropriate method of anaesthesia is employed.

Fetal acid–base

Normal functioning of the fetal enzyme systems depends on stability of the pH within the tissues. Derangements in pH may be primary due to respiratory or metabolic dysfunction, but the clinical picture is often mixed.

Normal gaseous exchange

- The placenta functions as the lung whilst the fetus is *in utero*.
- Free gaseous exchange depends upon normal flow of both maternal and fetal blood through the placental bed.
- High HbF concentration together with the higher affinity of HbF for O_2 ensures adequate amounts of O_2 are transferred to the fetus.
- Under normal conditions the fetus obtains the majority of energy by aerobic metabolism of glucose.
- Some of the waste product—CO_2—is carried in simple solution, but the vast majority is carried as dissociated hydrogen (H^+) and bicarbonate (HCO_3^-) ions. The H^+ ions are mainly buffered by Hb, and the HCO_3^- ions pass out into the extracellular fluid.
- At the placenta, the CO_2 in solution diffuses across to the maternal circulation. The CO_2 carried as H^+ and HCO_3^- ions is also released and transferred. Elimination of the CO_2 means the concentration of H^+ ions in the fetal blood is reduced.
- UA blood (from the fetus to the placenta) has a low pO_2, high CO_2 and a low pH (opposite of adult circulation).
- Umbilical venous blood (from the placenta to the fetus) has a high pO_2, low pCO_2 and a low pH (opposite of adult circulation).

Disturbance of normal gaseous exchange

Various factors can disturb normal gaseous exchange at the placenta.

- ***Maternal factors***. Hypotension from aorto-caval compression, regional analgesia or anaesthesia. Uterine contractions may produce high pressure, reducing uterine blood flow. Chronic impairment of uteroplaental blood flow, e.g. pre-eclampsia.
- ***Placental factors***. Placental abruption and abnormal placental circulation, e.g. pre-eclampsia.
- ***Fetal factors*** Umbilical cord compression, fetal anaemia and fetal arrhythmia.

Reduction of perfusion of the placenta from fetal vessels is manifest as variable decelerations, whilst a reduction in perfusion from the maternal circulation is manifest as late decelerations.

Consequences

Impaired gaseous exchange at the placenta has several consequences:

- *Respiratory acidosis.* During the early stages of reduced placental perfusion, CO_2 transfer across the placenta is reduced, leading to a high pCO_2 and a low pH. This may be transitory. If corrective measures are taken and the FHR improves, it may be treated conservatively. A degree of respiratory acidosis occurs in most uncomplicated labours.

- Further reduction in placental perfusion affects O_2 transfer, resulting in a low pO_2. Fetal adaptation occurs. Increased O_2 extraction with centralization of blood flow to brain and myocardium at the expense of other organs occurs. Physiological reserve of the fetus will determine how long this can be sustained, but will be reduced in high risk situations.
- *Metabolic acidosis.* If aerobic metabolism cannot be maintained because of reduced O_2 supply, anaerobic metabolism may supplement energy supplies, resulting in lactic acid formation. Lactic acid forms lactate and H^+ ions, some of which will be buffered by Hb and HCO_3^- ions. H^+ ions are not easily eliminated at the placenta and buffers have an infinite capacity, and eventually the pH and bicarbonate levels will fall, producing a metabolic acidosis with a low pO_2, low pH and low HCO_3^-. Metabolic acidosis is damaging to fetal tissues.

Base deficit

- Base deficit enables the physician to differentiate between a respiratory and a metabolic acidosis.
- Respiratory acidosis does not use up buffering capacity, whereas metabolic acidosis does.
- Base deficit measures how much available buffer has been used up, and is actually the amount of base (alkali) needed to add to the blood in order to restore the pH to normal.
- Base deficit is defined as the mmol/L of base required to titrate the blood back to a normal pH.
- A base deficit is negative and is calculated from the pH and the pCO_2.

Cord gas analysis

- Following delivery, cord gas analysis is a useful adjunct in assessing the overall condition of the newborn and deciding subsequent neonatal management.
- The UA cord blood result better reflects the condition of the fetus.
- Sampling the smaller UA can be technically difficult in comparison with the vein. It is good practice to sample both the UA and umilical vein and compare the two results to ensure that the UA has indeed been analysed.
- The mean difference in pH between the artery and vein is ~0.08 units.
- Table 20.2 shows the mean blood gas results from both the UA and umbilical vein.

Table 20.2 Mean blood gas results from umbilical artery and vein at delivery

Measurement	Umbilical artery	Umbilical vein
pH	7.26	7.35
pCO_2	7.3kPa	5.3kPa
Base deficit	2.3mmol/L	2.9mmol/L

Effect of analgesia and anaesthesia on the fetus

- The pain of labour causes hyperventilation, leading to respiratory alkalosis with resulting vasoconstriction and reduced placental blood flow and oxygen availability to the fetus.
- Many women request pharmacological methods of pain relief in labour, which may confer advantages to the fetus, but may also pose certain risks.
- Most systemic drugs given to the mother are transferred to the fetus. However, the amount transferred will depend on both maternal and fetal factors, as well as the characteristics of the drugs themselves.
- Blood levels of any transmitted drug are disproportionately higher in the fetal brain compared with other tissues.
- This is partly due to the high cerebral blood flow and relatively poor development of the blood–brain barrier in the fetus.
- Chronic fetal hypoxia further increases the levels in the fetal brain as a consequence of the redistribution of blood in favour of the cranial circulation.

Nitrous oxide

Nitrous oxide, in a 50:50 mixture with oxygen known as Entonox, is the most widely available inhalational analgesic for labour.

- Entonox rapidly crosses the placenta but is cleared quickly, resulting in minimal effect on the fetus or neonate.
- Neurobehavioural scores on babies exposed to *in utero* Entonox have shown little effect at 2 and 24h.
- Maternal hyperventilation, to achieve adequate analgesia, can lead to respiratory alkalosis in the mother, displacing the oxygen dissociation curve to the left, resulting in reduced oxygen availability to the fetus.
- Prolonged use may cause vasoconstriction within the placental bed and reduce uteroplacental blood flow, reducing fetal oxygenation.
- Entonox may reduce maternal respiratory drive, leading to periods of hypoventilation between contractions, with resulting hypoxia.

Systemic opioids

The opioids pethidine, diamorphine and, to a lesser extent morphine, are widely used to provide analgesia in labour.

Pethidine

- Rapidly crosses the placenta by passive diffusion, causing intrauterine sedation in the fetus.
- The effects are dependent on dose and timing, with maximal effects seen 2–3h after IM administration and with repeated doses. Fetal exposure can result in respiratory depression at birth, leading to lower Apgar scores, reduced oxygen saturations and increased CO_2 tensions.
- If given within 1h of delivery, neonatal effects are minimal.
- Fetal sedation can result in CTG alterations.
- Reduction in baseline variability and accelerations are seen 25min after IV and 40min after IM administration.

- Reduced variability can last longer than the 40min normally associated with the quiet or sleep phase.
- CTG interpretation can be more difficult after administration, so it is important that the preceding CTG is normal and reactive.
- A reduction in fetal movements, altered fetal EEG activity and reduced fetal scalp oxygen tensions have been observed, but these effects are of unknown clinical significance.
- Pethidine is a weak base, resulting in increased ionization and accumulation in the relatively more acidic fetal circulation.
- With fetal acidosis, this effect is further increased, making the pethidine less able to cross back into the maternal circulation (ion trapping).
- Norpethidine, the active metabolite of pethidine, compounds the neonatal effects and has proconvulsant properties.
- Neurobehavioural patterns are altered, with babies exposed to intrauterine pethidine tending to be sleepier, less attentive and slower to establish breastfeeding.
- Administration of naloxone to the neonate can reverse the effects of opiates although it is increasingly controversial. The painful stimulus of an IM injection is thought to be largely responsible for 'waking the baby up'. The opioid effect outlasts the short-acting effect of naloxone.

Morphine and diamorphine

- The fetal side effects of morphine and diamorphine are very similar to those of pethidine.
- Equianalgesic doses of pethidine cause less neonatal respiratory depression than either morphine or diamorphine.
- The metabolite, morphine-3-glucuronide, does not have the side effects of norpethidine.

Regional analgesia and anaesthesia

- Maternal hypotension can occur as a result of either sympathetic blockade or aorto-caval compression, which can be detrimental to the fetus.
- If left untreated, this will cause fetal hypoxia with a fall in fetal pH.
- Continuous fetal monitoring is therefore mandatory following regional techniques.
- However, provided maternal hypotension is avoided and uteroplacental perfusion maintained, regional techniques are well tolerated by the fetus.
- Regional techniques do not influence the resistance in uterine vessels, intervillous blood flow or flow velocity in the UA.
- Relief of pain achieved with regional techniques, by reducing circulating maternal levels of catecholamines, increases placental blood flow.
- Maternal body temperature increases after epidural analgesia. The mechanism is unclear, but marked hyperthermia may result in a fetal tachycardia not associated with significant fetal hypoxia and fetal pH is not affected. This can give rise to an erroneous diagnosis of fetal distress or to a false diagnosis of intrauterine infection, increasing the number of newborns investigated and treated with antibiotics.
- Placental transfer of opioids occurs rapidly after epidural administration and should be considered when delivery is imminent.

- Epidural or intrathecal fentanyl doses >100 micrograms may cause neonatal respiratory depression and have an effect on establishing breastfeeding.

General anaesthesia

- Approximately 20% of CSs are performed using GA.
- The ideal induction to delivery time is between 5 and 15min.
- Prolonged induction to delivery time increases the risk of fetal acidosis but can be minimized if both aorto-caval compression and hypotension are avoided.
- Lipid-soluble anaesthetic agents rapidly cross the placenta and a prolonged induction to delivery time allows progressive uptake by the fetus, resulting in neonatal sedation with low Apgar scores.

IV induction agents

- *Thiopental*: this is the most commonly used induction agent and at 4mg/kg the baby is protected from excessive sedation because of the fetal circulation through the liver. At 8mg/kg neonatal depression will occur.
- *Propofol*: doses >2.5mg/kg can cause neonatal depression. Although associated with rapid wakening in the adult, this advantage has not been observed in the neonate.
- *Ketamine*: at doses of 1mg/kg, the neonatal condition is comparable with thiopental. At 2mg/kg, neonatal depression and low Apgar scores will result.
- *Etomidate*: this is rapidly metabolized by a cholinesterase in the placenta and at 0.3mg/kg will cause minimal depression in the neonate. It significantly reduces neonatal plasma cortisol levels at 1h of age, which may be detrimental to an already compromised baby.
- *Benzodiazepines*: compared with thiopental induction doses, benzodiazepines double the time to sustained neonatal respiration. They can cause neonatal respiratory depression, lethargy, poor feeding, hypothermia, hypotonia and jaundice; should be avoided.

Neuromuscular-blocking agents

- These agents are ionized compounds at normal physiological pH. Under normal circumstances, placental transfer is minimal with no effect on the fetus or neonate.
- There are case reports of suxamethonium apnoea in an affected neonate after suxamethonium was administered to an affected mother.

Inhalation anaesthesia

- *Nitrous oxide*: it freely crosses the placenta and if >50% is used, may cause neonatal depression with low Apgar scores. High concentrations of nitrous oxide can cause diffusion hypoxia and fetal acidosis. A 50:50 mixture with oxygen should be administered prior to delivery of the baby.
- *Volatile anaesthetic agents*: isoflurane, enflurane, desflurane and sevoflurane are widely used for CS.
  - These lipid-soluble drugs cross the placenta causing a dose- and time-dependent neonatal depression.

- Using a 1 MAC equivalent with nitrous oxide and an induction–delivery interval of <11min, excessive neonatal depression is avoided.
- Sevoflurane and desflurane are safe but have no benefits over isoflurane.
- Sevoflurane metabolism is associated with fluoride ion production, causing an increase in neonatal serum fluoride 24h after delivery, the consequences of which are unknown.

Further reading

The Use of Electronic Fetal Monitoring. RCOG Press, 2001.

Chapter 21

Controversies in obstetric analgesia

Paul Clyburn, Anette Scholz and Gavin Sullivan

Feeding in labour

Feeding in labour is a contentious issue with no definitive proven answer. Opinions are often divided between anaesthetists, obstetricians and midwives on the best way to proceed. Starvation during labour is not popular with many midwives, and to a lesser extent many mothers; however, the dangers of GA in a woman with a full stomach should never be dismissed.

Risks of feeding

- The arguments for and against feeding during labour centre around the real worries of acid aspiration syndrome, also known as Mendelson's syndrome.
- This is caused by aspiration of acidic stomach contents into the lungs during GA, causing chemical pneumonitis.
- GA is sometimes necessary and, by its nature, it is difficult to predict the mothers who may require a GA.
- The aspiration of solid particles (i.e. partially digested chunks of food) into either the main or more distal bronchi is also a potential hazard and was the main cause of death of women in Mendelson's original study.
- Fortunately, acid aspiration is now rare as a result of increased use of regional anaesthesia techniques and also thought to be due to:
  - Application of cricoid pressure (Sellick's manoeuvre).
  - Greater awareness of risks among all grades of anaesthetists.
  - Better trained anaesthetic assistants.
  - The implementation of nil by mouth policies during labour.
- However, there is no proof that the widespread introduction of nil by mouth policies alone has affected maternal outcome.
- Is it time to institute more liberal feeding policies on the delivery suite given that the number of GAs currently administered in the UK is small and therefore the risk of acid aspiration even smaller?

Physiology of labour

- Labour is an active process, especially in the second stage, during which women utilize between 800 and1100kcal/h, the equivalent to moderate aerobic exercise.
- Labour can be prolonged, and it is known that labouring mothers develop high levels of ketones in their urine and are prone to hypoglycaemia.
- The uterus is a versatile organ and can metabolize ketones, fatty acids and glucose during active contractions, but it is also known that the uterus contracts better in a slightly alkaline milieu.
- During pregnancy, progesterone causes a reduction in lower oesophageal sphincter tone and a tendency towards reflux; a change that remains until ~48h postdelivery (although this is an estimate and by no means definite).
- Gastrin from the placenta increases the gastric volume and decreases gastric pH.

- Pain, anxiety and the use of parental, epidural or intrathecal opioids during labour can prolong gastric emptying, increase gastric residual volume and increase the frequency of vomiting.

This dichotomy of physiology in the labouring women presents a real problem when trying to institute a safe feeding policy for all mothers in labour.

Alternatives to nil by mouth policies

Starvation and dehydration during labour are not popular with mothers, and there is some contrary evidence that would suggest it may increase obstetric risk. Therefore, alternative strategies have been promoted and instituted in a number of hospitals.

Intravenous hydration

- Ketosis in the mother has been treated in the past by the use of IV 5% dextrose with definite improvement in the biochemistry of the mother.
- However, it was found that this predisposed the fetus to develop hyponatraemia, hyperinsulinaemia and rebound hypoglycaemia.
- This practice has now stopped.
- IV saline or Hartmann's solution is often administered during labour to prevent dehydration, particularly if labour is prolonged.

Clear oral fluids

- A policy that is becoming more widespread is allowance of clear fluids during labour, i.e. water, glucose drinks, tea (without milk) or pulpless fruit juice, such as apple juice.
- Recent interest has centred on the ingestion of isotonic sports drinks, which are rapidly absorbed from the stomach, provide a source of calories and offset any ketosis.
- 100–200mL/h of isotonic sport drink has been suggested as a safe nutritional alternative to solid food, without increasing gastric volume in women who have not received parenteral opioids.

Low residue diet

- Low residue, simple, carbohydrate-based foodstuffs, e.g. biscuits, are digested rapidly, and many advocate their being allowed during labour.
- High fibre, fatty or protein-based foodstuffs should be avoided, as these take much longer to empty from the stomach in the normal patient, let alone the parturient.
- Feeding women a low residue diet during labour has been shown to have no effect on the outcome of labour.

Risk assessment

- A rational approach to feeding in labour would be to differentiate feeding management based on a risk assessment of all mothers in labour.
- Low risk women, i.e. labour proceeding with normality and no opioid analgesia, may be offered a low residue diet and clear oral fluids.

- High risk women, i.e. opioid analgesia administered or labour not proceeding with normality and at risk of requiring operative delivery, should be restricted to water only and given antacid prophylaxis regularly during labour.
- Unfortunately, identifying women who are at high risk of operative delivery at a time early in their labour is not always straightforward.
- Policies that allow liberal feeding in labour in the uncomplicated parturient can be fraught with difficulties when an epidural, oxytocin augmentation or assistance during delivery is requested. To then render the woman nil by mouth at this stage, may well be too late to be useful.
- Whatever the situation, the safety of the mother should be the first priority. If in doubt about the progress and outcome of labour, it is preferable to adopt caution and restrict feeding.

Further reading

Scrutton MJL *et al.* Eating in labour. A randomized controlled trial assessing the risks and benefits. *Anaesthesia* 1999; **54**: 329–334.

Kubli M *et al.* An evaluation of isotonic 'sports drinks' during labor. *Anesthesia and Analgesia* 2002; **94**: 404–408.

Liu B *et al.* Does eating during labour influence obstetric outcome? *International Journal of Obstetric Anesthesia* 2007; 16 Suppl: S11.

Monitoring the mother and fetus with an epidural

Although the Royal College of Anaesthetists and Association of Anaesthetists of GB and Ireland guidelines state that for local or regional anaesthetic procedures, full monitoring should be instituted, this is not always practised in obstetric anaesthesia.

Basic principles

- Monitoring for epidurals requires not just standard physiological monitoring, but a system in which these are a part of the whole.
- A 24h epidural service requires the presence of an experienced anaesthetist who is trained and competent in the practice of regional anaesthesia and its complications, and the possible complications of normal labour.
- Similarly, midwives caring for the parturient with an epidural should be trained to be familiar with the technique and its potential pitfalls.
- As is the case with all regional anaesthetic techniques, access to resuscitation equipment and drugs is mandatory.

Monitoring requirements

- When performing an epidural for labour analgesia, access to the following monitoring should be available:
  - Non-invasive BP.
  - ECG.
  - Pulse oximetry.
- Specifically before embarking upon an epidural, the mother's pulse and BP should have been recorded, which provides a baseline and excludes hypertensive disease of pregnancy.
- The caveat to this is that a woman in active labour may have a systolic BP up to 30mmHg higher than usual.
- Following insertion of the epidural, the mother must be fully monitored throughout her labour, in respect of both her BP and fetal CTG.

Pitfalls

- The most hazardous time during the use of an epidural must be regarded as the time immediately after a 'top-up'.
- This is when there is highest risk of:
  - Hypotension.
  - IV injection.
  - Total spinal block.

- After an epidural top-up is given, the mother's BP should be measured every 5min for 15–20min and every 10–15min thereafter.
- The presence of a midwife is mandatory after an epidural has been sited. She should not be responsible for any other women on the delivery suite.

- Although midwives in many units are trained to administer epidural 'top-up' injections, the epidural and its effects are still the responsibility of the anaesthetist.

Effects of an epidural on the fetus

Epidural analgesia is an indication for continuous electronic fetal monitoring (EFM), according to the NICE and the Royal College of Obstetricians and Gynaecologists published guidelines.

Effects on CTG

- There is little evidence for any direct effects of epidural analgesia on FHR. However, indirect effects such as maternal hypotension can lead to placental hypoperfusion with its concomitant fetal bradycardia.
- In contrast, the 'stress' of childbirth, especially a prolonged or difficult delivery, will produce excess levels of catecholamines with detrimental effects on placental perfusion and uterine synchrony, with maternal tachypnoea leading to respiratory alkalosis and reduced oxygen delivery to the tissues and fetus.
- These consequences are all reduced by effective epidural analgesia, and an improvement in maternal progress in labour may ensue.
- However, midwifery staff will all have experienced detrimental changes in CTG traces following insertion of an epidural and presumed this to be the cause.
  - Placing the mother in the full left lateral position to relieve aorto-caval compression may well be helpful in these situations, together with the administration of oxygen by face mask.
  - Occasionally, administration of vasopressors may be required to treat maternal hypotension.

Continuous vs intermittent monitoring

- The ideal situation for the mother with an epidural is one where she retains motor function and remains mobile. This has been facilitated with the use of low dose LAs combined with opioids.
- Continuous fetal monitoring of a woman with an epidural should continue, and this may restrict a woman's movements.
- However, it is possible to perform continuous fetal monitoring when the woman is sitting, standing or walking around the delivery room.

Further reading

Clinical Effectiveness Support Unit. *The Use of Electronic Fetal Monitoring*. RCOG Press, 2001.

Mobilizing with an epidural

Ambulation in obstetric terms is used to describe walking, standing or sitting out in the chair during the course of labour.

Ambulatory epidurals are regional analgesic techniques that allow mothers requesting an epidural to walk during labour.

Why ambulation?

The following have been postulated as potential benefits of ambulation during labour:
- Upright position may increase pelvic dimension.
- May reduce aorto-caval compression.
- May improve maternal satisfaction, e.g. ability to void, feeling of self-control.
- Possible reduction of instrumental delivery.
- Possible reduction of duration of labour and need for epidural drugs.

Benefits

Whether any real benefits result from walking during labour is controversial.
- Better obstetric outcome has been claimed in association with ambulation during labour, but recent clinical investigations have shown that walking has no effect on labour or delivery.
- Some studies have shown that because ambulation has no disadvantage and improves maternal satisfaction, it does provide some benefit.
- Easy labour rather than a difficult one allows ambulation—women with greater pain or those with short duration labour do not ambulate.

Risks

Controversy persists regarding which criteria to predict safe ambulation.
- To date, only one fall has been reported in the literature.
- In a study of 110 patients who had CSE in labour and ambulated, none of them fell and 85% of them could safely stand by the bed after demonstrating a bilateral strong straight leg rise prior to walking.
- Walking requires adequate motor power, proprioception, vestibular function and visual acuity.
- Proprioceptive input from the joints via the dorsal columns is needed to maintain balance without falling.
- Somatosensory impairment with low dose epidural is possible in the presence of normal motor function, increasing the risk of stumbling.
- Dorsal column function tests may be necessary prior to ambulation.

Tests to evaluate dorsal column function include

- Manual joint displacement.
  - i.e. large toe or ankle to test joint position sense.
- Tuning folk.
  - To test vibrational sense.
- Romberg.

- Ask patient to stand with their feet together and to close their eyes. Visual input is removed and instability can be brought about due either to proprioceptor or vestibular lesion.
- Somatosensory evoked potentials (SEPs).
  - SEPs reflect conduction of an afferent volley along the peripheral nerve, dorsal columns, medial lemniscal pathway to the primary somatosensory cortex. They are obtained after stimulus of a peripheral nerve, e.g. post. tibial nerve, and recorded over spine and scalp.
- Computerized dynamic posturography (CDP).
  - Method of assessing individually the relative contribution of somatosensory, visual and vestibular input to maintain balance. The patient stands in front of a 3-sided visual surround on a pressure-sensitive forceplate which records the amount of patient sway during each of the test protocols.

- The degree of dorsal column function impairment depends on the concentration of LA used. The higher the concentration, the more abnormal the dorsal column function tests.
- To date, no difference in dorsal column transmission between patients with low dose CSEs and mothers without regional analgesia has been found, even when more complicated tests such as SEP and CDP have been used.

The relative contribution of dorsal column function, proprioception and muscle strength to overall balance remains incompletely understood.

The medical legal implication of allowing a patient to walk with an epidural in labour, if clinical tests demonstrate even minimal impairment of motor power and dorsal column function, is unclear.

Other risk factors for ambulation during labour

Postural hypotension

- Adequate fluid replacement, stable BP and adequate supervision are important. As yet, no significant BP changes have been reported with ambulatory epidurals.

Fetal monitoring

- Any patient with an epidural can ambulate, unless there is an obstetric reason for staying in bed.
- Continuous EFM is not an indication for remaining in bed, as the woman can sit in a chair or stand by the bed with the CTG attached.
- Telemetry (if available) is an additional option for monitoring.

Recommendations for safe ambulation during labour

- High acceptability of walking epidural amongst obstetric and anaesthetic staff.
- Low risk labour.
- Strong sustained bilateral straight leg raise ± simple dorsal column function tests.
- Mother feels confident to walk—ask her to put her feet to the ground, if the soles of her feet feel like cotton wool, then walking is usually not safe.
- Ask mother to perform a deep knee bend after standing with two people assisting, before she starts walking.
- Mother is accompanied at all times.
- Continuous fetal CTG monitoring should continue.
- Epidural 'top-ups' may be performed on the bed or whilst sitting in the chair.

LA concentrations for ambulatory epidurals

CSE

- Intrathecal injection of 2.5mg bupivacaine with 10 micrograms fentanyl or 2–4mL of low dose epidural mix injected intrathecally. e.g. 2–4mg bupivacaine with 4–8 micrograms fentanyl.
- 10–40 micrograms sufentanil intrathecally with or without LA is possible.
- Subsequent epidural boluses (10mL) with low dose epidural mix, e.g. 0.1% bupivacaine + 2 micrograms/mL fentanyl.

Epidural alone

- 15–30mL of low dose bupivacaine/fentanyl mixture (0.1% bupivacaine with 2 micrograms/mL fentanyl).
- 15–30mL of low dose ropivacaine/fentanyl mixture (0.1% ropivacaine with 2 micrograms/mL fentanyl).

Summary

- Optimum LA/opioid combination providing rapid analgesia with minimal side effects is unknown.
- Test doses with 3mL lidocaine 2% or bupivacaine 0.5% increases motor weakness and should be avoided when ambulating.
- Motor ± dorsal column function tests should be performed each time the patient gets out of bed, as increasing doses of LA can impair motor function.

Further reading

Simmons S *et al.* Combined spinal–epidural versus epidural analgesia in labour. *Cochrane Database of Systematic Reviews* 2007; Issue **3**: CD003401.

Wilson MJ *et al.* Randomized controlled trial comparing traditional with two 'mobile' epidural techniques: anesthetic and analgesic efficacy. *Anesthesiology* 2002; **97**: 1567–1575.

Buggy D, Fernando R. Controversies in obstetric anaesthesia: ambulation during regional analgesia for labour should be discouraged. *International Journal of Obstetric Anesthesia* 1999; **8**: 179–183.

Fever and regional anaesthesia

The diagnosis of fever and infection in pregnancy often raises questions about the safety of regional anaesthesia for pain relief in labour.

Definition

- Fever is an increase in core temperature above 38°C mediated by endogenous pyrogens, which is secondary to an increase in the hypothalamic set point.
- It can result from a variety of infectious micro-organisms, tissue trauma, malignancy, drug administration, endocrine and immunological disorders.
- Infection is the most common cause of fever in pregnancy.

Causes of infection in pregnancy

Bacterial
- UTI.
- Pneumonia.
- Chorioamnionitis.
- Endometritis.

Viral
- Papilloma virus.
- Human immunodeficiency virus (HIV).
- Hepatitis virus (types A–E).
- Herpes simplex virus (type 1 + 2).
- Measles.
- Chickenpox.
- Rubella.

- Overall incidence of maternal infection in labour is ~3.1%.
- UTIs are the most common infection in labour.
- Infection remains the leading cause of maternal morbidity and mortality worldwide.

Physiological changes in pregnancy and fever

- Pregnancy is associated with an increase in maternal basal metabolic rate.
- Fetal temperature is ~0.5°C higher than maternal temperature, leading to a better oxygen delivery.
- Urinary tract dilatation is one of the most significant changes during pregnancy, leading to urinary stasis and predisposing to UTIs.
- Pregnancy is associated with decreased immune system function; febrile diseases may therefore take a more severe course.
- Presence of bacteria in blood samples alone (unassociated with fever and/or infection) is common but clinical significance is unclear.

Bacterial infection and regional anaesthesia

The most common causal organisms are Gram-negative bacteria (95%).

Urinary tract infection

- Most common bacterial infection during pregnancy.
- Can be asymptomatic (10%) or lead to pyelonephritis (1–2%).
- Pyelonephritis needs prompt treatment and may lead to sepsis.
- Patients are often dehydrated due to fever, vomiting and anorexia, which needs correcting.
- There is no evidence that regional anaesthesia is detrimental in febrile patients with UTI, although antibiotic therapy is indicated before siting a regional anaesthetic technique.

Chorioamnionitis

- Incidence 0.5–10%.
- Symptoms include temperature, uterine tenderness, foul-smelling amniotic fluid.
- Complications include PPH, postpartum infection, sepsis and death.
- Accounts for 20–40% of neonatal sepsis and neonatal respiratory tract infections.
- No evidence that neuroaxial blocks are contraindicated in febrile mothers with amniotic infection.
- Antibiotics should be administered before starting labour regional analgesia.

Pneumonia

- Bacterial pneumonia is uncommon in healthy mothers.
- Alcohol, drug abuse and heavy smoking may predispose to respiratory infection.
- *Streptococcus* is the most common isolated pathogen.
- Physiological changes such as decreased functional capacity, increased oxygen consumption and deceased cellular immunity may predispose to pneumonia.
- Administration of epidural analgesia may reduce the increased oxygen consumption.
- IV antibiotics should be given prior to neuroaxial block.

Septic shock

- Occurs infrequently, usually in the postpartum period.
- Most common aetiologies are chorioamnionitis, pyelonephritis and endometritis.
- Diagnosis is often established by the development of pronounced hypotension and vasodilatation.
- Often leads to cardiovascular instability and multiorgan failure.
- Regional anaesthesia for pain relief and CS is contraindicated.

Summary of bacterial infection

- To date, no study has documented a causal relationship between neuroaxial block in the presence of bacteraemia and subsequent developent of complications such as epidural abscess and meningitis.
- Regional anaesthesia seems to have a low risk of neurological sequelae in febrile mothers when antibiotics have been administered and the presence of sepsis is excluded. Unfortunately, there is no good evidence to indicate when epidural analgesia is safe.
- A prudent management plan would be:
  - If WCC <20 and/or temperature <38°C, an epidural is probably safe to be inserted.
  - If WCC >20 and/or temperature >38°C, many anaesthetists would withhold an epidural until blood cultures have been taken, at least two consecutive doses of appropriate IV antibiotics given and there is evidence of an improvement in infection markers, i.e. decreasing WCC or C-reactive protein.
  - Spinal anaesthesia is considered to be safe unless there are signs of haemodynamic instability from sepsis.
- An isolated WCC >20 can be normal in labour if there are no other signs or markers of sepsis.
- Anaesthetic management of an infected patient should be based on an individual risk–benefit analysis, obstetric indication, urgency and route of delivery.

Viral infection and regional anaesthetic implication

Herpes simplex (HSV1 + HSV2)

- Differentiation between primary (initial) and secondary (reccurring) infection is important.
- Co-existence of genital lesions, fever, myalgia or headache suggests a primary lesion.
- Primary infection in the peripartum period has a very high risk of vertical transmission to the neonate due to viraemia.
- Administration of regional anaesthesia raises concern of neuroaxial spread.
- Safety of regional anaesthesia in primary infection with HSV has not been established.
- There is evidence that regional analgesia is safe in patients with secondary infection, because viraemia is rarely present.
- Active lesion at needle insertion site is a contraindication for both types of HSV infection.

Hepatitis

- Mild hepatitis does not alter anaesthetic management and pregnancy outcome.
- Preanaesthetic assessment should determine degree of hepatic impairment.
- Correction of dehydration and electrolyte abnormalities is recommended.
- History of IV drug abuse and HIV infection is common.

- Regional anaesthesia may be safely employed in febrile mothers with hepatitis provided thrombocytopenia is absent, and coagulation studies and BP are normal.
- Universal safety precautions are necessary.

Human immunodeficiency virus (HIV)

- A HIV-positive patient meets criteria for AIDS by definition if CD4 T-cell count falls below 200 cells/mL.
- High maternal viral load increases the likelihood of perinatal transmission of HIV.
- Evidence suggests that most perinatal HIV transmission occurs during labour and delivery.
- Elective CS and antiviral prophylaxis have an additive effect in prevention of vertical HIV transmission.
- HIV is a neurotopic virus, and CNS infection takes place in early stages of the disease process.
- It is well established that HIV infection does not preclude the administration of regional anaesthesia.
- HIV positivity alone should not determine the preferred method of anaesthesia.
- Anaesthetic management must be tailored to individual obstetric indications, urgency and co-existing diseases.
- Universal safety precautions are necessary.
- Risk of HIV transmission from needle stick injury with HIV-infected blood is ~0.32%.

Summary of viral infections

- If there is no localized infection at the site of needle insertion and no acute viraemia, the risk of causing CNS infection with regional anaesthesia is small.
- The risk has to be balanced against the problems arising from GA.

Additional risk factors for CNS infection via epidural/spinal

- Diabetes.
- Immunocompromise.
- Epidural equipment (contaminated by operator or imperfectly sterilized).
- Poor technique, multiple attempts at insertion.
- Prolonged epidural catheterization (organisms travel along catheter track and come from patient's own skin or from contaminated bed).
- Occlusive dressing.
- Hyperhydrosis.
- Lack of strict asepsis, e.g. mask.

Epidural analgesia and hyperthermia

Epidurals for labour analgesia have been reported to cause gradual increase in maternal core body temperature, resulting in hyperthermia.

- The mechanism for this remains unclear.
- Possible causes include:
  - cessation of hyperventilation after pain relief.
  - increased incidence of shivering.
  - decreased sweating.
  - thermoregulatory and vascular modification caused by the epidural.
  - inflammatory related to increased interleukin-6 levels in women who receive epidurals.
- An association between epidural analgesia and increased maternal temperature was found, independent of other risk factors such as prolonged labour and preterm rupture of membrane.
- In recent studies, hyperthermia was noted ~5h after initiation of block.
- Observed temperature increase in patients with labour epidurals averaged at 0.1°C/h.
- No maternal temperature changes were reported in parturients receiving parenteral opioids for labour pain.
- The clinical consequences of epidural-related hyperthermia for mother and fetus are unclear.
- There may or may not be an association between maternal fever and neonatal sepsis.

There is evidence that epidurals for labour analgesia cause a small temperature rise. The aetiology and consequences are unclear.

Other causes of fever, e.g. infection should always be considered and excluded.

Further reading

Kuczkowski KM, Reisner LS. Anesthetic management of parturient with fever and infection. *Journal of Clinical Anesthesia* 2003; **15**: 478–488.

Chapter 22

A–Z of conditions in obstetric anaesthesia

Rachel Collis, Elizabeth Duff,
Valerie Billing and Aravindh Jayakumar

Abdominal pregnancy

Characteristics

- Implantation of pregnancy outside the uterine cavity.
- Incidence of 10.9 per 100 000 births.
- Maternal mortality is up to 30%.
- Poor fetal outcome: 40–95% fetal mortality.
- Diagnosis can be difficult.
- Associated with massive haemorrhage due to placental attachment to intra-abdominal organs.

Key points

Delivery

- Best managed in a tertiary unit.
- Seek advice from a haematologist and have blood products immediately available.
- Placenta may not be completely excised and therefore at risk of sepsis after CS.
- GA ± invasive monitoring advised due to high risk of massive blood loss.
- Critical care facility for postoperative care.

Reference

Ramachandran K *et al.* Massive hemorrhage in a previously undiagnosed abdominal pregnancy presenting for elective Cesarean delivery. *Canadian Journal of Anaesthesia* 2004; **51**: 57–61.

Achondroplasia

Characteristics

- Spinal and craniofacial abnormalities include:
  - Large head, short limbs, saddle nose with normally proportioned trunk.
  - Kyphoscoliosis and lumbar lordosis.
  - Decreased neck movements.
  - Stenosis of foramen magnum and spinal canal.
  - Large tongue and mandible.
  - Atlantoaxial instability.
- May have restrictive lung disease with markedly decreased FRC.

Key points

Delivery

- Usually requires CS because of cephalopelvic disproportion.
- Associated with difficult intubation, therefore regional may be preferable.
- Difficult regional because of spinal deformities.
- Increased risk of dural puncture.
- Spinal canal stenosis can impair CSF flow, and dural puncture may be more difficult to recognize.
- CSE useful to control the block.

- May have unpredictable spread of LA in epidural space.
- No neurological complications of regional techniques are documented.
- If GA needed:
  - Ensure facilities for awake fibreoptic intubation are available.
  - May require smaller endotracheal tube.
  - IV access may de difficult.
  - Avoid hyperextension of the neck.
- Aorto-caval compression may be severe.
- Invasive arterial monitoring and blood gases may be required in patients with cardiorespiratory compromise.

References

Morrow MJ *et al.* Epidural anaesthesia for Caesarean section in an achondroplastic dwarf. *British Journal of Anaesthesia* 1998; **81**: 619–621.

Ravenscroft A *et al.* Spinal anaesthesia for emergency Caesarean section in an achondroplastic dwarf. *Anaesthesia* 1998; **53**: 1236–1237.

Acupuncture

Characteristics

- A technique of inserting and manipulating needles into acupuncture points on the body to restore health and well-being; has been used to treat pain.

Key points

Antenatal

- Has been used safely for the treatment of symphysis pubis dysfunction and lower back pain in pregnancy.

Delivery

- Acupuncture in labour can decrease pain and reduce the use of epidural analgesia.
- Some evidence for its use as an adjunct to conventional pain control.
- Further studies are required.

References

Elden H *et al.* Effects of acupuncture and stabilising exercises as adjunct to standard treatment in pregnant women with pelvic girdle pain: randomised single blind controlled trial. *British Medical Journal* 2005; **331**: 249–250.

Nesheim BI, Britt-Ingjerd R. Performance of acupuncture as labor analgesia in the clinical setting. *Acta Obstetrica et Gynecologica Scandinavica* 2006; **85**: 441–443.

Acute epiglottitis

Characteristics

- Inflammation of supraglottic structures.
- Serious, acute, life-threatening disease with the potential for sudden upper airway obstruction.
- Caused by a variety of organisms; most common is *Haemophilus influenza*.
- Causes sore throat, pyrexia, dysphagia, stridor and drooling.
- Cherry red epiglottitis on laryngoscopy.
- No reliable markers for prediction of need for invasive airway support.

Key points

- Supportive treatment, deliver oxygen and secure airway as required.
- May require intubation, which is likely to be difficult.
- In pregnancy there are increased problems because of congested mucus membranes and increased risk of aspiration.
- Flexible nasendoscope can be useful to diagnose and view larynx.
- ENT and Anaesthetic consultants need to be informed immediately.
- Treat with antibiotics, cefotaxime ± metronidazole.
- Full monitoring prior to induction.
- Awake fibreoptic intubation or head-up gas induction both described.
- ENT surgeon ready to perform immediate tracheostomy if required.
- IV ranitidine and metoclopramide pre-induction.

References

Ames WA *et al.* Adult epiglottitis: an under-recognized, life-threatening condition. *British Journal of Anaesthesia* 2000; **85**: 795–797.

Hunter KA, Malinow A. Acute epiglottitis in a gravid 19-year-old. *International Journal of Obstetric Anesthesia* 1996; **5**: 105–107.

Acute fatty liver of pregnancy

Characteristics

- Presents with nausea, vomiting and epigastric pain, usually in the third trimester.
- Causes progressive liver failure, coagulopathy, encephalopathy and ARF.
- Probably part of the spectrum of pre-eclampsia and HELLP syndrome.
- Rare, incidence 1 in 7000–15 000 deliveries.
- 10% maternal and perinatal mortality.
- Risk factors include nulliparity and multiple pregnancy.

Key points

Delivery

- Mother needs urgent delivery—balance of risk between induction of labour and CS.
- Causes coagulopathy, LFT abnormalities and low blood glucose.
- Regional techniques contraindicated if coagulopathy present.
- May require invasive monitoring and critical care support pre- and postdelivery.

Reference

Fesenmeier MF *et al.* Acute fatty liver of pregnancy in three tertiary care centers. *American Journal of Obstetrics and Gynecology* 2005; **192**: 1416–1419.

Addison's disease/crisis

Characteristics

- Adrenal insufficiency—either primary or secondary.
- Symptoms: weight loss, weakness, nausea, fatigue, abdominal pain, diarrhoea, postural hypotension.
- Can be life-threatening in pregnancy.
- Associated with fetal death *in utero* and postpartum adrenal crisis.
- Crisis more likely in labour, illness and during delivery.
- Difficult to diagnose in pregnancy due to altered cortisol levels.

Key points

Antenatal

- Continue with normal steroid replacement therapy in pregnancy.
- If nausea and vomiting, administer IV fluids and IV hydrocortisone.
- Monitor electrolytes in pregnancy.
- Stop mineralocortocoids if pre-eclampsia develops.
- Seek endocrine advice.

Delivery

- Consider extra dose of steroids during second stage.
- If CS—give 100mg hydrocortisone 6hly and IV saline for 24h. Decrease IV steroids over 3 days.
- Signs of crisis are hypotension, hypoglycaemia and raised potassium.
- Treat crisis with IV fluids and IV steroids, and correct hypoglycaemia and reduce potassium levels with IV dextrose and insulin infusion.

Reference

Gradden C *et al.* Addison's disease in pregnancy. *Lancet* 2001; **357**: 1197.

Advanced malignancies

Characteristics

- Tumour growth may be more rapid in pregnancy. Effects dependent on the primary tumour.
- Rare but most common are: breast cancer, cervical cancer, Hodgkin's disease, melanoma and leukaemia.

Key points

Delivery

- May be preterm to initiate chemo- or radiotherapy treatment of mother, although some chemotherapy agents are safe for the fetus.
- Check coagulation and platelets prior to regional technique.
- May have haemodynamic instability—CSE useful to minimize this.
- May require intra-arterial BP monitoring.
- Consider fluid preload.
- Critical care facility for postdelivery care.

Reference

Kutomi O *et al.* Intrathecal fentanyl/meperidine combined with low-dose epidural bupivacaine for Caesarean section in a patient with advanced Krukenberg tumors. *Acta Anaesthiologica Scandinavica* 2002; **46**: 1272–1275.

Alcoholism

Characteristics

- Defined as excess drinking leading to the impairment of the patient's health and social activities.
- May cause malnutrition, liver disease, pancreatitis, oesophageal varices, altered drug metabolism, coagulopathy, cardiomyopathy and central and peripheral neuropathy.
- Patients often conceal the extent of drinking.
- Acute withdrawal may last between 8h and 5 days. Characterized by tremor, hypertension, tachycardia, arrhythmias, nausea, vomiting, insomnia, confusion and hallucinations.

Key points

- Aim to assess extent of the problem.
- May require benzodiazepines for acute withdrawal.
- Patients may develop seizures, low blood glucose and dehydration.
- Check coagulation and platelets.
- Assess for signs of cardiomyopathy and arrhythmias.
- Regional anaesthesia is safe
  - Contraindications: infection, coagulopathy.
  - Relative contraindication: peripheral neuropathy.
  - Document carefully.
  - Will require fluid loading prior to procedure.
- Acute intoxication causes an increased aspiration risk.
- For GA, doses of IV agents and volatiles may need to be altered depending on liver function and degree of intoxication.

Reference

Kuczkowski KM. Anesthetic implications of drug abuse in pregnancy. *Journal of Clinical Anesthesia* 2003; **15**: 382–394.

Amphetamine abuse

Characteristics

- Amphetamines (speed) are sympathomimetic amines acting as indirect CNS stimulants.
- Effects last for 3–6h.
- May be ingested orally, smoked or injected IV.
- Symptoms of acute intoxication include: psychosis, paranoia, delirium, mania, decreased need for sleep, dilated pupils, raised HR and BP, nausea and vomiting, hyper-reflexia, respiratory depression, cardiac arrhythmias, seizures, coma, hyperpyrexia, proteinuria and confusion.
- Chronic abuse causes dopamine depletion, memory impairment and insomnia.
- High doses cause cardiovascular system collapse, myocardial infarction, cerebrovascular accident, seizures, renal failure, ischaemic colitis and hepatotoxicity.
- There is an increased incidence of suicides and accidents.

Key points

- Universal precautions if thought to be an IV user.
- Difficult venous access if IV user.
- Send urine for toxicology.
- Associated with fetal anomalies, IUGR, fetal distress and placental abruption.
- Regional block may cause severe hypotension.
- Response to vasopressors can be unpredictable. Direct-acting vasopressor may be more reliable.
- Need to rehydrate mother.
- If requires GA—acute ingestion increases MAC of volatile agents and chronic ingestion decreases it.

References

Kuczkowski KM. Anesthetic implications of drug abuse in pregnancy. *Journal of Clinical Anaesthesia* 2003; **15**: 382–394.

Kuczkowski KM Benumof JL. Amphetamine abuse in pregnancy: anesthetic implications. *Acta Anaesthiologica Belgica* 2003; **54**: 161–163.

Amyloidosis

Characteristics

- Abnormal deposits of protein in tissues.
- Can be primary or secondary.
  - Primary associated with deposits in tongue, GIT, heart, blood vessels, nerves, skin and mucous membranes.
  - Secondary disease occurs secondary to other chronic diseases, with deposits in the liver, spleen, lymph nodes, kidneys and adrenal glands.
- Cardiac and renal deposits can lead to organ failures.
- Macroglossia associated with failed intubations.
- Can have coagulation and platelet abnormalities with vascular fragility.
- Cardiac arrhythmias and compromised ventricular function can occur.

Key points

Antenatal

- Assess underlying pathologies and degree of organ dysfunction.
- Assess coagulation and platelet function.
- If suitable for regional technique, this may be safest.
- Assess airway—may require awake fibreoptic intubation.

Delivery

Invasive monitoring may be required if organ dysfunction severe.

Reference

Weir PS *et al.* Anaesthesia for caesarean section in a patient with systemic amyloidosis secondary to familial Mediterranean fever. *International Journal of Obstetric Anesthesia* 1998; **7**: 271–274.

Amyotrophic lateral sclerosis

Characteristics

- Progressive neurological disease of upper and lower motor neurons causing irreversible muscle weakness and spasticity.
- Often fatal within 3–5yrs.
- Rare in obstetric population.
- Maternal disease does not regress and may worsen due to increased respiratory and weight-bearing demands.
- Causes weakness, fasciculations, autonomic instability and cardiac denervation.
- Uterine muscles not involved in degeneration process and labour may be facilitated by pelvic floor weakness.

Key points

- Respiratory function may be a problem. Requires monitoring of oxygen saturation and blood gases in labour.
- Supportive care required.
- Bulbar reflexes may not be intact.
- Regional anaesthesia is possible. Spinal and GA have been used successfully for CS. CSE useful to control and avoid excessive height of block.
- Use suxamethonium with care. Increased sensitivity to non-depolarizing muscle relaxants.
- Requires critical care facility for postoperative care.

References

Leveck DE *et al.* Rapid progression of amyotrophic lateral sclerosis presenting during pregnancy: a case report. *Journal of Obstetrics and Gynaecology Canada* 2005; **27**: 360–362.

Lupo VR *et al.* Amyotrophic lateral sclerosis in pregnancy. *Obstetrics and Gynecology* 1993; **82**: 682–685.

Ankylosing spondylitis

Characteristics

- Chronic inflammatory arthropathy with systemic involvement.
- Onset 15–25yrs olds.
- Males >females.
- Causes fibrosis, ossification and ankylosis of joints, predominantly sacroiliac joints and the spine.
- 50% of patients have other joints involved.
- May be associated with psoriasis and inflammatory bowel disease.
- Can have restrictive lung defects and lung fibrosis.
- Decreased neck movements and risk of cervical spine fractures on minimal trauma to neck.
- Temperomandibular joint involvement.
- Can rarely affect cricoarytenoid joints.
- Can develop cardiovascular system disease—aortic and mitral regurgitation and conduction defects can occur.
- Massive ossification of the ligamentum flavum is very uncommon.

Key points

- May require oxygen saturation and blood gas monitoring in labour if lung disease present.
- ECG ± echocardiography is required during antenatal assessment. May require ECG monitoring in labour.
- Regional anaesthesia is possible:
  - Spinal may be difficult, but effective.
  - Increased risk of epidural haematoma.
  - Slowly titrate epidural to decrease risk of high block.
  - May be difficult to remove epidural after labour.
- If GA required, likely to be a difficult intubation and require awake fibreoptic intubation.
- Care with cervical spine positioning.
- Positioning of whole patient may be difficult.

Reference

Schelew BL *et al.* Ankylosing spondylitis and neuraxial anaesthesia-a 10 year review. *Canadian Journal of Anaesthesia* 1996; **43**: 65–68.

Antiphospholipid syndrome

Characteristics

- Syndrome of hypercoagulability, associated with autoimmune specific antibodies against phospholipids.
  - Increased risk of thrombosis in pregnancy.
  - Increased incidence of second trimester miscarriage.
- Can be primary or secondary to other systemic diseases, e.g. systemic sclerosis, SLE.
- Associated with venous and arterial thromboemboli.
- Causes raised APTT (not associated with bleeding risk—caused by lupus anticoagulant antibody interfering with assay) and decreased platelets.
- Can have adrenal insufficiency, pulmonary hypertension and systemic hypertension.
- May be associated with Budd–Chiari syndrome.
- Increased risk of DVT peripartum.
- Predisposition to pre-eclampsia and placental abruption.

Key points

- Keep patient warm and well hydrated.
- Often on SC heparin, usually LMWH, and aspirin, which is continued for 6/52 postpartum. Regional anaesthesia is possible, but needs to be timed carefully with anticoagulation therapy. Continue with aspirin, as it is not a contraindication to regional anaesthesia.
- Regional anaesthesia can be performed if normal PT, no significant decrease in platelets and an isolated raised APTT (as increase is secondary to lupus anticoagulant).

- May get occasional true clotting factor defects, which would contraindicate regional techniques.
- If emergency CS required and on heparin, GA should be used with protamine available (LMWH is incompletely reversed with protamine). Liaise with on-call haematologist.

Reference

Ralph CJ. Anaesthetic management of parturients with the antiphospholipid syndrome: a review of 27 cases. *International Journal of Obstetric Anesthesia* 1999; **8**: 249–252.

Antithrombin III deficiency (See Chapter 4, p 121)

Characteristics

- Antithrombin III is synthesized in the liver and endothelial cells, and its primary action is the inhibition of activated factor IIa (thrombin) and Xa.
- Antithrombin deficiency may be congenital or arise secondary to acquired disorders, e.g. liver dysfunction or sepsis.
- It is the most clinically important of the inherited thromboplilias, resulting in venous thromboembolism in the majority of affected individuals, which may be life-threatening during high risk periods such as pregnancy.

Key points

- Prophylactic anticoagulation is indicated during pregnancy and is best provided with LMWH ± low dose aspirin. Heparin acts by potentiation of antithrombin III; therefore, more heparin may be required for the desired effect if levels of antithrombin III are low.
- At the time of delivery, IV antithrombin III concentrate may be substituted or used with LMWH.
- Keep patient warm and well hydrated.
- Regional anaesthesia is possible, but needs to be timed carefully with anticoagulation therapy. Continue with aspirin, as it is not a contraindication to regional anaesthesia.
- Close liaison with the haematologist is essential.

Reference

Yamada T *et al.* Management of pregnancy with congenital antithrombin III deficiency: two case reports and a review of the literature. *Journal of Obstetrics and Gynaecology Research* 2001; **27**: 189–197.

Aortic dissection

Characteristics

- Rare.
- Associated with Marfan's disease, pre-eclampsia and aortic coarctation.
- 50% of dissections in women <40yrs old occur in pregnancy, more commonly in the later months.
- Diagnosis needs a high degree of clinical suspicion. Presents with back, chest or abdominal pains.
- Needs MRI/CT or Doppler echocardiogram to diagnose.
- Type A starts in the ascending aorta and needs surgical repair.
  - If <28 weeks gestation—surgical repair undertaken with the fetus *in situ*.
  - If >32 weeks gestation—surgical repair is undertaken after CS.
- Type B is in the descending aorta and usually treated medically.

Key points

- BP needs to be controlled to decrease the velocity of ventricular contraction. Treat with GTN infusion, labetalol, nifedipine or hydralazine.
- Epidural decreases the effect of vessel shear stress and wall tension by decreasing CO and BP in labour.
- For CS, the best method of anaesthesia is controversial. Consider invasive monitoring and large-bore IV cannulae. If the patient is anticoagulated, GA is the only option, and steps must be taken to obtund the pressor response to laryngoscopy.

Reference

Jayaram A *et al.* Pregnancy complicated by aortic dissection: caesarean delivery during extradural anaesthesia. *British Journal of Anaesthesia* 1995; **75**: 358–360.

Aortic stenosis (See Chapter 4, p 88)

Characteristics

- Narrowing of aortic valve. Symptoms occur when valve area <0.8cm^2 although sometimes earlier in pregnancy because of increased CO.
- Symptoms are of angina, shortness of breath, dizziness, collapse and sudden death.
- Ejection systolic murmur on auscultation radiating to carotids. If asymptomatic prepregnancy, will generally tolerate pregnancy well.

Key points

Antenatal

- Needs echocardiogram to assess severity in mid-trimester. If severe stenosis, echo needs to be repeated at 32–36 weeks gestation.
- Liaise with cardiologist.
- Can be associated with aortic root dilatation.
- Cardiac failure may be precipitated by the physiological increase in blood volume during pregnancy.

Delivery

- If severe (valve area <1cm^2), the patient has a fixed CO and does not tolerate fluid depletion, i.e. dehydration or bleeding, tachycardia, IVC compression or vasodilatation well. Extreme care avoiding all these factors and a very slow incremental low dose epidural for labour is recommended.
- Invasive arterial monitoring advisable.
- CS will require very careful epidural, CSE or cardiac-style GA, with invasive arterial and central venous monitoring.
- Effective left uterine displacement is important.
- Avoid bolus IV syntocinon; give as a slow syntocinon infusion instead.
- Use α agonists, rather than α and β agonists to maintain BP.

References

Ray P *et al.* Recognition and management of maternal cardiac disease in pregnancy. *British Journal of Anaesthesia* 2004; **93**: 428–439.

Brighouse D. Anaesthesia for Caesarean section in patients with aortic stenosis: the case for regional anaesthesia. *Anaesthesia* 1998; **53**: 107–108.

Colclough GW *et al.* Epidural anesthesia for a parturient with critical aortic stenosis. *Journal of Clinical Anesthesia* 1995; **7**: 264–265.

Arnold–Chiari malformations

Characteristics

- Structural defects in the skull, dura, brain, spine and spinal cord often associated with myelomeningocele.
- Different types of the condition exist.
- There is underdevelopment of cranial fossae and overcrowding of hindbrain structures.
- Risk of descent of hindbrain structures through foramen magnum.
- CSF outflow obstruction through the 4th ventricle.
- Associated with obstructive sleep apnoea, inspiratory stridor and scoliosis because of association with a syrinx in the spinal cord and syringomyelia.
- Sudden death may occur.
- May have abnormal autonomic nervous system control.
- Type II may have raised ICP and therefore at risk of coning; not always present in type I.
- May have a ventriculoperitoneal shunt *in situ*.

Key points

Antenatal

- Needs neurological assessment.

Delivery

- No absolute recommendations with regards to regional vs general anaesthesia and vaginal vs CS delivery if ICP not rasied.
- Safe use of regional anaesthesia is documented in type I.
- Avoid rises in ICP (i.e. hypercarbia, straining in labour).

- Avoid large boluses of solution into the epidural space (as this may increase ICP).
- Avoid spinal anaesthesia in patients with raised ICP.

References

Agustí M *et al.* Anaesthesia for caesarean section in a patient with syringomyelia and Arnold–Chiari type I malformation. *International Journal of Obstetric Anesthesia* 2004; **13**: 114–116.

Kuczkowski KM. Spinal anesthesia for Cesarean delivery in a parturient with Arnold–Chiari type I malformation. *Canadian Journal of Anaesthesia* 2004; **51**: 639.

Arthrogryposis multiplex congenital

Characteristics

- Non-progressive condition associated with multiple joint contractures, degeneration of anterior horn cells, skin and tissue abnormalities, micrognathia, cervical spine and joint stiffness.
- Increased risk of spina bifida occulta.
- Scoliosis may occur with respiratory compromise.
- Associated with tracheal and laryngeal clefts and stenoses.
- May rarely have cardiac or pulmonary disease.

Key points

Antenatal

- Antenatal review essential.
- Vascular access often limited and difficult, may require central venous access.
- Prone to bone fractures.
- Associated with difficult airway.

Delivery

- Can have a hypermetabolic response to GA. This responds to active cooling.
- Regional anaesthesia may be technically difficult. Abnormal vertebral anatomy can complicate siting and spread of epidural and spinal blocks.
- Breech and transverse lies are more common, with increased need for CS.

References

McGillivray K *et al.* Congenital arthrogryposis in pregnancy. *Journal of Obstetrics and Gynaecology* 2002; **22**: 218–219.

Quance DR. Anaesthetic management of an obstetrical patient with arthrogryposis multiplex congenital. *Canadian Journal of Anaesthesia* 1988; **35**: 612–614.

Automatic implantable cardioverters

Characteristics

- Devices used in the treatment of patients with recurrent tachyarrhythmias unresponsive to conventional drug therapies.
- Senses arrhythmias and delivers shocks accordingly.
- Risk of associated fetal arrhythmia is small; transient fetal arrhythmias have been reported. Direct current (DC) shocks appear to be safe.

Key points

Antenatal

- Need full electrophysiological review.
- Pregnancy does not increase the risk of major implantable cardioverter-related problems or result in a higher number of discharges.
- Hormonal changes and strong uterine contractions do not seem to precipitate arrhythmias or increase incidence of firing.

Delivery

- Leave device on for vaginal delivery.
- During CS, defibrillator device should be turned off, due to use of diathermy. Most have an additional pacing mode, which should be left on. Have external defibrillator pad on the anterior chest wall to provide immediate facility for defibrillator should an arrhythmia occur.
- General or regional anaesthesia is safe.

References

Tan HL *et al.* Treatment of tachyarrhythmias during pregnancy and lactation. *European Heart Journal* 2001; **22**: 458–464.

Natale A *et al.* Implantable cardioverter–defibrillators and pregnancy: a safe combination? *Circulation* 1997; **96**: 2808–2812.

Blalock–Taussig shunts

Characteristics

- Used to palliate cyanotic heart defects.
- Shunt between subclavian artery or carotid artery to the right pulmonary artery or from the right ventricle to the pulmonary artery.

Key points

Antenatal

- Increased risk of thrombosis during pregnancy, so often on LMWH.
- Need early cardiology assessment and echocardiography.
- No pulse in left arm.
- Often hypoxic and polycythaemic.

Delivery

- May need early delivery because of cardiac failure.
- Require endocarditis prophylaxis.
- Avoid hypotension and decreased SVR, as these will dramatically decrease pulmonary perfusion.

- Use very careful slow incremental low dose epidural, CSE or a cardiac GA with arterial monitoring.
- Use phenylephrine as vasopressor.

References

Iserin L. Management of pregnancy in women with congenital heart disease. *Heart* 2001; **85**: 493–494.

Khairy P *et al.* Pregnancy outcomes in women with congenital heart disease. *Circulation* 2006; **113**: 517–524.

Dob DP, Yentis SM. Practical management of the parturient with congenital heart disease (Review). *International Journal of Obstetric Anesthesia* 2006; **15**: 137–144.

Budd–Chiari syndrome

Characteristics

- Hepatic venous outflow obstruction.
- Rare in pregnancy.
- May occur in the postpartum period.
- Either acute or chronic:
  - The acute syndrome is due to a hypercoagulable state causing thrombosis of major hepatic veins resulting in liver cell necrosis.
  - Caused by pregnancy, HELLP, SLE, severe pre-eclampsia, thrombotic thrombocythaemia purpura, malignancy, antiphospholipid syndrome, protein C deficiency and factor V Leiden.
  - The chronic syndrome is usually due to an IVC web and results in liver fibrosis.
- Treatment is aimed at preservation of liver function using stents and shunts. If untreated, leads to liver failure and death.

Key points

- Syndrome causes hepatomegaly, portal hypertension, ascites and varices.
- There is poor platelet function and coagulopathy, therefore avoid regional techniques.
- Avoid suxamethonium due to decreased pseudocholinesterase levels and therefore an unpredictable neuromuscular block.
- Liaise with haematology.
- Treatment is with anticoagulation, shunts and liver transplantation.
- If acute presentation occurs in pregnancy and the fetus is adequately mature, a CS may be performed as a combined procedure with a liver transplant.
- If chronic with a shunt *in situ*, the patient will be on long-term warfarin, which may be converted to LMWH in pregnancy. Need LFTs and coagulation checked throughout pregnancy and regular monitoring of liver blood flow via ultrasound scanning. Severe cases should be managed in major hepatic units.

References

Valentine JM *et al.* Combined orthotopic liver transplantation and caesarean section for the Budd–Chiari syndrome. *British Journal of Anaesthesia* 1995; **75**: 105–108.

Segal S *et al.* Budd–Chiari syndrome complicating severe preeclampsia in a parturient with primary antiphospholipid syndrome. *European Journal of Obstetetrics, Gynecology and Reproductive Biology* 1996; **68**: 227–229.

Cardiac tamponade

Characteristics

- Accumulation of fluid in the pericardial sac impeding cardiac function.
- Causes are iatrogenic, trauma, connective tissue disorders, malignancy and infection.

Key points

- Signs are tachycardia, hypotension, raised JVP and increased SVR.
- Acutely will require resuscitation and assessment of airway, breathing and circulation, with associated supportive care.
- Will require pericardiocentesis and may require pericardial window formation under GA. This would require invasive monitoring, continuous fetal monitoring, critical care postoperatively and facilities for immediate CS if required.

Reference

Webster JA *et al.* Anesthesia for pericardial window in a pregnant patient with cardiac tamponade and mediastinal mass. *Canadian Journal of Anaesthesia* 2003; **50**: 815–818.

Cardiomyopathy (dilated)

Characteristics

- Rare.
- Similar to peripartum cardiomyopathy (see next section), but is reserved for patients who do not meet the exact criteria for peripartum cardiomyopathy.
- Can occur in the second trimester.

Key points

- Need to optimize maternal status medically until the fetus can be delivered.
- Worse outcome than peripartum cardiomyopathy.
- Diuretics, nitrates and β-blockers acceptable. ACE inhibitors known to cause severe fetal problems.

Reference

Ray P *et al.* Recognition and management of maternal cardiac disease in pregnancy. *British Journal of Anaesthesia* 2004; **93**: 428–439.

Cardiomyopathy (peripartum)

Characteristics

- Rare disorder—1 in 1500–4000 live births.
- High rate of mortality.
- Aetiology unknown with poorly understood pathology.
- Defined as onset of cardiac failure with no identifiable cause within the last month of pregnancy or within 5 months after delivery, in the absence of heart disease before the last month of pregnancy.

- Associated with older maternal age, greater parity, Afro-Caribbean race and multiple gestation.
- Symptoms are fatigue, dyspnoea, pedal oedema, paroxysmal nocturnal dyspnoea, nocturnal cough, new regurgitant murmur, raised JVP, hepatomegaly and pulmonary crackles.

Key points

- High degree of suspicion important.
- Low threshold for echocardiogram. ECG may be normal, sinus tachycardia, LV hypertrophy, inverted T waves or non-specific ST changes. Echo will show new LV systolic dysfunction.
- CXR shows cardiomegaly.
- Treatment involves salt restriction, diuretics and vasodilators.
- If the ejection fraction is <35%, LMWH therapy is indicated.
- Fetus should be delivered once mature enough.
- Need input from the cardiologists.
- Epidural good for labour but beware if anticoagulated.
- Regional or GA suitable for CS, dependent on maternal status and anticoagulation.
- If GA, should be a cardiostable anaesthetic with invasive monitoring. Avoid tachycardia and swings in BP. Phenylephrine as vasopressor if tachycardic. Obtund pressor response to intubation.
- Early critical care referral essential.
- ACE inhibitors are beneficial in the postpartum period.

References

Ray P *et al.* Recognition and management of maternal cardiac disease in pregnancy. *British Journal of Anaesthesia* 2004; **93**: 428–439.

Abboud J *et al.* Peripartum cardiomyopathy: a comprehensive review. *International Journal of Cardiology* 2007; **118**: 295–303.

Pryn A *et al.* Cardiomyopathy in pregnancy and caesarean section: four case reports. *International Journal of Obstetric Anesthesia* 2007; **16**: 68–73.

Cauda equina syndrome

Characteristics

- Damage to the cauda equina causing low back pain, unilateral or bilateral sciatica, saddle sensory disturbance, bowel and bladder dysfunction and variable lower limb motor and sensory deficits.
- Caused by trauma, lumbar disc compression, abscess, spinal anaesthesia (more common in association with spinal catheters, but can occur with single-shot spinals), tumours and idiopathic.
- Rare in pregnancy.

Key points

Antenatal

- Can occur during pregnancy and requires urgent decompression surgery.
- Will require gastric acid prophylaxis. GA with rapid sequence induction usually used, but has been performed under a regional technique.

- Position ideally in left lateral position with abdomen supported, to avoid aorto-caval and fetal compression.
- Usual monitoring with the addition of fetal heart monitoring.
- Avoid hypotension, hypoxia and severe anaemia.
- Aim to protect maternal safety, avoid fetal asphyxia and prevent premature labour.
- Most anaesthetic agents are thought to be safe.
- Neurological assessment before regional techniques and careful explanation of risks in antenatal period with review of notes and MRI.

Delivery
- Regional techniques can be difficult, with increased complications associated with previous surgery.
- Labour is not contraindicated.

References

Tsen LC. Neurologic complications of labor analgesia and anesthesia (Review). *International Anesthesiology Clinics* 2002; **40**: 67–88.

Kathirgamanathan A *et al.* Lumbar disc surgery in the third trimester—with the fetus in utero. *International Journal of Obstetric Anesthesia* 2006; **15**: 181–182.

Cell salvage

Characteristics

- Already established in general and orthopaedic surgery to decrease need for allogenic blood transfusion.
- Limited use in obstetric practice due to worries over AFE. Blood washing has been found to eliminate the active tissue factor from amniotic fluid.

Key points

- The use of leukodepletion filters at CS has been shown to decrease particulate contaminants significantly to a concentration equivalent to that found in maternal blood.
- Risks decrease by using two suction units, one for the amniotomy and the other for blood losses.
- Some evidence for use in patients in extremis or Jehovah's Witnesses.
- More randomized controlled studies needed.

Reference

Catling SJ *et al.* Clinical experience with cell salvage in obstetrics: 4 cases from one UK centre. *International Journal of Obstetric Anesthesia* 2002; **11**: 128–134.

Cerebral tumours/craniotomy

Characteristics

- Cerebral tumours are rare in pregnancy, but symptoms such as headaches and vomiting may be mistaken for those of pregnancy itself.
- Needs multidisciplinary care. Management must be on an individual basis, with careful balance between maternal and fetal physiology.
- May remove tumour during the pregnancy or wait to deliver the fetus and perform a craniotomy at the same time.

Key points

- If craniotomy is required in pregnancy, use antacid prophylaxis, rapid sequence with cricoid pressure, maintain BP within 10% of normal during the procedure, obtund pressor response to laryngoscopy and maintain left lateral tilt.
- Invasive BP monitoring is required and critical care postoperatively.

Delivery

- If CS with tumour still *in situ*—GA.
- If any doubt about ICP—need recent MRI/CT scan and neurological review.
- Epidural may increase ICP when boluses given.
- Dural tap may cause acute deterioration and coning.

References

Chang L *et al.* Anesthesia for cesarean section in two patients with brain tumours. *Canadian Journal of Anaesthesia* 1999; **46**: 61–65.

Balki M *et al.* Craniotomy for suprasellar meningioma in a 28-week pregnant woman without fetal heart rate monitoring. *Canadian Journal of Anaesthesia* 2004; **51**: 573–576.

Cerebral venous sinus thrombosis

Characteristics

- Varied presentation.
- Features include headache, nausea and vomiting, decreased level of consciousness, seizures, focal neurological deficits and cranial nerve palsies.
- Causes cerebral infarction secondary to tissue congestion and may be complicated by cerebral haemorrhage.
- Caused by infection, trauma, idiopathic and hypercoagulable states, e.g. pregnancy and the puerperium. Diagnosed by MRI/CT and contrast studies.

Key points

- Avoid lumbar puncture.
- Supportive care required.
- Local thrombolysis may be given.
- Anticoagulation.
- May require open thrombectomy.
- Should be nursed in a critical care environment.
- Low risk of recurrence in further pregnancy.

Reference

Kimber J. Cerebral venous sinus thrombosis (Review). *Quarterly Journal of Medicine* 2002; **95**: 137–142.

C1 esterase deficiency/angioneurotic oedema

Characteristics

- Autosomal dominant condition.
- Causes episodic local SC and submucosal oedema involving the upper respiratory tract and GIT.
- Episodes associated with stress, ovulation, menstruation, trauma and infection.
- Does not respond to steroids or antihistamines.
- Disease is worse during pregnancy.

Key points

Antenatal

- A comprehensive plan is essential.

Delivery

- Inform senior staff on admission.
- Epidural suitable for labour to decrease stress.
- Patient must be turned regularly to alter pressure areas.
- Request C1 inhibitor concentrate from blood bank once patient is in labour.
- If CS, give dose of the C1 inhibitor concentrate.
- Regional better than GA if possible.
- Avoid upper airway instrumentation; if necessary use a smaller endotracheal tube than usual.
- High risk of developing oedema postpartum; therefore, have a low threshold for a further dose of inhibitor at this time.
- Nurse in a high dependency area as oedema can occur some hours after stress.

References

Nathani F *et al.* Pregnancy and C1 esterase inhibitor deficiency: a successful outcome. *Archives of Gynecology and Obstetrics* 2006; **274**: 381–384.

Griffiths RJ, O'Sullivan G. C1-esterase inhibitor deficiency and elective caesarean section. *International Journal of Obstetric Anesthesia* 2005; **4**: 263–264.

Chagas disease

Characteristics

- Tropical disease, endemic in Latin America, caused by infection with *Trypanosoma cruzi*.
- Transmission occurs through bites or through mucosal surfaces.
- 10–30% go on to develop chronic disease.
- Presents with cardiac and gastrointestinal symptoms.
- Infection can transmit to the fetus.
- May have chronic disease years after initial infection.
- Severity of disease must be considered.

Key points

- Causes atrophy of cardiac and gastrointestinal tissues, cardiac dilation, thinning of ventricular walls, damage to the cardiac conduction system (causing RBBB and left anterior fascicular block progressing to complete AV block), and destruction of autonomic ganglia in the gut causing megacolon and megaoesophagus.

Antenatal

- No drug treatment.
- ECG, echo ± cardiology review antenatally.

Delivery

- May require ECG monitoring in labour.
- Epidural suitable for labour but with slow incremental top-ups if severe cardiac disease.
- May require invasive monitoring during CS.

Reference

Gilson GJ *et al.* Chagas disease in pregnancy. *Obstetrics and Gynecology* 1995; **86**: 646–647.

Charcot–Marie–Tooth disease

Characteristics

- Autosomal dominant condition causing chronic peripheral motor and sensory neuropathy.
- Characterized by muscle wasting, causing diaphragmatic weakness and respiratory insufficiency.
- Disease often exacerbated in pregnancy.
- May require increased respiratory support as pregnancy progresses.
- Diaphragmatic splinting occurs in late pregnancy.

Key points

Antenatal

- Careful antenatal assessment of the disease.
- Assessment of respiratory function essential, particularly in patients with upper limb involvement.
- May use non-invasive ventilation at home.
- Monitor respiratory function in pregnancy and labour.

Delivery

- Increased risk of operative delivery.
- Cautious use of suxamethonium due to risk of hyperkalaemia.
- Prolonged action of non-depolarizing muscle relaxants.
- No evidence of increased risk of malignant hyperpyrexia.
- Low dose CSE useful for CS.
- GA may be required dependent on severity of disease; admission to critical care may be required postoperatively ± ventilator support.

Reference

Reah G *et al.* Anaesthesia for Caesarean section in a patient with Charcot–Marie–Tooth disease. *Anaesthesia* 1998; **53**: 586–568.

Chorioamnionitis

Characteristics

- More common during long labour or prolonged rupture of membranes.
- Can initiate premature labour or occur intra-partum.
- Characterized by fever >37.8°C, HR >120, fetal tachycardia>160, purulent amniotic fluid or vaginal discharge, abdominal tenderness, WCC >15 and increased risk of placental abruption.

Key points

- Systemic infection is a relative contraindication to a regional anaesthetic technique.
- Absolute risk of epidural or spinal abscess in the obstetric population is low.
- Risk/benefit ratio to mother must be weighed up for each individual case.
- After administration of IV antibiotics, a regional anaesthetic technique can be justified. Spinal anaesthesia may be safer than epidural because no foreign body is left *in situ*.

References

Hinchliffe D *et al.* Management of failed intubation in a septic parturient. *British Journal of Anaesthesia* 2002; **89**: 328–330.

Cohen Y *et al.* Epidural analgesia and maternal fever. *Canadian Journal of Anaesthesia* 2002; **49**: 760.

Cirrhosis

Characteristics

- Chronic damage to the liver causing irreversible fibrosis and loss of function.
- Caused by autoimmune disease, alcohol abuse and infections (e.g. hepatitis B and C).
- Problems in pregnancy depend on severity of condition. May be uneventful.
- If decompensated, increased risk of premature labour, stillbirth, liver failure in pregnancy and variceal bleeding, particularly in the second trimester.

Key points

Antenatal

- Early assessment and gastroenterology review.
- Universal precautions for staff if infective cause.
- May have anaemia, coagulation abnormalities, low platelet count or decrease in liver function.

Delivery

- Regional technique may be contraindicated.
- If GA—carefully titrate doses of IV agents.
- May precipitate encephalopathy.

- Close attention to fluid and electrolyte status. Avoid dehydration and maintain oxygen-carrying capacity.
- Care with suxamethonium, as plasma cholinesterase levels may be low.

References

Duke J. Pregnancy and cirrhosis: management of hematemesis by Warren shunt during third trimester gestation. *International Journal of Obstetric Anesthesia* 1994; **3**: 97–102.

Chen KH *et al.* Anesthetic management of a pregnant living related liver donor. *International Journal of Obstetric Anesthesia* 2006; **15**: 149–151.

Coarctation of the aorta

Characteristics

- Narrowing of a section of the aorta, usually immediately beyond the origin of the left subclavian artery or at or just distal to the insertion of the ligamentum arteriosum.
- Associated with a bicuspid aortic valve.
- Most are surgically corrected in childhood and will not be problematic in pregnancy.
- May still have hypertension.
- May re-stenose.
- Associated with aortic dissection, increased risk of ischaemic heart disease and sudden death.
- Uncorrected maternal mortality is between 3 and 9%.
- Increased risk of LVF, aortic rupture and endocarditis.

Key points

Antenatal

- Early echocardiogram and cardiology review.
- SV may be limited, therefore increase CO by an increase in HR.

Delivery

- Endocarditis antibiotic prophylaxis.
- If uncorrected, decreases in SVR are not well tolerated.
- Avoid bradycardia and maintain left ventricular filling pressure.
- Carefully titrated epidural with opioids is suitable for vaginal delivery.
- CS—GA ± invasive monitoring with remifentanil useful to obtund pressor response to intubation. Alternative is carefully tirated CSE or epidural anaesthesia.

References

Ray P *et al.* Recognition and management of maternal cardiac disease in pregnancy. *British Journal of Anaesthesia* 2004; **93**: 428–439.

Findlow *et al.* Congenital heart disease in adults. *British Journal of Anaesthesia* 1997; **78**: 416–430.

Dob DP, Yentis SM. Practical management of the parturient with congenital heart disease (Review). *International Journal of Obstetric Anesthesia* 2006; **15**: 137–144.

Cocaine abuse

Characteristics

- Cocaine prolongs adrenergic stimulation by blocking presynaptic uptake of sympathomimetic neurotransmitters.
- Causes euphoria, hypertension, tachycardia, arrhythmias, seizures, hyper-reflexia, fever, dilated pupils, oedema, proteinuria and emotional instability.
- Withdrawal causes fatigue, depression and craving.
- Pregnancy causes increased cardiovascular sensitivity to cocaine.
- Patients may deny abuse.
- Increased risk of premature labour, fetal distress and IUGR, abruption, uterine rupture, hepatic rupture, cerebral ischaemia/infarction and death.

Key points

Antenatal

- Perform a urine toxicology screen.
- May have decreased platelet count.

Delivery

- Regional anaesthesia if possible.
- May develop ephedrine-resistant hypotension—phenylephrine probably a better option.
- May still have pain perception, despite adequate spinal or epidural sensory level.
- Prone to cardiovascular system instability. Esmolol infusion may help with cocaine-induced tachycardia, but may increase risk of cocaine-induced coronary vasospasm.
- Labetalol, GTN and hydralazine may be useful to treat hypertension.
- Propofol and thiopental appear safe and effective. Volatile agents may increase risk of arrhythmia.

Reference

Kuczkowski KM. Peripartum care of the cocaine-abusing parturient: are we ready? (Review). *Acta Obstetrica et Gynecologica Scandinavica* 2005; **84**: 108–116.

Cockayne syndrome

Characteristics

- Rare autosomal recessive condition causing failure of DNA repair.
- Presents as dwarfism, microcephaly, photosensitivity, telangectasia and mental retardation.
- Normally fatal in adolescence, but some with mild disease survive to adulthood with normal intelligence. In the mild form of the disease, features are less severe and later in onset.
- Often cachexic, and short stature.
- Due to size of patient and small pelvis, likely to require CS.

Key points

- Due to stature, the gravid uterus may impair respiratory function. Monitor respiratory function in pregnancy.
- If regional technique, use low dose spinal ± epidural.
- May be a difficult intubation.

Reference

Rawlinson SC *et al.* Spinal anaesthesia for caesarean section in a patient with Cockayne syndrome. *International Journal of Obstetric Anesthesia* 2003; **12**: 297–299.

CREST syndrome

Characteristics

- Calcinosis, Raynauds phenomenon, Oesophageal dysmotility, Sclerodactyly and Telangectasia. Systemic autoimmune condition.
- May be complicated by aspiration and pulmonary disease, gastrointestinal bleeding, pulmonary hypertension, fibrosis of myocardium and arrhythmia, primary biliary sclerosis, renal disease and entrapment neurological symptoms.
- May be taking NSAIDs and steroids.
- Increased risk of premature labour.

Key points

Antenatal

- Pregnancy may worsen the disease; those with renal, cardiac and pulmonary complications are most at risk.
- May be difficult to differentiate between the disease itself and pre-eclampsia.

Delivery

- Difficult venous access.
- May be a difficult intubation and prone to oral bleeding, consider an awake fibreoptic intubation.
- Epidural and spinal possible after performing a coagulation screen. CSE may be useful, as a lower dose spinal may be required.
- Care with positioning.
- Keep patient warm and well hydrated.

Reference

Bailey AR *et al.* Spinal anaesthesia for Caesarean section in a patient with systemic sclerosis. *Anaesthesia* 1999; **54**: 355–358.

Cushing's syndrome

Characteristics

- Excess production of corticosteroids from the adrenal gland or by their exogenous administration.
- In general, most cases caused by an ACTH-secreting pituitary adenoma, but in pregnancy more are caused by adrenal adenomas.
- Increased maternal morbidity and mortality due to raised BP, hypokalaemia, diabetes, excessive weight gain, pre-eclampsia, cardiac failure and poor wound healing.
- Treatment of the cause in pregnancy seems to improve outcome.

Key points

- Difficult venous access and generally obese.
- Difficult control of blood sugar.
- Increased risk of difficult intubation.
- Muscle weakness may predispose to respiratory failure.
- May require steroid supplementation.
- May need surgical treatment in pregnancy. Laparoscopic adrenalectomy has been described.

References

Mellor A *et al.* Cushing's disease treated by trans-sphenoidal selective adenomectomy in mid-pregnancy. *British Journal of Anaesthesia* 1998; **80**: 850–852.

Tejura H *et al.* Cushing's syndrome in pregnancy. *Journal of Obstetrics and Gynaecology* 2005; **25**: 713–714.

Lindsay JR *et al.* Cushings syndrome during pregnancy: personal experience and review of literature. *Journal of Clinical Endocrinology and Metabolism* 2005; **90**: 3077–3083.

Cyanotic heart disease (See Chapter 4, p 83–84)

Characteristics

- Any congenital heart defect involving a right- to left-sided shunt.
- If surgically corrected, there is no increased risk to mother or fetus.
- Patients with uncorrected tetralogy of Fallot have an increased risk of morbidity and mortality, due to decreased SVR and increased right to left shunt.
- Success of pregnancy determined by functional status of RV.
- High mortality if pulmonary hypertension present.

Key points

Antenatal

- Careful antenatal assessment and early cardiology review.
- Continue with usual medications during pregnancy.
- At risk of arrhythmias, hypoxaemia, increased risk of thrombosis and decreased exercise capacity.

Delivery

- May require endocarditis prophylaxis.
- Air and particulate filters essential on all IV lines in patients with intracardiac shunts.
- Avoid anything that will decrease SVR.
- Avoid myocardial depression, hypovolaemia and decreases in VR.
- Avoid increases of PVR.
- Maintain normal or slightly increased RV filling pressure and SVR.
- Aim for a vaginal delivery with an assisted second stage.
- O_2 saturation, BP and ECG should be monitored in labour.
- Deliver oxygen via face mask.
- Epidural analgesia may be used with caution, with slow incremental low dose top-ups/infusion, fluid loading and careful use of vasopressors.
- Ensure no air enters the venous lines.
- GA preferred for CS with invasive monitoring or very cautious CSE or epidural anaesthesia. GA with IPPV may increase right to left shunt.
- Care with oxytocin; no IV bolus, give by infusion, and avoid ergometrine.
- Will require critical care admission postoperatively.

References

Findlow D *et al.* Congenital heart disease in adults. *British Journal of Anaesthesia* 1997; **78**: 416–430.

Ray P *et al.* Recognition and management of maternal cardiac disease in pregnancy. *British Journal of Anaesthesia* 2004; **93**: 428–439.

Dob DP, Yentis SM. Practical management of the parturient with congenital heart disease (Review). *International Journal of Obstetric Anesthesia* 2006; **15**: 137–144.

Cystic fibrosis (See Chapter 4, p 105)

Characteristics

- Autosomal recessive condition.
- Affects exocrine glands causing abnormal mucociliary transport.
- Increasing numbers of patients surviving to adulthood.
- Problems are of chronic respiratory difficulty (pulmonary hypertension and right heart failure, and respiratory failure), malabsorption, liver cirrhosis and pancreatic failure.
- Outcome dependent on severity of disease.
- Pregnancy usually well tolerated.
- Increased risk of postpartum respiratory complications.

Key points

Antenatal

- Multidisciplinary antenatal assessment of all systems.
- Optimize pulmonary function.
- Perform regular pulmonary function tests and blood gases.
- Regular physiotherapy.

Delivery

- Ideally use regional anaesthesia. CSE useful with cautious top-ups.
- May require non-invasive ventilation during CS delivery and postnatally.

- May need elective CS, as labour may not be possible due to poor respiratory reserve.
- Cautious use of epidural opioids.

Reference

Cameron AJ, Skinner TA. Management of a parturient with respiratory failure secondary to cystic fibrosis. *Anaesthesia* 2005; **60**: 77–80.

Demyelinating disease

Characteristics

- Multiple sclerosis is the most common.
- Due to abnormalities of the myelin sheath.
- Causes limb weakness, visual disturbances, paraesthesia, inco-ordination, spasticity, hyper-reflexia, pain, mild dementia and dysarthria, respiratory muscle weakness and bulbar weakness.
- Has a remitting and relapsing course.
- Exacerbations are related to stress, trauma and infection.
- Exacerbations occur less frequently in pregnancy and increase in the first 3 months postpartum.

Key points

Antenatal

- Antenatal assessment of condition.
- Document neurological deficit prior to regional technique and needs fully informed consent.

Delivery

- Epidural and spinal not contraindicated.
- Neither type of delivery nor anaesthesia related to relapse.
- May experience prolonged anaesthesia with epidural, particularly if *in situ* for a long period of time.
- Maximum safe dose of LA is lowered due to loss of blood–brain barrier.
- No evidence that volatile inhalation agents affect disease.
- May require postoperative respiratory support if GA used.
- Avoid suxamethonium as may cause hyperkalaemia.
- Avoid pyrexia.
- Needs careful follow-up and early referral to neurologist if problems.

References

Drake E *et al.* Obstetric regional blocks for women with multiple sclerosis: a survey of UK experience. *International Journal of Obstetric Anesthesia* 2006; **15**: 115–123.

Whitaker JN. Effects of pregnancy and delivery on disease activity in multiple sclerosis. *New England Journal of Medicine* 1998; **339**: 339–340.

Devic's syndrome

Characteristics

- Bilateral acute optic neuritis and transverse myelitis (causing functional transection of the spinal cord).
- Triggered by infection and autoimmune disease.
- Symptoms of back pain and progressive paraparesis.
- Increased risk of UTI, anaemia and premature labour.

Key points

- Risk of autonomic hyper-reflexia causing hypertension, bradycardia, sweating and cerebral haemorrhage.
- Epidural and spinal effective at preventing autonomic hyper-reflexia.
- Epidural easier to control with small incremental doses and regular assessment. May require smaller dose of LA than usual to provide adequate regional block. Avoid adrenaline in epidural.
- Avoid suxamethonium. Use non-depolarizing muscle relaxants as normal.

Reference

Gunaydin, B *et al.* Epidural anaesthesia for Caesarean section in a patient with Devic's syndrome. *Anaesthesia* 2001; **56**: 565–567.

Duchenne muscular dystrophy

Characteristics

- X-linked recessive disease of skeletal and cardiac muscle usually affecting males, causing progressive muscle weakness.
- Female carriers usually asymptomatic, but rarely can manifest signs and symptoms of the disease.
- A male fetus has a 50% chance of Duchenne muscular dystrophy.

Key points

- Perioperative complications include: cardiac arrhythmias and failure, cardiac arrest, malignant hyperpyrexia.
- Increased risk of cardiac arrhythmias.
- Avoid suxamethonium and volatile anaesthetics (rocuronium and total IV anaesthesia).
- Regional anaesthesia advisable (CSE for surgery, early siting of labour epidural).
- Prenatal administration of anaesthesia should not harm the male affected fetus.

Reference

Molyneux MK. Anaesthetic management during labour of a manifesting carrier of Duchenne muscular dystrophy. *International Journal of Obstetric Anesthesia* 2005; **14**: 58–61.

Dysfibrogenaemia

Characteristics

- May be congenital or acquired.
  - *Acquired* is secondary to abruption, intrauterine death, AFE and massive haemorrhage.
  - *Congenital* syndrome is rare.
- May be asymptomatic.
- Some patients have increased bleeding and some have a thrombotic tendency.
- Most will be under care of a haematologist because of personal or family history of bleeding or thrombosis.

Key points

Antenatal

- Patients with congenital dysfibrogenaemia—liaise with haematologist preferably with an interest in haemostasis and thrombosis.
- Assess coagulation screen.

Delivery

- Increased risk of PPH and thrombosis.
- May need to treat with fibrinogen and/or heparin.

References

Meldrum DJ *et al.* Spinal anaesthesia and dysfibrinogenaemia. *International Journal of Obstetric Anesthesia* 2001; **10**: 64–67.

Bolton-Maggs PH *et al.* The rare coagulation disorders—review with guidelines for management from the United Kingdom Haemophilia Centre Doctors' Organisation. *Haemophilia* 2004; **10**: 593–628.

Ebstein's anomaly

Characteristics

- Congenital anomaly in which the tricuspid valve is displaced apically and usually incompetent, so called atrialization of RV.
- If asymptomatic, usually well tolerated in pregnancy.
- Can be associated with an ASD or Wolf–Parkinson–White syndrome—in this situation arrhythmias and cyanosis may occur.
- In severe cases can get a right to left shunt through an ASD, and cardiac failure may develop.

Key points

Antenatal

- ECG and echocardiogram as part of antenatal review with a cardiology opinion.

Delivery
- Epidural safe in labour, but use with slow, incremental doses to avoid profound decrease in SVR.
- Maintain pre- and afterload.
- Avoid increases to PVR.
- For patients with right to left shunt, see cyanotic heart disease, page 606.

References

Groves ER, Groves JB. Epidural analgesia for labour in a patient with Ebstein's anomaly. *Canadian Journal of Anaesthesia* 1995; **42**: 77–79.

Connolly HM, Warnes CA. Ebstein's anomaly: outcome of pregnancy. *Journal of the American College of Cardiology* 1994; **23**: 1194–1198.

Misa VS, Pan PH. Evidence-based case report for analgesic and anesthetic management of a parturient with Ebstein's anomaly and Wolff–Parkinson–White syndrome. *International Journal of Obstetric Anesthesia* 2007; **16**: 77–81.

Ehler's–Danlos syndrome

Characteristics

- Heterogenous group of hereditary connective tissue disorders.
  - Classic types (type I, II and III) cause joint hypermobility, skin hyperelasticity, easily bruised, poor skin healing, excess bleeding, pneumothorax and valvular prolapse. May have decreased response to LA agents. Pregnancy is likely to be uncomplicated.
  - Type IV is due to abnormal type III collagen in the GIT, vascular tissue and uterus. Much poorer prognosis. Can have spontaneous rupture of bowel, major vessels and uterus. Likely to have elective CS due to increased risk of uterine rupture. Sudden death in pregnancy reported.

Key points

Antenatal
- Careful assessment and discuss risks and benefits of GA vs regional techniques.
- Type IV is a major concern.

Delivery
- GA usually preferable due to possible increased bleeding diathesis and risk of major bleed.
- Avoid sudden increases in BP.
- May have C-spine problems, therefore care with intubation necessary.
- Clotting usually normal but can be altered, and platelets may be low.

References

Glynn JC, Yentis SM. Epidural analgesia in a parturient with classic type Ehlers–Danlos syndrome. *International Journal of Obstetric Anesthesia* 2005; **14**: 78–79.

Kuczkowski KM. Ehlers–Danlos syndrome in the parturient: an uncommon disorder–common dilemma in the delivery room. *Archives of Gynecology and Obstetrics* 2005; **273**: 60–62.

Campbell N, Rosaeg OP. Anesthetic management of a parturient with Ehlers Danlos syndrome type IV. *Canadian Journal of Anaesthesia* 2002; **49**: 493–496.

Eisenmenger's syndrome (See also Chapter 4, page 84–5)

Characteristics

- Associated with congenital heart defects, pulmonary hypertension, reversed shunt (right to left) and peripheral cyanosis.
- Prognosis depends on severity of pulmonary hypertension, but overall poor.
- PVR is fixed and the subsequent decrease in SVR in pregnancy increases the right to left shunt.

Key points

Antenatal

- Pulmonary vasodilators have been described during pregnancy.
- Regular cardiology assessment important.

Delivery

- Often by CS delivery early in the third trimester because of poor fetal growth and deteriorating maternal condition.
- Avoid increased HR, SV and oxygen consumption as may get RV compromise.
- Avoid decreases in SVR and VR.
- Avoid hypercarbia, acidosis and low oxygen saturations.
- Air and particulate filters essential on all IV lines in patients with intracardiac shunts.
- Epidural must be titrated carefully to avoid large drops in SVR.
- GA advised for CS.
- Low dose CSE for CS has been described.
- Arterial line monitoring mandatory, CVP ± CO monitoring might be useful.
- Avoid oxytocin IV bolus, use a slow oxytocin infusion instead.
- Increased risk of thrombosis, therefore, will require prophylactic heparin.
- Will require monitoring for 7 days postoperatively.

References

Ray P *et al.* Recognition and management of maternal cardiac disease in pregnancy. *British Journal of Anaesthesia* 2004; **93**: 428–439.

Cole PJ *et al.* Incremental spinal anaesthesia for elective Caesarean section in a patient with Eisenmenger's syndrome. *British Journal of Anaesthesia* 2001; **86**: 723–726.

Lacassie HJ *et al.* Management of Eisenmenger syndrome in pregnancy with sildenafil and L-arginine. *Obstetrics and Gynecology* 2004; **103**: 1118–1120.

Epidermolysis bullosa

Characteristics

- Rare, inherited group of skin disorders.
- Causes blisters, pronounced scarring of skin and mucous membranes after minor trauma.
- Pregnancy occurs rarely in these patients.
- Vaginal delivery is first choice, although in severe cases this may not be possible because of contractures.
- Varying degrees of severity.
- May have microstomia due to severe facial scaring.

Key points

Antenatal

- Assessment of airway and venous assess.

Delivery

- Care with dressings; use paraffin gauze and light crepe bandages for IV cannulae. Never use adhesive dressings. Use minimal manual venous occlusion. Difficult venous access.
- Suxamethonium and non-depolarizing muscle relaxants are safe.
- Care with pressure points and eyes. Care with monitoring, e.g. saturation prose, BP Cuff and ECG electrodes. Invasive arterial BP monitoring may be useful.
- Tracheal intubation can be safe, with minimal examples in the literature of mucosal trauma. Lubricate laryngoscopes and oropharyngeal airways. May be a difficult intubation with very limited mouth opening.
- Care with oral suctioning.
- Spinal and epidurals are safe.
- PR analgesia can be used.

Reference

Ames WA *et al.* Anaesthetic management of epidermolysis bullosa (Review). *British Journal of Anaesthesia* 1999; **82**: 746–751.

Epilepsy/pseudoseizures

Characteristics

- Many different types of seizures; grand mal associated with increased risk to mother and fetus.
- Pseudoseizures characterized by resistance to open eyes, maintenance of papillary reflexes, response to pain, psychiatric history or previous episodes, seizure lasting >90s without cyanosis.

Key points

- Minimize risk of seizures antenatally if possible.
- May have increased seizure frequency in pregnancy.
- Changes in blood volume and poor compliance affect medication.
- If seizures in labour or delivery—protect and secure airway, support ventilation and deliver fetus.
- Check blood sugar.

- No contraindication to regional techniques.
- If on long-term anticonvulsants, may have altered response to anaesthetic drugs.

References

Kalviainen R, Tomson T. Optimizing treatment of epilepsy during pregnancy. *Neurology* 2006; **67** (Suppl 4): S59–S63.

Kuczkowski KM. Labor analgesia for the parturient with neurological disease: what does an obstetrician need to know? *Archives of Gynecology and Obstetrics* 2006; **274**: 41–46.

Factor V Leiden (See Chapter 4, p 122)

Characteristics

- Mutation in gene for factor V, producing abnormal factor V that is resistant to the action of activated protein C, which therefore cannot stop factor V Leiden making excess fibrin.
- Seven times greater risk of DVT/PE in pregnancy.

Key points

Antenatal

- If had DVT/PE in the past, needs to be treated with LMWH in pregnancy.
- Best managed in a joint haematology/high risk obstetric clinic.

Delivery

- Need to wait 24h after therapeutic dose of enoxaparin before regional anaesthesia, i.e. >40mg enoxaparin BD or equivalent. Wait 4h after procedure before the next dose.
- TED (thromboembolism deterrent) stocking in labour.
- Early mobilization and good hydration.
- Consider changing to IV unfractionated heparin before 38th week to allow flexibility if recent thrombosis needing full anticoagulation.

References

Harnett MJ *et al.* The use of central neuraxial techniques in parturients with factor V Leiden mutation. *Anesthesia and Analgesia* 2005; **101**: 1821–1823.

Murphy PT. Factor V Leiden, pregnancy complications and adverse outcomes. *Quarterly Journal of Medicine* 2006; **99**: 639.

Factor XI deficiency

Characteristics

- Inherited coagulation disorder.
- History of increased bleeding with dental extractions, trauma, surgery and mennorrhagia.
- Causes prolongation of APTT.

Key points

Antenatal

- Needs early review by haematologist and clear delivery plan in place.

Delivery

- Regional techniques contraindicated.
- For labour analgesia, avoid IM injections. Use IV opioids ± Entonox.
- Factor XI concentrate or viral-inactivated FFP will be needed to cover operative delivery.
- Use antifibrinolytics.

References

Christiaens F *et al.* Anaesthetic management of a parturient with severe congenital factor XI deficiency undergoing Caesarean section for triplet pregnancy. *International Journal of Obstetric Anesthesia* 1998; **7**: 50–53.

Bolton-Magga PH *et al.* The rare coagulation disorders—review with guidelines for management from the United Kingdom Haemophilia Centre Doctors' Organisation (Review). *Haemophilia* 2004; **10**: 593–628.

Familial hypokalaemic periodic paralysis

Characteristics

- Calcium channel disorder.
- Periods of paralysis associated with seemingly normal muscle function in between.
- Paralysis precipitated by stress, cold, carbohydrate load and fasting. Lasts from hours to days. Associated with hypokalaemia.
- Rarely death occurs from respiratory failure or pulmonary aspiration.
- Diaphragm and cranial nerves not usually involved.

Key points

Delivery

- Avoid hypokalaemia and triggers of paralysis. Keep patient warm.
- Epidural and spinal safe ± arterial line for easier sampling. Epidural helps to decrease the stress associated with labour.
- Continuous ECG monitoring.
- Respiratory support rarely required.
- Suxamethonium causes generalized muscle rigidity.
- Possible increased risk of malignant hyperpyrexia; monitor temperature if using trigger agents.
- Use small doses of non-depolarizing muscle relaxant and monitor response with peripheral nerve stimulator, as may cause prolonged weakness.
- Postoperative monitoring on critical care facility useful, and continuing monitoring of potassium advised.

Reference

Robinson JE *et al.* Familial hypokalemic periodic paralysis and Wolff–Parkinson–White syndrome in pregnancy. *Canadian Journal of Anaesthesia* 2000; **47**: 160–164.

Familial Mediterranean fever

Characteristics

- A chronic inflammatory condition affecting serosal surfaces such as peritoneum, pleura and joints.
- Associated with amyloidosis.
- Repeat bouts of fever associated with inflammation of serosal surfaces.
- Most common in patients of Mediterranean and Middle Eastern origin.
- Uncomplicated Familiar Mediterrean Fever causes no additional problems for the anaesthetist.
- Renal failure most common cause of death. May have had renal transplant.
- In the presence of amyloid nephropathy, pregnancy has a deleterious effect on renal function.
- Cardiac disease causes LVF, conduction defects and restrictive cardiomyopathy.
- High incidence of pre-eclampsia, thromboembolism, anaemia and IUGR.

Key points

Antenatal

- Assessment in a multidisciplinary clinic assessing renal and cardiac function.

Delivery

- Regional techniques good option but may need to be carefully titrated because of multisystem disease.
- If cardiac disease present—requires invasive monitoring.
- May require critical care support postpartum.

Reference

Weir PS, McLoughlin CC. Anaesthesia for caesarean section in a patient with systemic amyloidosis secondary to familial Mediterranean fever. *International Journal of Obstetric Anesthesia* 1998; **7**: 271–274.

Fontan's procedure

Characteristics

- Palliative procedure for patients with a functional or anatomical single ventricle permitting diversion of systemic VR to the pulmonary arteries. There is no functional RV, therefore pulmonary flow is entirely passive.
- Improves cyanosis and volume overload, but patients have a limited capacity to increase their CO.
- Patients are at risk of arrhythmias and thromboembolism.
- At risk of paradoxical thromboembolism of the Fontan if fenestrated.
- Progressive decrease in ventricular function.
- Hepatic dysfunction and cyanosis will eventually occur.
- Usually anticoagulated.

Key points

Antenatal

- Will require meticulous cardiac, obstetric and haematological supervision during pregnancy.
- Most will be anticoagulated with warfarin.

Delivery

- Vaginal delivery is possible.
- Invasive arterial monitoring may be useful.
- Endocarditis prophylaxis needed at the onset of active labour.
- Anticoagulation needs to be stopped for shortest time possible.
- Epidural can be used with care and with good fluid preloading, provided anticoagulation reversed.
- Air and particulate filters essential on all IV lines in patients with intracardiac shunts.
- Labour best in left lateral position because pulmonary flow entirely reliant on passive VR.
- Postpartum will require critical or coronary care monitoring.

References

Findlow D, Doyle E. Congenital heart disease in adults (Review). *British Journal of Anaesthesia* 1997; **78**: 416–430.

Cohen AM, Mulvein J. Obstetric anaesthetic management in a patient with the Fontan circulation. *British Journal of Anaesthesia* 1994; **73**: 252–255.

Ray, P. *et al.* Recognition and management of maternal cardiac disease in pregnancy. *British Journal of Anaesthesia* 2004; **93**: 428–439.

Friedreich's ataxia

Characteristics

- Autosomal recessive condition.
- Progressive degeneration of the spinocerebellar and corticospinal tracts.
- Mixed upper and lower motor neuron disease with cerebellar symptoms.
- Associated with scoliosis and hypertrophic cardiomyopathy.
- Prone to cardiac arrhythmias.

Key points

Antenatal

- Multidisciplinary antenatal assessment.
- Echocardiogram and 24h ECG will be helpful.
- Careful assessment of scoliosis.

Delivery

- Elective CS may decrease the cardiovascular stress associated with labour.
- May have impaired respiratory function.
- Preserve pre- and afterload and avoid tachycardia.
- Avoid suxamethonium due to risk of hyperkalaemia.
- No evidence of increased sensitivity to non-depolarizing muscle relaxants.

- Ideally avoid GA if possible.
- CSE useful for CS ± invasive monitoring.

Reference

Wyatt S, Brighouse D. Anaesthetic management of vaginal delivery in a woman with Friedreich's ataxia complicated by cardiomyopathy and scoliosis. *International Journal of Obstetric Anesthesia* 1998; **7**: 185–188.

Gaucher's disease

Characteristics

- Autosomal recessive lysosomal storage disorder caused by enzyme deficiency managed with long-term enzyme replacement.
- Leads to accumulation of glycosphingolipids and multiple end-organ dysfunction.
- Types I–III, with type I (and type II rarely) surviving to reproductive age. Extremely heterogenous in onset and organ involvement.

Key points

Antenatal

- Hepatosplenomegaly, thrombocytopenia, isolated clotting factor deficiency (factor IX and von Willebrand's disease) and anaemia.
- Risk of excessive bleeding; full haematological work-up required.
- Does not preclude regional technique after careful assessment.
- Skeletal involvement, i.e. osteopenia, pathological fractures, therefore care with positioning and transferring.
- Associated with lung parenchymal disease and pulmonary hypertension (rare), and neurological dysfunction, e.g. bulbar involvement, seizures, chronic aspiration.
- Difficult intubation associated with skeletal abnormalities and trismus.

Reference

Ioscovich A *et al.* Anesthesia for obstetric patients with Gaucher disease: survey and review. *International Journal of Obstetric Anesthesia* 2004; **13**: 244–250.

Gilbert's disease

Characteristics

- Autosomal dominant, benign condition with mildly elevated (up to 50mcmol/L) unconjugated serum bilirubin.
- Mild jaundice occurs with stress, infection, starvation or surgery.
- Liver function otherwise normal.

Key points

Delivery

- Not associated with HELLP syndrome.
- Stress of long labour/hyperemesis can precipitate attack.
- Postdelivery jaundice may occur.

- Avoiding long starvation times and use of IV dextrose minimizes risk of jaundice.
- Not associated with abnormal clotting, therefore regional analgesia useful.
- Use morphine and paracetamol more cautiously due to delayed metabolism.
- Nicotinic acid has been used to increase serum unconjugated bilirubin.

References

Taylor S. Gilbert's syndrome as a cause of postoperative jaundice. *Anaesthesia* 1984; **39**: 1222–1224.

Zusterzeel PL *et al.* Gilbert's syndrome is not associated with HELLP syndrome. *British Journal of Obstetrics and Gynaecology* 2001; **108**: 1003–1004.

Glanzmann's thrombasthenia

Characteristics

- Rare, autosomal recessive platelet disorder caused by lack of glycoprotein IIb–IIIa.
- Diagnosed in childhood, usually presenting with marked mucocutaneous bleeding.
- Normal platelet numbers, but platelet function and aggregation are severely impaired.
- Women should be counselled about the high risk of severe peripartum bleeding before deciding whether to conceive.
- Late severe PPH at 7–21 days is recognized even after apparently adequate platelet transfusion at the time of delivery.
- Multiple platelet transfusions can lead to antiplatelet antibody production and a reduced effectiveness of further platelet transfusions.
- Neonatal alloimmune thrombocytopenia, due to fetal platelets inducing GpIIb–IIIa antibodies in the mother, may result in thrombocytopenia in the neonate.

Key points

Antenatal

- Must be managed jointly with a haemophilia centre.

Delivery

- Regional anaesthesia absolutely contraindicated for labour and CS.
- Other treatments include immunoglobulins to dampen the antiplatelet response, plasmaphoresis, single donor platelet/HLA-matched platelet transfusion, oxytocin infusion and recombinant factor VIIa.

References

Montes S, Lyons G. Peri-partum management of a patient with Glanzmann's thrombasthenia using Thrombelastograph. *British Journal of Anaesthesia* 2002; **88**: 734–738.

Bolton-Maggs PH *et al.* A review of inherited platelet disorders with guidelines for their management on behalf of the UKHCDO. *British Journal of Haematology* 2006; **135**: 603–633.

Guillain–Barré syndrome

Characteristics

- Acute or subacute ascending demyelinating polyradiculoneuritis classically following viral infection, e.g. Epstein–Barr virus, leading to pain, paraesthesia and paralysis extending proximally.
- Management involves symptomatic relief, thromboprophylaxis, nutrition and physiotherapy, and regular monitoring of respiratory function (forced vital capacity).
- IV immunoglobulin and plasmapharesis are reserved for severe cases.

Key points

Antenatal

- Full neurological assessment and respiratory function tests.
- Careful explanation of regional techniques.

Delivery

- GBS has no effect on uterine contraction or cervical dilatation, hence vaginal delivery preferred.
- May require assisted instrumental delivery.
- In cases with significant neurological deficit who require regional techniques for labour or CS, there is an increased sensitivity to LAs and autonomic instability. For this reason, care is necessary with spinal anaesthesia.
- Suxamethonium can cause hyperkalaemia.
- There is increased sensitivity to non-depolarizing neuromuscular blockers.
- Postoperative ventilation may be required following GA.

References

Brooks, H *et al.* Pregnancy, anaesthesia and Guillain Barre. *Anaesthesia* 2000; **55**: 894–898.

Karnad DR, Guntupalli KK. Neurologic disorders in pregnancy (Review). *Critical Care Medicine* 2005; **33** (10 Suppl): S362–S371.

Haemophilia A/haemophilia carrier

(See Chapter 4, p 119)

Characteristics

- X-linked recessive disorder of coagulation (factor VIII deficiency).
- Females are carriers, with 50% chance of male offspring having haemophilia.

Carriers

- Genetic testing for definitive carrier identification.
- Most women have no increased risk of bleeding, but male babies may have haemophilia and should be delivered in a hospital with comprehensive haemophilia services.
- 10–20% of women will have reduced factor VIII (<40U/dL) and are at risk of bleeding during pregnancy and delivery. Factor VIII increases in pregnancy, thus uncomplicated vaginal delivery with levels >40U/dL may not require blood product replacement. For CS, factor VIII concentrate required to achieve >50U/dL. Levels need to be maintained for 4–5 days postoperatively.

Key points

Antenatal

- Preconception counselling should be offered.
- Managed in a haemophilia centre with regular monitoring of factor VIII levels if low.

Delivery

- In women with normal factor VIII levels, regional techniques are not contraindicated.
- Vaginal delivery preferable, but instrumental delivery contraindicated for male babies.
- For women with low factor VIII levels, give factor VIII concentrate (recombinant) and DDAVP according to haematological advice.
- Regional techniques may be safe after replacement (specialist advice required).
- Postoperative monitoring of coagulation vital.
- Avoid IM injections.

Acquired haemophilia

- Rare acquired bleeding disorder associated with pregnancy.
- Can present with severe bleeding in pregnancy and the perpuriem with abnormal clotting.
- Requires urgent referral to haemophilia centre for immunomodulation therapy.

Reference

Walker ID *et al.* Haemostasis and Thrombosis Task Force. *Journal of Clinical Pathology* 1994; **47**: 100–108.

Heart block

Characteristics

- Congenital or acquired (ischaemic heart disease, cardiomyopathy, drugs, spinal and epidural anaesthesia), acute or chronic.
- Types I–III, with types II, III being more serious.
- Symptoms can include chest pain, shortness of breath, fatigue and heart failure.
- Congenital type III degree heart block associated with maternal anti-R*o* antibodies. Usually known prior to pregnancy but may be asymptomatic and noticed because of abnormally slow pulse for pregnancy or syncope because of increased cardiovascular demands of pregnancy.

Key points

Antenatal

- Full cardiological assessment including echocardiography.
- May require pacing in pregnancy. Most young people now fitted with DDDI (physiological) pacemaker.
- Responds well to physiological demands of pregnancy.
- Pacemaker check required in antenatal period.

Delivery

- Paced women with DDDI pacemaker usually require routine care only.
- In unpaced heart block, regional anaesthesia advised with caution.
- Invasive monitoring may be needed for CS delivery with a high block.
- α and β agonists, vagolytics and external pacing should be available.

Reference

Ray P *et al.* Recognition and management of maternal cardiac disease in pregnancy. *British Journal of Anaesthesia* 2004; **93**: 428–439.

Adekanye O *et al.* Bradyarrhythmias in pregnancy: a case report and review of management. *International Journal of Obstetric Anesthesia* 2007; **16**: 165–170.

Heart–lung transplant

Characteristics

- There are an increasing number of post-transplant patients of reproductive age who generally have a good outcome in pregnancy.
- Immunosuppressive therapy is responsible for increased risk of maternal and fetal complications including hypertension, pre-eclampsia, low birth weight, prematurity and infection.
- Immunosuppressive therapy continues in pregnancy with the minimal dosage possible.
- Pregnancy does not increase the risk of graft rejection.

Key points

Antenatal

- Denervated heart is devoid of functional autonomic innervation.
- The transplanted heart responds to haemodynamic changes seen in pregnancy by Frank–Starling mechanism.
- Upregulation of adrenoreceptors leads to increased sensitivity to circulating catecholamines.

Delivery

- Haemodynamic changes in labour are well tolerated.
- Mode of delivery is based on obstetric indication alone.
- Regional techniques are not contraindicated.

Reference

Padhan P. Pregnancy in recipients of solid-organ transplants. *New England Journal of Medicine* 2006; **354**: 2726–2727.

Hereditary neuropathy

Characteristics

- Herditary neuropathy with liability to pressure palsies (HNPP).
- Autosomal dominant with variable penetrance and well-defined genetic defect leading to abnormal myelin formation.
- Presents at any age with self-limiting, painless, focal neuropathies at entrapment sites following trauma or compression.
- Some reports of chronic neuropathy.
- *Hereditary neuralgic amyotrophy (HNA):* painful brachial plexopathy reported after childbirth. No clear genetic defect.

Key points

Antenatal

- History suggestive of recurrent entrapment neuropathies may indicate a hereditary neuropathy. Seek neurological advice.
- Counselling and documentation in case of regional techniques.

Delivery

- Regional techniques are not contraindicated, but great care is required with positioning of mother.

Reference

Peters G, Hinds NP. Inherited neuropathy can cause postpartum foot drop. *Anesthesia and Analgesia* 2005; **100**: 547–548.

Hereditary spherocytosis

Characteristics

- Autosomal dominant disorder causing early destruction of erythrocytes in the spleen.
- Patients suffer with haemolytic anaemia, marrow hyperplasia, splenomegaly, jaundice and gallstones.
- Splenectomy is the treatment of choice in severe cases, improving Hb and platelet levels.
- Increased cholesterol levels may have detrimental effects on the patient (myocardial infarction, stroke).
- Pregnancy can be complicated by anaemia and haemolytic crises.

Key points

- Careful observation in pregnancy with folic acid supplementation, prevention of infection and haematological input.
- Postsplenectomy patients should have prophylaxis against infection.

Reference

Pajor A *et al.* Pregnancy and hereditary spherocytosis. Report of 8 patients and a review. *Archives of Gynecology and Obstetrics* 1993; **253**: 37–42.

Herpes simplex infection

Characteristics

- Herpes simplex infection is common and can be in an active or inactive state.
- Patients may be immunocompromised due to co-existing disease and medication.

Key points

- CS delivery recommended in presence of active perineal infection.
- Regional anaesthesia is not contraindicated.
- Reports of epidural morphine being associated with reactivation of the infection and pruritus.

Reference

Crosby ET *et al.* Epidural anaesthesia for Caesarean section in patients with active recurrent genital herpes simplex infections: a retrospective review. *Canadian Journal of Anaesthesia* 1989; **36**: 701–704.

HIV infection

Characteristics

- Women of reproductive age are the fastest growing group of HIV sufferers.
- A multiorgan disease affecting cell-mediated immunity, which can be complicated by opportunistic infections, tumours, antiretroviral therapy and substance abuse. The following manifestations have been reported:
  - Neurological (intracranial tumours, abscesses, neuropathies, myopathies).
  - Pulmonary (infections, tuberculosis, lymphomas).
  - Cardiac (myocarditis, pulmonary hypertension, cardiomyopathy, coronary artery disease).
  - Gastrointestinal (gastroparesis, hepatitis).
  - Haematological (hypercoagulable states, bone marrow failure).
- Monitoring of disease state with viral load and CD4 counts now commonplace.
- Vertical transmission to the fetus *in utero* (4.5%), during childbirth (60%) and breastfeeding (35%) can occur. Transmission rates lower with antiretroviral therapy.

Key points

- High infection risk with high viral load; universal precautions essential.
- CS lessens the risk of transmission to the unborn baby. Antiretroviral therapy given prior to vaginal or caesarean delivery to reduce vertical transmission.
- HIV and drug therapy have minimal effect on complications associated with pregnancy and, in turn, pregnancy does not have a detrimental effect on HIV disease process.

- Anaesthetic technique is governed by systemic effects of disease.
- Regional techniques and blood patch are safe.

References

Evron S *et al.* Human immunodeficiency virus: anesthetic and obstetric considerations (Review). *Anesthesia and Analgesia* 2004; **98**: 503–511.

Bevacqua BK, Slucky AV. Epidural blood patch in a patient with HIV infection. *Anesthesiology* 1991; **74**: 952–953.

Horner's syndrome

Characteristics

- A triad of miosis, ptosis and enophthalmus with facial flushing and anhydrosis.
- The patient complains of blurred vision, strange feeling over face, nasal stuffiness and the sensation of respiratory difficulty (as a result of both high epidural and spinal anaesthesia).
- Paralysis of sympathetic pathways from C6 to T1 leads to unopposed parasympathetic tone producing the clinical signs.

Key points

- Most common after regional techniques with excessive sympathetic block.
- Symptoms usually benign and resolve spontaneously but, if prolonged, exclusion of other causes of Horner's syndrome is important (intracranial pathology). Patient reassurance required.

Reference

Theodosiadis PD *et al.* A case of unilateral Horner's syndrome after combined spinal epidural anesthesia with ropivacaine 10mg/mL for cesarean section. *International Journal of Obstetric Anesthesia* 2005; **15**: 68–70.

Hypertrophic obstructive cardiomyopathy

Characteristics

- Genetically transmitted cardiac disease with LV hypertrophy and poor LV compliance.
- Pregnancy can be well tolerated depending on prenatal NYHA functional status.
- Reduction in preload and afterload results in poor LV filling (fixed CO state).

Key points

Antenatal

- Regular cardiology assessment with echocardiography.
- β-blockers frequently prescribed as tachycardia of pregnancy increases functional obstruction.

Delivery

- Caution with regional anaesthesia due to effect on afterload, although there are reports of successful use for labour analgesia and CS.
- Invasive monitoring required.
- Phenylephrine vasopressor of choice, avoiding large swings in afterload.

References

Spirito P, Autore C. Management of hypertrophic cardiomyopathy (Review). *British Medical Journal* 2006; **332**: 1251–1255.

Ray P *et al.* Recognition and management of maternal cardiac disease in pregnancy. *British Journal of Anaesthesia* 2004; **93**: 428–439.

Hypothyroidism/hyperthyroidism

Characteristics

Hypothyroidism

- Most common cause is autoimmune thyroiditis, which can affect 2.5% of pregnant women.
- Usually subclinical, with those affected being picked up by screening programmes.
- Evidence for impaired neuron intellectual development in the unborn child supports thyroid hormone replacement in these women.

Hyperthyroidism

- Autoimmune (Grave's disease) is not common in pregnancy and treatment depends on the severity of the disease.
- Antithyroid drugs (propothiouracil) can control the disease with good outcomes.
- Surgery may be indicated and is safe in the second trimester.
- Maternal complications include preterm labour, miscarriage, placental abruption, pre-eclampsia, cardiac failure and thyroid storm.
- Thyroid antibodies can cross the placenta causing fetal abnormalities, IUGR and neonatal hyperthyroidism.

Key points

- Early involvement of endocrinologist to control and monitor disease process.
- Pregnancy may ameliorate autoimmune thyroid disease.
- Surgery in the presence of uncontrolled hyperthyroidism is associated with a high mortality.

Reference

Lazarus JH. Thyroid disorders associated with pregnancy: etiology, diagnosis, and management (Review). *Treatments in Endocrinology* 2005; **4**: 31–41.

Hypoplastic anaemia

Characteristics

- Rare in pregnancy, with bone marrow failure and pancytopenia in peripheral blood posing a risk of infection and bleeding to the mother.
- Other complications include IUGR, fetal death, chorioamnionitis and preterm delivery.
- Pregnancy may have a detrimental effect on the disease.
- Patients can present with bleeding gums and bruising.

Key points

- Appropriate replacement therapy of red cells, white cells and platelets is required under haematological guidance.
- Platelet antibody production can result in ineffective transfusions.

Delivery

- Mode of delivery will depend on obstetric indication and severity of disease process.
- Regional anaesthesia may be contraindicated if severe thrombocytopenia.
- Anxiety regarding epidurals and infection.

Reference

Wong AY *et al.* Anesthetic management of Cesarean delivery in a patient with hypoplastic anemia and severe pre-eclampsia. *Canadian Journal of Anaesthesia* 2004; **51**: 923–927.

Implanted intrathecal pump

Characteristics

- Intrathecal opioid-delivering pumps are used for the treatment of severe refractory malignant and non-malignant pain.
- Implantation of an intrathecal catheter involves tunnelling the catheter and attaching it to an SC pump in the abdomen or thorax.
- Patients may be on multiple other medications.
- No reports of utilizing the pump alone for management of labour analgesia, but some discussion on a possible plan for its use in this setting.
- Pumps can be dislodged in the pregnant abdomen.

Key points

- Seek expert advice on use of pump and position of catheter (imaging).
- Use of pump may be hazardous, and complications can include difficulty in finding the pump port, flushing of concentrated opioids through the catheter, and infection (antibiotic prophylaxis).
- Device does not preclude regional techniques for labour/delivery (with caution). Epidural space may be scarred and spread of LA unpredictable, and attempts at epidural insertion should be made at a remote site to avoid shearing.

Reference

Tarshis J *et al.* Labour pain management in a parturient with an implanted intrathecal pump. *Canadian Journal of Anaesthesia* 1997; **44**: 1278–1281.

Intracranial mass/cyst

Characteristics

- Tumours and epidermoid cysts are rare in pregnancy, and growth may be increased by hormone excess.
- Patients present with symptoms of raised ICP (headache, seizures).
- Patients with stable neurology may progress to term with regular neurosurgical evaluation.

Key points

- Mode of delivery depends on tumour size and location, being largely led by a multidisciplinary approach to management.
- Epidural analgesia and spinal anaesthesia are potentially hazardous because of tentorial herniation and increases in ICP, but both have been safely reported.
- Meningitis after rupture of epidermoid cyst can occur.
- GA should include avoidance of fluctuation in ICP and maintenance of stable haemodynamics (remifentanil, topical anaesthesia of larynx, local infiltration of surgical site). Sufficient depth of anaesthesia and rapid recovery required with multimodal analgesia and minimizing opioid use.

Reference

Imarengiaye C *et al.* Goal oriented general anesthesia for Cesarean section in a parturient with a large intracranial epidermoid cyst. *Canadian Journal of Anaesthesia* 2001; **48**: 884–889.

Isaac's syndrome

Characteristics

- Continuous muscle fibre activity syndrome is a very rare peripheral motor neuron disease with a possible autoimmune origin.
- Stiffness, delayed relaxation, continual muscle movements and ataxia.
- Treated with phenytoin, carbamazepine and acetazolamide.

Key points

- No contraindication to regional blockade.
- Possible increased sensitivity to neuromuscular-blocking drugs.

Reference

Morgan PJ. Peripartum management of a patient with Isaacs' syndrome. *Canadian Journal of Anaesthesia* 1997; **44**: 1174–1177.

Jehovah's Witness

Characteristics

- Patients will not accept the transfusion of blood or blood products on religious grounds.
- Ethical, moral, legal and practical issues make cases complicated, and each should be tackled with respect for the patient, with full informed consent and clear ideas about the patient's wishes.
- Patients can refuse stored whole blood, minor blood fractions (clotting factors, albumin) and non-stored autologous blood (cell salvage) to varying degrees.

Key points

Antenatal

- Detailed patient consent in presence of a witness including availability and acceptability of cell salvage techniques.
- Preoperative measures to optimize Hb levels: dietary, iron supplements (oral or IV), erythropoietin.

Delivery

- Early warning of obstetric/anaesthetic staff on admission.
- Delivery in consultant-led unit (recommendation of Jehovah's Witness Association).
- IV and early use of oxytocins postdelivery.
- Limit blood sampling and excessive blood loss (surgical technique, haemodilution, aprotinin, tranexamic acid, DDAVP).
- Morbidity/mortality results from inadequte circulating volume, oxygen carriage, low platelets and coagulation failure, oncotic pressure and immune status.
- Epidural blood patch may be refused.

Reference

Rasanayagam SR, Cooper GM. Two cases of severe postpartum anaemia in Jehovah's witnesses. *International Journal of Obstetric Anesthesia* 1996; **5**: 202–205.

King–Denborough syndrome

Characteristics

- Rare disease of unknown inheritance.
- Presents with progressive myopathy, congenital skeletal and facial deformities.
- Marked kyphoscoliosis with respiratory failure which can be exaggerated in pregnancy.
- Increased physiological demands in labour can lead to significant cardiorespiratory compromise.

Key points

Antenatal

- Assessment of respiratory function and skeletal abnormalities.

Delivery

- Regional technique desirable if anatomically possible.
- Epidural beneficial in labour, with likely instrumental assistance for delivery.
- Craniofacial deformity can result in airway problems.
- Invasive monitoring may be useful, with serial arterial blood gas analysis.
- Avoid suxamethonium as susceptible to malignant hyperpyrexia.
- Ephedrine and oxytocin safe.
- Good postoperative care required.

Reference

Habib AS. Anesthetic management of a ventilator-dependent parturient with the King–Denborough syndrome. *Canadian Journal of Anaesthesia* 2003; **50**: 589–592.

Klippel–Fleil syndrome

Characteristics

- Inherited condition with skeletal, cardiac and genitourinary abnormalities.
- Fusion of cervical vertebra can lead to progressive neurological damage and spinal cord anomalies. Scoliosis is common and other abnormalities of any vertebra including spina bifida.
- Cardiac abnormalities include PDA, coarctation of aorta and/or mitral valve prolapse.
- Maxillofacial abnormalities and deafness may occur.
- Obstructive sleep apnoea is reported.

Key points

- Difficult intubation, hypermobility and neurological complications.
- Full radiological assessment of cervical spine and airway.
- Regional anaesthesia preferred.
- Awake fibreoptic reported for CS under GA.

References

Dresner MR, Maclean AR. Anaesthesia for caesarean section in a patient with Klippel–Feil syndrome. The use of a microspinal catheter. *Anaesthesia* 1995; **50**: 807–809.

Singh D *et al.* Anaesthetic management of labour in two patients with Klippel–Feil syndrome. *International Journal of Obstetric Anesthesia* 1996; **5**: 198–201.

Klippel–Trenaunay–Weber syndrome

Characteristics

- Rare, non-hereditary syndrome consisting of superficial and deep haemangiomata, hypertrophy of soft tissue and bone with extremity overgrowth and varicose veins.
- Can affect the trunk and epidural space.
- Cerebral and spinal cord arteriovenous fistulae predispose to haemorrhage and increased risk of DIC.

Key points

- Coagulation screen to eliminate chronic DIC.
- Regional techniques are not contraindicated if MRI evaluation of the epidural space is made.
- Mode of delivery depends on site of venous abnormalities.
- Multidisciplinary antenatal care with provision for cell salvage and alert to risk of haemorrhage/DIC.

References

Dobbs P *et al.* Epidural analgesia in an obstetric patient with Klippel–Trenaunay syndrome. *British Journal of Anaesthesia* 1999; **82**: 144–146.

Sivaprakasam MJ, Dolak JA. Anesthetic and obstetric considerations in a parturient with Klippel–Trenaunay syndrome. *Canadian Journal of Anaesthesia* 2006; **53**: 487–491.

Laparoscopic surgery in pregnancy

Characteristics

- Up to 2% pregnancies complicated by surgery.
- Laparoscopy is a safer option than open techniques for all gestational ages.
- Pneumoperitoneum and positional changes have exaggerated cardiovascular and respiratory effects in pregnancy.

Key points

- Maintain uteroplacental blood flow, oxygenation and normal end-tidal CO_2.
- Avoid teratogenic drugs.
- Position changes should be made gradually.
- Fetal monitoring pre- and postoperatively.
- Invasive monitoring only if otherwise indicated.

Reference

O'Rourke N, Kodali BS. Laparoscopic surgery during pregnancy (Review). *Current Opinion in Anesthesiology* 2006; **19**: 254–259.

Larsen syndrome

Characteristics

- Rare congenital condition inherited or caused by spontaneous mutation.
- Collagen malformation results in skeletal deformities; dislocated hips, knees and elbows, abnormal hands and feet, short stature and cervical spine instability.
- Potential airway difficulties from: abnormal facies, tracheomalacia, laryngomalacia, subglottic stenosis.
- Cardiac defects: VSD, ASD, PDA, aortic dilatation, mitral valve prolapse.

Key points

Antenatal

- Assesment of airway, respiratory function and spine.
- Kyphoscoliosis can result in restrictive lung disease.

Delivery

- Epidural anaesthesia advisable if possible.

Reference

Michel TC *et al.* Obstetric anesthetic management of a parturient with Larsen syndrome and short stature. *Anesthesia and Analgesia* 2001; **92**: 1266–1267.

Laryngeal papillomatosis/tracheal stenosis

Characteristics

- Recurrent laryngeal benign tumours caused by the human papillomavirus (HPV).
- Patients present with hoarseness, stridor and airway obstruction.
- Pregnancy may lead to activation of HPV and worsening symptoms.
- Repeated surgical excision required.
- Vertical transmission to fetus can occur.

Key points

Antenatal

- Multidisciplinary approach (ENT, obstetrics, anaesthetics).
- Risk of complete airway obstruction, hypoxia, aspiration, fetal distress and preterm labour.
- Preoperative nasal fibreoptic assessment of airway.
- May require resection in the third trimester of pregnancy.
- May require open airway technique.
- Minimize risk of aspiration with antacid prophylaxis and head-up position.

Delivery

- Regional techniques if possible.
- May need to use microlaryngeal tube for GA.

Reference

Tripi PA *et al.* Anesthetic management for laser excision of recurrent respiratory papillomatosis in a third trimester parturient. *Journal of Clinical Anesthesia* 2005; **17**: 610–613.

Latex allergy

Characteristic

- An increasing problem amongst patients and healthcare workers.
- Reactions can be immediate (type I) or delayed (type IV).
- Certain groups are more at risk: repeated catheterization, multiple surgery, occupational exposure, history of atopy.
- Can cause anaphylaxis due to airborne latex particles.

Key points

Antenatal

- Detailed allergy history.
- Plans for totally latex-free hospital environment to simple avoidance of latex gloves and catheters depending on type and severity.
- All staff made aware and patient put first on elective surgery list.
- Diagnosis based on formal testing.

References

Dakin MJ, Yentis SM. Latex allergy: a strategy for management. *Anaesthesia* 1998; **53**: 774–781.

Eckhout GV, Ayad S. Anaphylaxis due to airborne exposure to latex in a primigravida. *Anesthesiology* 2001; **95**: 1034–1035.

Lipomyelocele

Characteristics

- An intraspinal lipoma associated with disruption of the meninges, displacement of neural material and spina bifida.

Key points

- Epidural space anatomy can be unpredictable, but well-planned regional anaesthesia for labour and CS has been reported.
- Radiological assessment of lesion required—MRI in second trimester ideal. Detailed patient consent.

Reference

Thompson MD *et al.* Epidural blockade for labour and Caesarean section with associated L4–5 lipomyelocele. *Anesthesiology* 1999; **30**: 1217–1218.

Long QT syndrome

Characteristics

- Rare genetic condition affecting the ion channels in the heart, with risk of Torsades de Pointe, ventricular tachycardia, ventricular fibrillation and death.
- Symptomatic patients give history of syncope, seizures and cardiac arrest.
- ECG changes and family history of sudden cardiac death may be present.
- Treatment includes β-blockers, pacemaker, automatic internal defibrillator and sympathectomy (see automated implantable cardioverters, page 608).

Key points

Antenatal

- Detailed cardiac history and early involvement of cardiologist.
- Ensure all electrolytes are normal.
- Continue β-blockers, avoid class Ia, Ic and III antiarrhythmics, and minimize catecholamine release.
- Automated defibrillators should be checked.

Delivery

- Because tachycardias are associated with catecholamine release, some recommend elective caesarean delivery.
- Thiopental, suxamethonium and ephedrine can all prolong the QT interval.
- Avoid hypothermia.
- Regional anaesthesia recommended.
- Defibrillator should be turned off but pacing mode left on.
- Use bipolar diathermy.
- External defibrillator immediately available.

Reference

Al-Refai A *et al.* Spinal anesthesia for Cesarean section in a parturient with long QT syndrome. *Canadian Journal of Anaesthesia* 2004; **51**: 993–996.

Ludwig's angina

Characteristics

- Rapidly spreading infection of submandibular, sublingual and submental spaces precipitated usually by dental infection.
- Patients may have associated medical disease (diabetes, HIV, drug abuse).
- Present with bilateral swelling, induration of neck, dysphagia, trismus, and upper airway obstruction.
- Can develop bacteraemia, empyema, mediastinitis, retropharyngeal abscess.

Key points

- Difficult intubation with sudden total airway obstruction.
- Reports of awake fibreoptic intubations and trachesotomy.
- Early and aggressive management required.
- Early management in pregnancy essential because of increased airway difficulties.

References

Loughman TE, Allen DE. Ludwig's angina. The anaesthetic management of nine cases. *Anaesthesia* 1985; **40**: 295–297.

Niederhauser A *et al.* Ludwig's angina in pregnancy. *Journal of Maternal and Fetal Neonatal Medicine* 2006; **19**: 119–120.

Lymphangioleiomyomatosis

Characteristics

- Rare idiopathic lung disease affecting women of reproductive age.
- Presents with cough, shortness of breath, bloody sputum, pleural effusions and spontaneous pneumothoraces resulting in severe lung impairment.
- Diagnosis by lung biopsy.

Key points

- Detailed preoperative assessment.
- Regional anaesthesia technique of choice.

Reference

McLoughlin L *et al.* Pregnancy and lymphangioleiomyomatosis: anaesthetic management. *International Journal of Obstetric Anesthesia* 2003; **12**: 40–44.

Lymphocytic hypohysitis

Characteristics

- Autoimmune disorder associated with pregnancy where pituitary is infiltrated with lymphocytes.
- Can present at any stage ante- or postpartum.
- Symptoms relate to mass effect (visual disturbance, headaches), hyperprolactinaemia or pituitary insufficiency.
- Can be self-resolving after delivery of the baby or a more chronic problem.
- Patients may require hormone replacement, steroid therapy or surgery.

Key points

- Multidisciplinary approach with neurosurgeons and endocrinologists to confirm diagnosis.
- Regional anaesthesia if raised ICP has been excluded (CT/MRI).
- Increased risk of developing pituitary necrosis (Sheehan's syndrome) from severe hypotension.
- PDPH may be difficult to diagnose.

Reference

Buckland RH, Popham PA. Lymphocytic hypophysitis complicated by postpartum haemorrhage. *International Journal of Obstetric Anesthesia* 1998; **7**: 263–266.

Malignant hyperthermia

Characteristics

- Rare pharmacogenetic condition of complex inheritance affecting muscle metabolism.
- Presents with tachycardia, arrhythmias, rising temperature and end-tidal CO_2 levels after exposure to certain triggers.
- Definitive diagnosis by caffeine–halothane contracture test.
- Aggressively treated with dantrolene sodium.

Key points

Antenatal

- Careful history and evaluation of susceptible patients or those with a strong family history.
- Plan for regional anaesthesia (with explanation to patient).
- Volatile-free anaesthetic machine available in case of emergency.

Delivery

- Regional anaesthesia advised.
- Dantrolene crosses placenta, so prophylaxis only for those with previous severe reaction and undergoing GA.
- Suitable volatile-free anaesthetic machine available (flushed with oxygen, change CO_2 absorber and rubber components).
- Monitor temperature and end-tidal CO_2: invasive only if other indication.
- Sodium citrate, ephedrine, thiopental, propofol, atracurium, oxytocin and amide LAs are safe in malignant hyperthermia. Avoid suxamethonium and volatiles.
- Continue monitoring postoperatively.
- Fetus may have malignant hyperthermia.
- Total IV propofol anaesthesia for CS has been described.

References

Lucy SJ. Anaesthesia for Caesarean delivery of a malignant hyperthermia susceptible parturient. *Canadian Journal of Anaesthesia* 1994; **41**: 1220–1226.

Macfarlane AJR *et al.* Caesarean section using total intravenous anaesthesia in a patient with Ebstein's anomaly complicated by supraventricular tachycardia. *International Journal of Obstetric Anesthesia* 2007; **16**: 155–159.

Marfan's syndrome

Characteristics

- Autosomal dominant disorder of connective tissue causing the following abnormalities:
  - Cardiovascular—mitral valve prolapse and regurgitation, aortic valve regurgitation and root dilatation, aortic dissection and aneurysm.
  - Musculoskeletal—tall with long limbs and digits, pectus excavatum, joint laxity, kyphoscoliosis, high arched palate.
  - Dural ectasia (ballooning of the lumbosacral dural sac) occurs in 60–90% and can lead to unpredictable spinal block.

Key points

Antenatal

- Regular cardiology assessment with echocardiography to identify early risk of increasing aortic root dilatation.
- Treatment with β-blockers for patients with aortic root dilatation >4cm or dissection to avoid sheer stress.

Delivery

- CS usually recommended if evidence of aortic root dilatation.
- Maintenance of cardiovascular stability with careful titration of regional/general anaesthesia.
- Dural ectasia makes single-shot spinal unreliable: CSE recommended.

Reference

Lacassie HJ *et al.* Dural ectasia: a likely cause of inadequate spinal anaesthesia in two parturients with Marfan's syndrome. *British Journal of Anaesthesia* 2005; **94**: 500–504.

Mediastinal masses

Characteristics

- Masses can be carcinoma, lymphoma (hormone sensitive), thyroid or thymus in origin, or neurogenic.
- Patients can present with dyspnoea, haemoptysis, oedema, dilated neck veins and cough.
- CT imaging of the thorax and rigid bronchoscopy are definitive investigations.

Key points

- Multidisciplinary approach to management in tertiary centre.
- Consider treatment options to reduce size of mediastinal mass if appropriate, e.g. radiotherapy or chemotherapy predelivery.
- Risk of cardiovascular collapse and complete airway obstruction on induction of GA (loss of bronchial tone, lower lung volumes).
- Difficulty in lying flat can make regional anaesthesia a difficult but safe option.
- Reports of successful awake fibreoptic intubation.

References

Boyne IC. Awake fibreoptic intubation, airway compression and lung collapse in a parturient: anaesthetic and intensive care management. *International Journal of Obstetric Anesthesia* 1999; **8**: 138–141.

Dasan J *et al.* Mediastinal tumour in a pregnant patient presenting as acute cardiorespiratory compromise. *International Journal of Obstetric Anesthesia* 2002; **11**: 52–56.

Motor neuron disease (amyotrophic lateral sclerosis)

Characteristics

- A progressive degenerative disease of the motor system of unknown aetiology.
- It involves upper and lower motor neurons and presents with weakness and fasciculations.

Key points

Antenatal

- Careful respiratory monitoring required.
- Increased physiological demands results in the disease presenting or deteriorating during pregnancy.

Delivery

- Fetal growth not usually affected.
- CS and vaginal birth reported.
- Severe hyperkalaemia with suxamethonium. Increased sensitivity to non-depolarizing muscle relaxants.
- May require prolonged invasive or non-invasive postoperative ventilation. Regional techniques have been safely described.

Reference

Chio A *et al.* Amyotrophic lateral sclerosis associated with pregnancy: report of four new cases and review of the literature. *Amyotrophic Lateral Sclerosis and Other Motor Neuron Disorders* 2003; **4**: 45–48.

Moyamoya disease

Characteristics

- Stenosis of internal carotid arteries with hazy collateral circulation around base of brain. Most common in Japan.
- Risk of cerebral haemorrhage and ischaemia increased in pregnancy.
- Surgical (revascularization) and medical (antiplatelet, anticoagulant, vasodilator) treatment.

Key points

Delivery

- Most case reports describe CS delivery.
- Normotension and normocapnoea important to maintain cerebral flow.
- Vaginal delivery requires good analgesia and instrumental assistance.
- Epidural and low dose CSE described with mild sedation.

Reference

Kato R. *et al.* Anesthetic management for Caesarean section in moyamoya disease: a report of five consecutive cases and a mini-review. *International Journal of Obstetric Anesthesia* 2006; **15**: 152–158.

Multiple endocrine neoplasia

Characteristics

- A group of inherited conditions (MEN1, 2A, 2B) with tumours in multiple endocrine glands (parathyroid, thyroid, pituitary, pancreas, adrenal medulla).
- Symptoms may be related to hyperparathyroidism, pituitary disease and phaeochromocytoma.
- Most problems in pregnancy related to phaeochromocytoma—part of MEN 2A and 2B syndrome. Presents with hypertension (at any time during pregnancy), headaches, sweating and palpitations, and can be mistaken for pre-eclampsia. There is no proteinuria with phaeochromocytoma.

Key points

- Antenatal diagnosis improves outcome for mother and fetus.
- Avoidance of hypertensive crises, which can lead to cardiac failure and death, is goal in pregnancy.
- Elective CS delivery with perioperative α-blockade and β-blockade is recommended after 24 weeks gestation, followed by tumour resection after a recovery period.

References

Ahn JT *et al.* Atypical presentation of pheochromocytoma as part of multiple endocrine neoplasia IIa in pregnancy. *Obstetrics and Gynecology* 2003; **102**: 1202–1205.

Dugas G *et al.* Pheochromocytoma and pregnancy: a case review and report of anesthetic management. *Canadian Journal of Anaesthesia* 2004; **51**: 134–138.

Myasthenia gravis

Characteristics

- Autoimmune disruption of postsynaptic acetylcholine receptors at the neuromuscular junction.
- Muscle fatigue (bulbar, pharyngeal, laryngeal and respiratory muscles).
- Requires long-term anticholinesterase therapy. Continue in labour; higher dose may need to be IM.
- Pregnancy can alter course, with relapses most likely in first trimester and postpartum.
- 30% of infants are born with transient myasthenic syndrome.
- Myasthenic and cholinergic crises (stress, exertion, infection) are differentiated by an edrophonium test.

Key points

Antenatal

- Thorough assessment of respiratory and bulbar function.

Delivery

- Vaginal delivery with assistance in second stage to reduce fatigue, with close monitoring of respiratory function intrapartum.
- Analgesia: epidural/spinal. Care with opioids. Very sensitive to non-depolarizing muscle relaxants (10% of standard dose recommended) and magnesium, which prolonges their effect. Suxamethonium can be used safely.
- Critical care support postdelivery is vital.

Reference

Rolbin WH *et al.* Anesthetic considerations for myasthenia gravis and pregnancy. *Anesthesia and Analgesia* 1978; **57**: 441–447.

Djelmis J *et al.* Myasthenia gravis in pregnancy: report of 69 cases. *European Journal of Obstetrics, Gynecology and Reproductive Biology* 2002; **104**: 21–25.

Myelodysplastic syndrome

Characteristics

- A group of haematological disorders with dysplastic haemopoiesis and blast cells present in peripheral blood and bone marrow.
- Present with anaemia and thrombocytopenia to varying degrees.
- Antiplatelet antibodies from multiple transfusions may be suppressed by immunoglobulins and steroids.

Key points

- Mode of delivery depends on obstetric indication and degree of thrombocytopenia.
- Maternal antibodies may cross placenta with unknown effect on fetus (intracranial haemorrhage during vaginal delivery).
- Regional anaesthesia contraindicated in severe thrombocytopenia.
- Nitrous oxide implicated in bone marrow suppression.

Reference

Christiaens F *et al.* Anaesthetic management of Caesarean section in a parturient with acute myelodysplastic syndrome. *International Journal of Obstetric Anesthesia* 1997; **6**: 270–273.

Myocardial ischaemia (See Chapter 4, p 76–78)

Characteristics

- Uncommon in pregnancy (1:10 000 deliveries), usually in last trimester or puerperium.
- High mortality.
- Coronary artery dissection is most common cause of death, with 78% of mothers having no risk factors for coronary artery disease.
- Consider early angiography.
- Coronary stenting or bypass grafting is treatment of choice immediately postpartum.
- Tissue plasminogen activator does not cross placenta, so suitable for thrombolysing after early postpartum period.

Key points

- Consider differential diagnoses: aortic dissection, pulmonary emboli, pre-eclampsia, haemorrhage, sickle crisis, sepsis.
- Use of anticoagulant or antiplatelet drugs will affect the choice of anaesthetic for labour or surgical delivery.
- Caution with ergometrine in mothers at risk of ischaemic heart disease.

Reference

Ray P *et al.* Recognition and management of maternal cardiac disease in pregnancy. *British Journal of Anaesthesia* 2004; **93**: 428–439.

Myotonic dystrophy

Characteristics

- Autosomal dominant multisystem degenerative condition affecting skeletal, smooth and cardiac muscle.
- Pregnancy is rare due to ovarian failure.
- Presents early in childhood with weakness and wasting of face, extremities and respiratory muscles.
- Cardiac involvement commonly leads to destruction of the conducting system, heart block and sudden death.
- Patients may be on oral anticoagulation.
- Cardiomyopathy and heart failure can also occur in pregnancy.
- Complications in pregnancy include polyhydramnios, premature labour, breech presentation, ineffective uterine contractions, retained placenta and PPH.
- High risk of neonatal death.

Key points

Antenatal

- Thorough preoperative assessment to include cardiorespiratory investigation and airway assessment.

Delivery

- Sensitive to premedicants, opioids, non-depolarizing neuromuscular-blocking agents and induction agents.
- Both regional and general anaesthesia can induce myotonia.
- Myotonia particularly associated with suxamethonium.
- Gastroparesis increases risk of aspiration.
- Higher incidence of difficult intubation.
- CSE is technique of choice for caesarean delivery.
- Ensure good surgical technique, and that theatre and fluids are warm to avoid myotonia.
- Respiratory failure is a frequent cause of postoperative morbidity.
- Higher risk of thromboembolism.

References

Campbell AM, Thompson N. Anaesthesia for Caesarean section in a patient with myotonic dystrophy receieving warfarin therapy. *Canadian Journal of Anaesthesia* 1995; **42**: 409–414.

O'Connor PJ *et al.* Urgent caesarean section in a patient with myotonic dystrophy: a case report and review. *International Journal of Obstetric Anesthesia* 1996: **5**: 272–274.

Needle phobia

Characteristics

- Abnormal, sometimes temporary, reaction that causes the thought of encountering a needle to trigger a panic reaction.
- May affect up to 10% of the population.
- Issues include consent, ethics and clinical aspects.

Key points

- A competent mother may refuse a procedure.
- Full explanation of the risks is required.
- Reports of successful use of inhalational GA for CS.
- It is useful to spend time talking through these issues in the antenatal period.

Reference

Simon GR *et al.* Sevoflurane induction for emergency Caesarean section: two case reports in women with needle phobia. *International Journal of Obstetric Anesthesia* 2002; **11**: 296–300.

Neurofibromatosis

Characteristics

- Autosomal dominant condition with variable expressivity: types I and II.
- A multisystem disorder with multiple neurofibromata and café au lait spots.
- Respiratory system: kyophoscoliosis, pulmonary fibrosis, pulmonary hypertension and right heart failure.
- Cardiovascular system: hypertension, renovascular disease, phaeochromocytoma, coarctation of aorta and mediastinal tumours.
- CNS: learning difficulties, epilepsy.
- Associated with carcinoid tumours.
- Full antenatal multidisciplinary assessment required.

Key points

- Pregnancy associated with increase in size and number of neurofibromata.
- Close monitoring of hypertension in pregnancy.
- Association with HELLP syndrome.
- Tumours in larynx and cervical cord can lead to airway management problems.
- Regional anaesthesia: CT/MRI of spinal cord late in pregnancy to evaluate spinal tumours and ICP.
- No clear evidence of abnormal response to any neuromuscular-blocking drugs.

References

Hirsch NP. Neurofibromatosis: clinical presentations and anaesthetic implications (Review). *British Journal of Anaesthesia* 2001; **86**: 555–564.

Sakai T *et al.* A parturient with neurofibromatosis type 2: anesthetic and obstetric considerations for delivery. *International Journal of Obstetric Anesthesia* 2005; **14**: 332–335.

Noonan's syndrome

Characteristics

- Non-chromosomal syndrome resembling Turner's syndrome affecting both males and females.
- Females have normal fertility.
- Features include short stature, joint contractures, webbed neck which may be fused, chest deformity and typical facial appearances (flattened face, high arched palate, micrognathia, dental malocclusion).
- Congenital cardiac defects are classically right sided, pulmonary stenosis being most common. Others include ASDs, septal hypertrophy, PDA, aortic stenosis and cardiomyopathy.
- Clotting derangement (hepatosplenomegaly) can occur, but bleeding tendency is usually mild.
- Renal dysfunction, dermatological problems, hearing and visual abnormalities also reported.

Key points

- Early involvement of anaesthetic and obstetric team in pregnancy to investigate and formulate plan of care.
- Assessment by cardiologist and haematologist.
- Cardiac defects must be fully quantified and invasive monitoring considered.
- Regional technique desirable but can be difficult to site with unpredictable spread from kyphoscoliosis.
- If bleeding abnormality severe, regional may be contraindicated.
- Potentially difficult intubation.
- Chest deformity can be associated with kyphoscoliosis and respiratory compromise.

References

McLure HA, Yentis SM. General anaesthesia for caesarean section in a parturient with Noonan's syndrome. *British Journal of Anaesthesia* 1996; **77**: 665–668.

McBain J *et al*. Epidural labour analgesia in a parturient with Noonan syndrome: a case report. *Canadian Journal of Anaesthesia* 2006; **53**: 274–278.

Oesophageal varices

Characteristics

- Extrahepatic (normal liver function, risk of variceal bleeding) or intrahepatic (risk of acute hepatic failure; encephalopathy, hyponatraemia, deranged clotting, metabolic acidosis) in origin.
- Increased portal pressure in normal pregnancy with up to 60% developing transient varices.

Key points

Antenatal

- Risk of massive variceal haemorrhage (Sengstaken–Blakemore tube, vasopressin and blood products).
- Antenatal multidisciplinary care with option of early endoscopic banding.
- Full haematological assessment of clotting.

Delivery

- Assisted vaginal delivery with epidural analgesia to avoid straining is recommended.

Reference

Heriot JA *et al.* Elective forceps delivery and extradural anaesthesia in a primigravida with portal hypertension and oesophageal varices. *British Journal of Anaesthesia* 1996; **76**: 325–327.

Opiate addiction

Characteristics

- Increased risk to mother and baby with high demand on obstetric anaesthetic services.
- Poor historians with varied ingestion of illicit substances (orally/IV).
- Often associated with poor venous access and viral blood-borne disease (hepatitis and HIV).
- Analgesia can be difficult (high pain scores) and unpredictable, with withdrawal and anxiety symptoms common.

Key points

Antenatal

- Comprehensive anaesthetic review with the help of a substance misuse midwife very useful to plan obstetric analgesia and venous access.
- Unpredictable response to drugs may highlight use of other substances.
- Cocaine misuse is a particular hazard, with increased risk of hypertension and abruption.

Reference

Cassidy B, Cyna AM. Challenges that opioid-dependent women present to the obstetric anaesthetist. *Anaesthesia and Intensive Care* 2004; **32**: 494–501.

Osler–Weber–Rendu (hereditary haemorrhagic telangectasia)

Characteristics

- Autosomal dominant condition with variable penetrance affecting vascular endothelium.
- Symptoms include: nose bleeds, gastrointestinal bleeding and iron deficiency anaemia, with telangectasia on oral mucosa, lips and fingertips.
- Arteriovenous malformations (AVMs) of pulmonary (30%), cerebral (20%), spinal (2%) and hepatic (30%) circulations can be asymptomatic.

Key points

- Pulmonary AVMs can increase in size during pregnancy.
- Regional technique preferred, MRI spinal cord to exclude AVM.
- Avoid trauma to mucous membranes.
- Risk of haemorrhage.

Reference

Waring PH *et al.* Anesthetic management of a parturient with Osler–Weber–Rendu syndrome and rheumatic heart disease. *Anesthesia and Analgesia* 1990; **71**: 96–99.

Osteogenesis imperfecta

Characteristics

- Rare, inherited disorder of connective tissue with variable severity.
- Types I–IV, with I and IV (autosomal dominant) capable of reproducing.
- Bone fragility (multiple fractures), short stature, blue sclera and deafness.

Key points

- Care with positioning and transferring patient, BP cuff placement (fractures) and laryngoscopy (risk of breaking teeth, fracturing mandible, hyperextending neck).
- Reports of suxamethonium fasiculations causing fractures.
- Tendency to non-malignant hyperthermia (cooling blankets and fluids).
- Chest deformities can affect lung function.
- Platelet function should be checked.
- Regional anaesthesia can be technically difficult but remains technique of choice.

References

Cho E *et al.* Anaesthesia in a parturient with osteogenesis imperfecta. *British Journal of Anaesthesia* 1992; **68**: 422–423.

Yeo ST, Paech MS. Regional anaesthesia for multiple caesarean sections in a parturient with osteogenesis imperfecta. *International Journal of Obstetric Anesthesia* 1999; **8**: 284–287.

Paroxysmal nocturnal haemoglobinuria

Characteristics

- Acquired defect of haemopoietic stem cells.
- Deficiency of cell surface proteins that regulate activation of complement.
- Haemolytic anaemia, severe thrombocytopenia, nocturnal haemolysis, haemoglobinuria, intra-abdominal and intracerebral thrombosis, infection and haemorrhage can occur.
- Aim to maintain Hb >10g/dL, folate and iron supplementation. Excess iron may precipitate haemolytic episode.

Key points

- Issues relate to infection control, drug-induced complement activation, peripartum anticoagulation and obstetric haemorrhage.
- Due to increased risk of thrombosis, frequently on LMWH.
- Attention to timing of epidural catheter insertion and removal, and the timing of subsequent redosing with heparin.
- Maintain normothermia, normovolaemia and acid–base homeostasis (acidosis may precipitate haemolysis), attention to asepsis, avoidance of stress responses and use of drugs and fluids that are unlikely to activate complement release.

- Irradiated, leukocyte-depleted RBCs are preferable for transfusion.
- GA may be required due to thrombocytopenia.

Reference

Paech MJ, Pavy TJ. Management of a parturient with paroxysmal nocturnal haemoglobinuria. *International Journal of Obstetric Anesthesia* 2004; **13**: 188–191.

Pemphigus vulgaris

Characteristics

- Immune-mediated bullous dermatosis.
- Autoantibodies against desmoglein 3, a desmosome transmembrane glycoprotein belonging to the cadherin family.
- Blisters due to loss of cell–cell adhesion in the basal and suprabasal layers of the deeper epidermis.

Key points

Antenatal

- Pregnancy may precipitate or aggravate disease.
- High dose prednisolone (60–360mg/day) for several weeks and gradual tapering to a maintenance dose.
- Some immunosurpressive drugs may need to be considered in pregnancy.
- Plasmapheresis has been proposed as a treatment option.
- The method of choice for delivery is vaginal, although local trauma may result in extension and worsening of local erosions.
- Delayed wound healing due to disease process and steroid therapy.

Delivery

- Skin very fragile; airway instrumentation and adhesive skin dressings problematic.
- Regional anaesthesia described.

References

Fainaru O *et al.* Pemphigus vulgaris in pregnancy: a case report and review of literature. *Human Reproduction* 2000; **15**: 1195–1197.

Abouleish El *et al.* Spinal anesthesia for Cesarean section in a case of pemphigus foliaceous. *Anesthesia and Analgesia* 1997; **84**: 449–550.

Pneumomediastinum and pneumothorax (Hamman's syndrome)

Characteristics

- Occurs in young primiparous women during the second stage of labour.
- Hamman's syndrome consists of substernal pain, SC and retroperitoneal emphysema, obliteration of cardiac dullness, crunching sounds over the heart synchronous with the heart beat (Hamman's sign), increased mediastinal pressure, dyspnoea, cyanosis, engorged veins and circulatory failure, pneumothorax, and roentgenographic evidence of air in the mediastinum.

Key points

- Surgical emphysema of the neck and face is pathognomonic.
- Conservative management with reassurance, oxygen supplementation and analgesics.
- Shortening the second stage of labour may help.
- The use of nitrous oxide and oxygen mixture is contraindicated.
- Epidural anaesthesia avoids further exertion.
- High subarachnoid block may compromise respiratory function.
- If GA is indicated, facilities for insertion of a chest drain should be immediately available.
- Usually resolve spontaneously within 2 weeks, and the pneumothorax rarely needs to be drained.

References

Reeder SR. Subcutaneous emphysema, pneumomediastinum, and pneumothorax in labor and delivery. *American Journal of Obstetrics and Gynecology* 1986; **154**: 487–489.

Miguil M, Chekairi A. Pneumomediastinum and pneumothorax associated with labour. *International Journal of Obstetric Anesthesia* 2004; **13**: 117–119.

Polychondritis

Characteristics

- Relapsing polychondritis is characterized by episodic inflammation and degeneration of cartilage and connective tissue involving the upper airway.
- Diagnosis confirmed when 3 of the 6 features are present: bilateral auricular chondritis, non-erosive seronegative inflammatory arthritis, nasal chondritis, ocular inflammation, respiratory tract chondritis and audiovestibular damage, and histological confirmation.

Key points

Antenatal

- The following can occur.
  - Respiratory failure due to collapse of portions of the tracheobronchial tree.
  - Aortic or mitral valvular insufficiency, vasculitis, life-threatening aneurysms, systemic vasculitides.
  - Spondyloarthropathy.
  - Connective tissue diseases.
  - Haematological diseases.
- Multidisciplinary management required (rheumatology, haematology and obstetric anesthesia).

Delivery

- Early epidural analgesia to decrease the stress.
- Regional anesthesia is preferred.
- Keep second stage of labour short.
- GA problems include propensity for gastro-oesophageal reflux; cricoid pressure may be relatively contraindicated if the woman has tracheal tenderness. A smaller tracheal tube may be required.

Reference

Douglas MJ, Ensworth S. Anaesthetic management of the parturient with relapsing polychondritis. *Canadian Journal of Anaesthesia* 2005; **52**: 967–970.

Polycythaemia rubra vera

Characteristics

- Overproduction of phenotypically normal myeloid cell lines independent of physiological stimulus.
- Characterized by: splenomegaly, generalized pruritus, increased blood viscosity and thrombotic events of the liver, heart, brain and lungs.
- Phlebotomy and cytotoxic chemotherapy (radioactive phosphorus, chlorambucil, hydroxyurea and interferon α) are treatment options.

Key points

Antenatal

- Pregnancy-induced hypertension, spontaneous abortion, maternal venous thromboembolism and perinatal death are associated.
- Pregnancy is associated with spontaneous control of the disease.
- No specific treatment is required except careful observation.
- Maintenance of the Hb level at 12g/dL to avoid the thrombotic complications.
- Phlebotomy and low dose empirical acetylsalicylic acid treatment avoid teratogenic effects of cytotoxic agents.
- May be on LMWH.

Delivery

- Regional anaesthesia not contraindicated. Care because of LMWH therapy.

Reference

Robinson S *et al.* The management and outcome of 18 pregnancies in women with polycythemia vera (Review). *Haematologica* 2005; **90**: 1477–1483.

Porphyria

Characteristics

- Acute hepatic porphyrias are genetic diseases.
- Acute neurological symptoms, sometimes fatal, triggered by different factors including pregnancy and many anaesthetic drugs.

Key points

- Inhalational agents, opioids, depolarizing and non-depolarizing muscle relaxants, LAs and anticholinergic drugs are considered safe.
- Epidural analgesia described for labour.
- Avoid diazepam, although midozolam considered safe. Avoid thiopental.

References

Rigg JD, Petts V. Anaesthesia for the porphyric patient. *Anaesthesia* 1993; **48**: 1009–1010.
Kantor G *et al.* Acute intermittent porphyria and Caesarean delivery. *Canadian Journal of Anaesthesia* 1992; **39**: 282–285.

Portal hypertension

Characteristics

- 400 times increased risk of mortality due to variceal bleeding or acute hepatic failure depending on cause of portal hypertension.
- Splenic artery aneurysm rupture can also occur.

Key points

- Shunt procedures, sclerotherapy or banding in second trimester to reduce chances of bleeding may be required.
- Effective epidural analgesia and avoid straining during second stage.
- Bloody tap common in sitting position due to engorged epidural veins.
- Invasive monitoring, large-bore IV cannulae, blood and blood products, Sengstaken–Blakemore tube and IV vasopressin should be available.
- GA if thrombocytopenia is present.

Reference

Heriot JA *et al.* Elective forceps delivery and extradural anaesthesia in a primigravida with portal hypertension and oesophageal varices. *British Journal of Anaesthesia* 1996; **76**: 325–327.

Protein C and S deficiency (See Chapter 4, p 121)

Characteristics

- Protein C is a vitamin K-dependent physiological inhibitor of coagulation.
- Heterozygous protein C deficiency associated with increase in thrombotic tendency especially in pregnancy.

Key points

- Can be cause of IUGR.
- LMWH and UFH have been used.
- Activated protein C has been successfully used.
- Caution with regional anaesthesia—timing of antithrombotic prophylaxis with relation to regional techniques should be considered.

References

Nelson SM, Greer IA. Thrombophilia and the risk for venous thromboembolism during pregnancy, delivery and puerperium. *Obstetric and Gynecology Clinics of North America* 2006; **33**: 413–427.

Sekiyama K *et al.* Successful management of a pregnant woman with heterozygous protein C deficiency using activated protein C concentrate. *Journal of Obstetrics and Gynaecology Research* 2003; **29**: 412–415.

Pseudoxanthoma elasticum

Characteristics

- Rare inherited disorder (autosomal dominant and autosomal recessive) of connective tissue, involves skin, Bruch's membrane in eyes and cardiovascular system.
- Elastic fibres are calcified and fragmented.
- Visual loss from subretinal haemorrhage, gastrointestinal haemorrhage, angina, hypertension and intermittent claudication.

Key points

Delivery

- Regional techniques described. Theoretical risk of epidural haematoma but no case reports. Low dose CSE or epidural for caesarean delivery with gradual onset of sympathetic block and lower risk of hypotension.
- Shortening the second stage of labour may decrease retinal bleeding secondary to heavy straining.

Reference

Douglas MJ *et al.* Anesthesia for the parturient with pseudoxanthoma elasticum. *International Journal of Obstetric Anesthesia* 2003; **12**: 45–47.

Pulmonary hypertension (See Chapter 4, p 96)

Characteristics

- Primary pulmonary hypertension is rare with very poor long-term prognosis.
- A peripartum mortality of >50% has been reported, and the recommendation to women with primary pulmonary hypertension is to avoid pregnancy.

Key points

Antenatal

- Regular assessment by cardiologist and pulmonary physician.
- Pulmonary vasodilators increasingly described; ileoprost and sildenafil.

Delivery

- Frequently need CS delivery.
- Regional and general anaesthesia described.
- Avoid stress in labour with effective analgesia and shortened second stage of labour.
- Avoid increase in PVR caused by hypoxia, acidosis, anxiety and fear.
- Controlled ventilation reduces VR.
- LAs to reduce pain from punctures and cannulation.
- Avoid sudden fall in SVR by slow induction of epidural balanced with vasoconstrictor support.
- An arterial line is absolutely indicated. Avoid overshoot of BP with strain on the LV.
- A calcium channel blocker (nifedipine) moderates PVR.
- Short-acting vasodilators (nitroglycerine, nitroprusside, adenosine, prostaglandins) have been recommended.
- Use of nitric oxide has been described.

References

Olofssen C *et al.* Cesarean section under epidural ropivacaine 0.75% in a parturient with severe pulmonary hypertension. *Acta Anaesthesiologica Scandinavica* 2001; **45**: 258–260.

Barnett CF, Machado RF. Sildenafil in the treatment of pulmonary hypertension. *Vascular Health Risk Management* 2006; **2**: 411–422.

Decoene C *et al.* Use of inhaled nitric oxide for emergency Cesarean section in a woman with unexpected primary pulmonary hypertension. *Canadian Journal of Anaesthesia* 2001; **48**: 584–587.

Quadriplegia with autonomic hyper-reflexia

Characteristics

- Life-threatening complication associated with labour in parturient with spinal cord injury at or above T6, uncontrolled reflex sympathetic activity in response to a stimulus below the level of the lesion.
- Higher incidence of premature labour especially if lesion is above T5.
- Transection of the cord above the level of T10 may result in painless labour.

- The first indication of labour may be development of autonomic hyper-reflexia.
- Control of autonomic hyper-reflexia in labour without an epidural block has been unsatisfactory.

Key points

- Early establishment of regional anaesthesia to interrupt reflex arc and prevent triggering of autonomic hyper-reflexia.
- In spinal anaesthesia, block height cannot always be predicted.
- In high lesions the ability both to vasoconstrict the splanchnic bed (T5–L2) and to increase HR via the cardioaccelerator fibres (T1–4) is lost.
- Caution with vasopressors.
- Graded incremental boluses via epidural with arterial line has advantages. Height of block assessed by ability to elicit muscle spasms in response to ethyl chloride spray or observing the level at which spastic paraparesis becomes flaccid.
- Epidural catheter for prevention and treatment of postoperative episodes of autonomic hyper-reflexia has been effective.

References

Burns R, Clark VA. Epidural anaesthesia for caesarean section in a patient with quadriplegia and autonomic hyperreflexia. *International Journal of Obstetric Anesthesia* 2004; **13**: 120–123.

Hambly PR, Martin B. Anaesthesia for chronic spinal cord lesions (Review). *Anaesthesia* 1998; **53**: 273–289.

Recombinant factor VIIa

Characteristics

- Recombinant activated factor VIIa has been successfully used to prevent or control bleeding in thrombocytopenia, platelet function disorders, impaired liver functions, extensive surgery and severe trauma with profuse bleeding.
- The haemostatic effect of recombinant activated factor VII mediated by enhanced rate of thrombin generation leading to a full thrombin burst and a fully stabilized fibrin plug with a tight fibrin structure, making it resistant to premature lysis.

Key points

- Acute management of PPH involves restoration of blood volume and control of bleeding.
- Therapies to control bleeding include oxytocin, ergot alkaloids, prostaglandins, uterine packing, uterine artery or internal iliac artery ligation, selective arterial embolization and hysterectomy.
- There is a potential role for recombinant activated factor VII in the treatment of major postpartum haemorrhage unresponsive to conventional treatments but must be given in conjunction with adequate fibrin and platletet replacement.
- Close collaboration between anaesthetist, obstetrician and haematologist is essential.

Reference

Ahoneu J, Jokela R. Recombinant factor VIIa for life-threatening post-partum haemorrhage. *British Journal of Anaesthesia* 2005; **94**: 592–595.

Retinal haemorrhage

Characteristics

- Retinal haemorrhages are pathological, and the degree of visual disability varies according to the area of retina involved.
- Causes include trauma, vascular obstruction, vasculitis, diabetes mellitus, hypertension, blood diseases and severe subarachnoid haemorrhage.
- Ophthalmic management is conservative, and in most cases of retinal venous haemorrhage there will be a complete recovery of vision in a few months.

Key points

- Epidural with care, i.e. slow incremental bolus.
- Avoid straining during vaginal delivery.
- Avoid increase in ICP due to coughing or straining.
- Retinal venous pressure may be increased by large epidural bolus dose, whereas fractionated epidural doses might decrease pressure in retinal veins by systemic venodilatation.

Reference

Chidley KE *et al.* Caesarean section following a recent retinal haemorrhage. *Anaesthesia* 1998; **53**: 483–485.

Rheumatoid arthritis

Characteristics

- Rheumatoid arthritis (Still's disease) is a chronic systemic disease with synovitis and extra-articular manifestations.
- Involvement of cervical spine with flexion deformities and atlantoaxial subluxation, temporomandibular and cricoarytenoid joints has implications for the management of the airway.

Key points

Antenatal

- Full assessment of airway and spine with appropriate X-rays if necessary.
- Systemic review for other manifestations of systemic disease.

Delivery

- Caesarean delivery may be necessary with severe hip problems. Although there is an argument for securing the airway with the patient awake in all who present with a known difficult airway, it is a logical approach to perform a spinal or epidural block for elective CS.
- Spinal or CSE techniques have been used.
- Stiff hips and scoliosis may complicate neuraxial anaesthetic technique and efficacy.
- Careful positioning of the patient is necessary.

Reference

Popat MT *et al.* Awake fibreoptic intubation following failed regional anaesthesia for Caesarean section in a parturient with Still's disease. *European Journal of Anaesthesiology* 2000; **17**: 211–214.

Ross procedure

Characteristics

- Replacement of diseased aortic valve with own pulmonary valve and replacement of pulmonary valve with an aortic cadaver homograft.
- It circumvents anticoagulation-related fetal loss, valve deterioration etc., which are associated with other valve replacement options.

Key points

- With a successful procedure, pregnancy can be uncomplicated, but management requires an understanding of the original valvular defect and corrective cardiac surgery procedure sequelae to that procedure.
- Patients with significant multivalvular heart disease require careful preoperative, multidisciplinary assessment and anaesthetic planning before delivery, to optimize cardiac function during the peripartum period and make informed decisions regarding mode of delivery and anaesthetic technique.

Reference

Campbell N *et al.* Anaesthetic management of a parturient with pulmonary stenosis and aortic incompetence for Caesarean section. *British Journal of Anaesthesia* 2003; **90**: 241–243.

Sarcoidosis

Characteristics

- Systemic disease with non-caseating granulomata in tissues with fibrosis.
- Hilar lymphadenopathy, pleural and alveolar fibrosis, bronchial stenosis, atelectasis, RVF, conduction anomalies, cardiomyopathy and hypercalcaemia can occur.
- Disease progression/relapse not clearly associated with pregnancy.

Key points

Antenatal

- Pulmonary and cardiac status should be evaluated.
- Airway involvement may present with difficult intubation.

Delivery

- May need increased steroid cover due to long-term use.
- Regional anaesthesia preferred if lung involvement is severe.
- Calcium should be maintained at normal level.
- Good postoperative analgesia after CS to avoid pulmonary sequelae.

Reference

Euliano TY *et al.* Sarcoidosis in a pregnant woman. *Journal of Clinical Anesthesia* 1997; **9**: 78–86.

Scoliosis/corrected spinal surgery

(See Chapter 4, p 104–105)

Characteristics

- Untreated severe scoliosis can lead to death due to cardiorespiratory failure.
- Pregnancy and labour aggravate cardiorespiratory compromise.
- Surgical correction with instrumentation such as Harrington rods, or fusion surgeries with bone grafts, is usually conducted as an adolescent.

Key points

Antenatal

- Serial assessment of respiratory function is important.
- X-ray evaluation of previous surgery, if possible, looking at length of instrumentation and presense of bone grafts is very useful to guide management planning.
- Neurological examination and documentation before regional technique is essential.

Delivery

- Complicated epidural placement, with higher risk of failure, inadequate analgesia and increased risk of dural puncture.
- Continuous spinal anaesthesia for labour and CS has been reported.
- Ultrasound-guided epidural placement has been successful.
- A one-shot spinal anaesthetic may be successful below instrumentation even if an epidural is not.

Reference

Yeo ST, French R. Combined spinal–epidural in the obstetric patient with Harrington rods assisted by ultrasonography. *British Journal of Anaesthesia* 1999; **83**: 670–672.

Sickle cell disease

Characteristics

- Autosomal recessive disorder with sickling crises in infancy and chronic organ failure.
- Maternal mortality per pregnancy ranges between 1 and 2% and perinatal mortality remains as high as 5–6%.
- May cause preterm delivery, fetal growth retardation, anaemia, acute organ failure, UTIs, thrombosis and sepsis.

Key points

Antenatal

- Systemic review of multisystem disease.
- Sickling crisis manifests as acute bone pain, chest syndrome, fever, leukocytosis or abdominal pain.
- Precipitating factors include cold, hypoxia, stress and/or intercurrent infection.
- Intravaginal prostaglandins can precipitate a sickle crisis.

Delivery

- Regional analgesia is preferable.
- Keep mother well oxygenated and hydrated in labour.
- Avoid aorto-caval compression to improve circulation.
- Avoid GA if possible.

References

Faron G *et al.* First sickle cell crisis triggered by induction of labor in a primigravida. *European Journal of Obstetrics, Gynecology and Reproductive Biology* 2001; **94**: 304–306.

Finer P *et al.* Epidural analgesia in the management of labor pain and sickle cell crisis—a case report. *Anesthesiology* 1988; **8**: 799–800.

Spina bifida

Characteristics

- Group of conditions that are categorized into spina bifida occulta and spina bifida cystica.
- Occulta is common (10–20%) and usually asymptomatic.
- Cystica is failed closure of the neural arch with herniation of the meninges (meningocele) or meninges and neural elements (myelomeningocele).
- Abnormal or tethered spinal cord may occur in spina bifida cystica, including the more unusual thoracic and cervical varieties (spinal dysraphism).

Key points

- Patients with all degrees of spina bifida should be assessed in the antenatal period, so that analgesia and anaesthesia can be planned.
- Spinal bifida occulta involves failure of fusion of only one arch, no external lesion and the spinal cord and nerves are normal. In these cases, spinal or epidural techniques are usually uncomplicated. An epidural should be performed above the level of the lesion and a spinal as low as possible.
- Patients with neurological abnormalities, cutaneous manifestations or involvement of more than one lamina may have a tethered cord and it is necessary to understand the extent of the defect before performing neuraxial anaesthesia. An MRI can be performed in pregnancy.

Reference

Ali L, Stocks GM. Spina bifida, tethered cord and regional anaesthesia. *Anaesthesia* 2005; **60**: 1149–1150.

Spinal muscular atrophy type III (Kugelberg–Welander disease)

Characteristics

- Degeneration of the anterior horn cells of the spinal cord.
- Proximal muscle weakness especially of lower limbs, muscle wasting, fasciculation, wheelchair bound, waddling, wide-based flat-footed gait with positive Gowers sign.
- Normal intellect, facial movements, sensation, autonomic and sphincter function.
- Scoliosis and chest wall muscle weakness predispose to pulmonary dysfunction and restrictive pulmonary deficit.

Key points

Antenatal

- Muscle weakness may worsen in pregnancy.

Delivery

- Often leads to prolonged or premature labour; assisted vaginal delivery or CS with slow postpartum recovery.
- Difficulty positioning on the operating table and gaining surgical access to the lower abdomen with fixed flexion contractures of the hips.
- Spinal anaesthesia may precipitate decompensation if compromised pulmonary function.
- Prolonged neuromuscular blockade after non-depolarizing drugs can lead to postoperative muscle weakness, impaired cough, reduced respiratory reserve and compromised baseline pulmonary function.
- Suxamethonium may precipitate acute hyperkalaemia.

Reference

McLoughlin L, Bhagvat P. Anaesthesia for Caesarean section in spinal muscular atrophy type III. *International Journal of Obstetric Anesthesia* 2004; **13**: 192–195.

Sturge–Weber syndrome

Characteristics

- Sturge–Weber syndrome (encephalotrigeminal angiomatosis) is a rare phakomatosis, with facial haemangioma encompassing at least part of cutaneous trigeminal nerve distribution and ipsilateral intracranial venous malformation.

Key points

- The leptomeningeal angiomatosis is predominantly venous. Arterial malformations are rare.
- The venous plexus may be extensive, causing the adjacent cortex to become atrophic.
- Intracranial haemorrhage and focal or generalized convulsions can occur.

- Difficult intubation has been described.
- The effects of pregnancy on this rare disorder remain undefined but of concern.

Reference

Batra RK *et al.* Anaesthesia and the Sturge–Weber syndrome. *Canadian Journal of Anaesthesia* 1994; **41**: 133–136.

Subarachnoid haemorrhage

Characteristics

- Incidence of subarachnoid haemorrhage from aneurysms and AVMs in pregnancy is between 0.01 and 0.05%.
- Negative angiography does not exclude aneurysm with absolute certainty.

Key points

Antenatal

- History of clipped aneurysm does not preclude vaginal delivery, although a shortened second stage with epidural analgesia may be recommended.
- Assessment of neurological function should be carried out.

Delivery

- Spinal or epidural anaesthesia not contraindicated with a stable history.
- Following a recent event, epidural analgesia, because of fluid in lumbar extradural space, may increase ICP.
- Dural puncture and CSF leak may dislodge the clot and cause further bleeding.
- Invasive arterial pressure monitoring is recommended.

Reference

Levy DM, Jaspan T. Anaesthesia for caesarean section in a patient with recent subarachnoid haemorrhage and severe pre-eclampsia. *Anaesthesia* 1999; **54**: 994–998.

Subdural haematoma

Characteristics

- Subdural haematoma following dural puncture is rare and may be cranial or spinal. Persistent headache and deterioration of neurological status should elicit suspicion.
- Cranial subdural haematomas may present acutely, subacutely or chronically, with headache, altered level of consciousness, seizures or psychiatric symptoms.

Key points

- Cause of subdural haematoma following dural puncture is low CSF pressure leading to traction and tearing of thin-walled meningeal blood vessels.

- The management of subdural haematoma is either conservative, i.e. clinical observation with possible ICP monitoring, or surgery.
- Haematomas <5mm often resolve spontaneously.

Reference

Kayacan N *et al.* Acute subdural haematoma after accidental dural puncture during epidural anaesthesia. *International Journal of Obstetric Anesthesia* 2004; **13**: 47–49.

Superior vena cava obstruction

Characteristics

- Rare and usually complicates tumours in the mediastinum.
- Affects venous drainage of the airway, leading to shortness of breath, stridor and cough.

Key points

- Spinal anaesthesia with rapid sympathectomy and haemodynamic decompensation might be disastrous due to combined obstructed VR from the upper extremities, and obstruction from the lower extremities by the gravid uterus.
- Epidural anaesthesia is preferred with titration of vasopressors and IV fluids.
- GA with rapid sequence induction and femoral–femoral access to institute immediate cardiopulmonary bypass if intubation or ventilation were not possible has been described.
- IV drugs and fluids should be administered through an IV cannula in the lower limb.
- Intra-arterial monitoring is essential.
- CVP monitoring is unreliable.

Reference

Buvanendran A *et al.* Perioperative management with epidural anesthesia for a parturient with superior vena caval obstruction. *Anesthesia and Analgesia* 2004; **98**: 1160–1163.

Supraventricular tachycardia

Characteristics

- Defined as any tachyarrhythmia with an HR >120bpm, requiring atrial or atrioventricular junctional tissue for its initiation and maintenance.
- Precipitated by associated haemodynamic, hormonal, autonomic and emotional changes.
- Peripartum oxytocic, tocolytic and anaesthetic drugs can induce supraventricular tachycardia.

Key points

- Care with the use of oxytocin and ephedrine.
- Reduced atrial filling caused by regional anaesthesia may increase arrhythmogenicity.

- Pharmacological treatment if haemodynamic changes, severe symptoms or sustained arrhythmias.
- Valsalva manoeuvre and facial ice immersion are well tolerated and aid diagnosis.
- β-blockers, verapamil and synchronized electrical cardioversion have been used.
- Adenosine is safe in pregnancy and labour.

Reference

Robins K, Lyons G. Supraventricular tachycardia in pregnancy. *British Journal of Anaesthesia* 2004; **92**: 140–143.

Suxamethonium apnoea

Characteristics

- Prolonged neuromuscular blockade caused by altered enzymatic activity of plasma cholinesterase.
- May be inherited or acquired.
- Pregnancy itself is associated with reduced plasma cholinesterase activity, although not clinically relevant.
- Cholinesterase activity is investigated by measurement of the enzyme concentration and dibucaine number. However, this test may be unreliable in pregnancy due to its associated reduced cholinesterase level.

Key points

- Strategies used include giving suxamethonium and anticipating a prolonged period of postoperative ventilation, or administration of rocuronium 0.9mg/kg, which has been shown to have a similar onset time to suxamethonium, but a problem in the event of failed intubation.
- Intubation using alfentanil in varying doses and propofol without neuromuscular-blocking drugs has been described.
- Administering alfentanil at a dose >25 micrograms/kg would require an opioid antagonist to the mother to reverse its effects in the event of failed intubation, and would also result in neonatal respiratory depression.
- The combination of thiopental and remifentanil is also reported.

Reference

Alexander R, Fardell S. Use of remifentanil for tracheal intubation for Caesarean section in a patient with suxamethonium apnoea. *Anaesthesia* 2005; **60**: 1036–1038.

Syringomyelia

Characteristics

- Progressive degenerative disease with cystic cavities within the spinal cord that cause severe neurological deficits.
- The clinical diagnosis is based on the triad: (1) loss of pain and temperature sensations with preservation of touch sensation over the neck, shoulders and arms; (2) amyotrophy; and (3) thoracic scoliosis.

Key points

Antenatal

- Preanaesthetic assessment to document neurological deficit and assess respiratory function.

Delivery

- Autonomic dysfunction if present necessitates invasive arterial monitoring and attention to normothermia.
- Caution with neuromuscular-blocking agents. Suxamethonium may cause hyperkalaemia.
- Syringobulbia (the extension of a syrinx into the brainstem) increases the risk of aspiration.
- Foramen magnum abnormalities may cause craniospinal pressure dissociation. A relatively higher CSF pressure in the head and lower pressure in the spine contraindicates the use of subarachnoid anaesthesia.
- Epidural anaesthesia may be considered for patients with anticipated difficult intubation, but accidental dural puncture may be hazardous.

Reference

Nel MR *et al.* Extradural anaesthesia for Caesarean section in a patient with syringomyelia and Chiari type I anomaly. *British Journal of Anaesthesia* 1998; **80**: 512–515.

Systemic lupus erythematosus

Characteristics

- Multisystem inflammatory disorder characterized by autoantibody production and immune-mediated tissue injury.
- Clinical features depend on the severity of damage to organ systems such as musculoskeletal, renal, haematological, neurological, cardiac and respiratory.

Key points

Antenatal

- Co-operation between the rheumatologist, obstetrician, neonatologist and anaesthetist is important
- Increased incidence of fetal loss, hypertension and pre-eclampsia.
- Associated with antiphospholipid syndrome and thrombosis, may need anticoagulation with LMWH. Lupus anticoagulant may cause isolated increase in APTT, not associated with increase bleeding risk.

Delivery

- Management includes all types of anaesthesia, depending on severity of the organ involvement.
- Important to time regional techniques with LMWH administration.
- Ulcers on nasal and oral mucous membranes may increase trauma with tracheal intubation.
- Raynaud's phenomena complicates placement of arterial lines.
- Peripheral neuropathies or fixed neurological deficits should be documented before regional anaesthesia.

- A coagulation screen including PT should be done.
- Antibiotic prophylaxis for valvular lesions and prosthetic joints.

Reference

Davies SR. Systemic lupus erythematosus and the obstetrical patient—implications for the anaesthetist *Canadian Journal of Anaesthesia* 1991; **38**: 790–795.

Systemic sclerosis

Characteristics

- Multisystem disease of unknown aetiology, causing overproduction and growth of collagen, widespread vascular damage, microvascular obliteration and Raynaud's phenomenon.

Key points

Antenatal

- Careful assessment of multisystemic condition.
- Review of cardiac function and exclusion of pulmonary hypertension, with assessment of airway and peripheral veins.
- Difficult venous access due to thickened skin, flexion contractures impair indirect BP measurement. Direct arterial cannulation may cause vasospasm and distal necrosis.
- Microsomia, nasal and oral telangiectasiae, oesophageal dysmotility and sphincter incompetence, pulmonary fibrosis, pulmonary hypertension, myocardial fibrosis, pericarditis, arrhythmias and conduction defects may occur.

Delivery

- Gradual regional technique may avoid profound hypotension.
- Prolonged sensory and motor blockade.
- Careful positioning—padding to avoid pressure necrosis, wrapping of limbs, warmth to avoid vasoconstriction.
- Avoid prolonged application of a pulse oximeter probe to one digit.

Reference

Bailey AR *et al*. Spinal anaesthesia for Caesarean section in a patient with systemic sclerosis. *Anaesthesia* 1999; **54**: 355–358.

Takayasu's disease

Characteristics

- Pulseless disease-occlusive thromboaortopathy is a rare inflammatory panendarteritis causing thrombosis and occlusion of systemic and pulmonary arteries.
- Cerebrovascular ischaemia occurs in one-third of patients, making maintenance of cerebral blood flow vital.
- Complications include hypertension, heart failure and peripartum cerebral haemorrhage.

Key points

- Regional anaesthesia is a safe technique especially in cerebrovascular disease, which mandates monitoring for cerebral ischaemia.
- When regional anaesthesia is prohibited, short-acting opioid and relaxant drugs allow rapid awakening and easy assessment of cerebral function. The use of processed EEG monitoring, whilst not absolutely sensitive or specific, may be better than no monitor when the patient is asleep.

References

Kathirvel S *et al.* Anesthetic management of patients with Takayasu's arteritis: a case series and review. *Anesthesia and Analgesia* 2001; **93**: 60–65.

Henderson K, Fludder P. Epidural anaesthesia for Caesarean section in a patient with severe Takayasu's disease. *British Journal of Anaesthesia* 1999; **83**: 956–959.

Thalassaemia

Characteristics

- Inherited disorder of Hb synthesis, excess α chains precipitate in RBC precursors.
- Defective erythroid precursor maturation and shortened red cell survival.
- Hypertrophy of the bone marrow; skull and long bone changes and hepatosplenomegaly all result.
- Iron overload from transfusions damages myocardium, liver and endocrine glands.

Key points

- Hypertransfusion therapy corrects anaemia and suppresses hyperactive erthryopoiesis.
- Hb maintained above 10g/dL during gestation.
- Leukocyte-depleted RBC concentrate prevents febrile non-haemolytic transfusion reactions, cytomegalovirus infections and reduces immunomodulatory effect of transfusions.
- Regular folic acid supplementation.
- Intraoperative cell salvage is useful.
- Regional anaesthesia is contraindicated in patients with hypersplenic crises and thrombocytopenia.
- Severe maxillofacial deformities may present difficult airway problems.
- Osteoporosis, osteopenia and scoliosis are common.

Reference

Butwick A *et al.* Management of pregnancy in a patient with beta thalassaemia major. *International Journal of Obstetric Anesthesia* 2005; **14**: 351–354.

Thalidomide deformities

Characteristics

- Large spectrum of malformations including limb, gastrointestinal, reproductive and spinal abnormalities.
- Problems include venous access, analgesia, BP monitoring, type of delivery and postpartum difficulties handling the newborn baby.

Key points

- Multidisciplinary group of obstetricians, anaesthetists and midwives.
- Early IV access. Large-bore cannulae or central venous line under ultrasound guidance. Subclavian veins may be poorly formed.
- Epidural analgesia has been used, though caution in spinal deformities.
- BP monitoring in amelic patients needs considerable ingenuity. Invasive monitoring by cannulation of a suitable peripheral artery remains an alternative.

Reference

Barrett PJ *et al.* Anaesthesia and thalidomide-related abnormalities. *International Journal of Obstetric Anesthesia* 1992; **1**: 235–236.

Thoracic aortic aneurysm

Characteristics

- Incidentally diagnosed ascending aortic aneurysm and/or dissection are rare but potentially fatal.
- Risk factors include systemic hypertension, Marfan's syndrome, other congenital cardiovascular abnormalities and pregnancy-induced changes in vessel wall.

Key points

- Epidural is preferred for caesarean delivery to avoid risk of hypertension associated with rapid sequence induction.
- If patient needs immediate cardiothoracic intervention, there is risk of life-threatening uterine haemorrhage during and after cardiopulmonary bypass.
- Oxytocin infusion and aprotinin have been used.

Reference

Ecknauer E *et al.* Emergency repair of incidentally diagnosed ascending aortic aneurysm immediately after Caesarean section. *British Journal of Anaesthesia* 1999; **83**: 343–345.

Thrombocytopenia (See Chapter 4, p 116)

Characteristics

- Idiopathic thrombocytopenia (ITP) is common and, in addition, there are pregnancy-related causes, e.g. gestational thrombocytopenia and pre-eclampsia/HELLP syndrome.
- The lowest platelet count at which one can safely administer neuraxial anaesthesia for labour and delivery is controversial.

Key points

- Low platelet counts in the antenatal period should be investigated by a haematologist and full discussion with mother about analgesia and anaesthesia options in labour given.
  - ITP—platelet counts may be very low, the patient may be on immunosuppressants and have undergone splenectomy. Early destruction of platelets in life cycle, but remaining platelets function well. Fetus may also be affected.
  - Gestational thrombocytopenia—modest reduction in platelet numbers.
  - Pre-eclampsia/HELLP syndrome—rapid fall in platelet numbers.
- Platelet number of 80×10^{12} is considered reasonable for an epidural, possibly as low as 50×10^{12} for spinal anaesthesia.
- There is discussion whether a laboratory abnormality alone, such as thrombocytopenia without a positive bleeding history, should preclude a patient from receiving a neuraxial block.
- No single coagulation test has been established as a reliable predictor of haematoma after neuraxial block.
- TEG will identify global abnormalities in the coagulation system. A normal TEG tracing may be utilized as laboratory evidence to support the clinical impression of normal coagulation and the decision to conduct a neuraxial technique.

References

Frenk V *et al.* Regional anesthesia in parturients with low platelet counts. *Canadian Journal of Anaesthesia* 2005; **52**: 114.

Beilin Y *et al.* Safe epidural analgesia in thirty parturients with platelet counts between 69,000 and 98,000 mm^{-3}. *Anesthesia and Analgesia* 1997; **85**: 385–388.

Frolich MA *et al.* Thromboelastography to assess coagulation in the thrombocytopenic parturient. *Canadian Journal of Anaesthesia* 2003; **50**: 853.

British Committee for Standards in Haematology. Guidelines for the investigation and management of idiopathic thrombocytopenic purpura in adults, children and in pregnancy. *British Journal of Haematology* 2003; **120**: 574–596.

Thrombotic thrombocytopenic purpura

Characteristics

- TTP is a severe multisystem disorder affecting the microcirculation of many organ systems, with significant maternal and fetal morbidity.
- Comprises classic pentad of fever, severe thrombocytopenia, microangiopathic anaemia, neurological symptoms or signs and renal failure.
- Pregnancy can be an initiating event for acute TTP or produce a high risk of relapse if previously diagnosed.
- Can be mistaken for severe pre-eclampsia or HELLP syndrome at initial presentation.

Key points

- Close liaison with haemoatologist is essential.
- Treatment options include low dose aspirin, anticoagulation with LMWH, immunosuppression and/or repeated plasma exchange.
- Analgesia/anaesthetic technique for delivery dictated by platelet count and anticoagulation therapy.
- High dependency care may be required following delivery.

Reference

Scully M *et al.* Successful management of pregnancy in women with a history of thrombotic thrombocytopenic purpura. *Blood Coagulation and Fibrinolysis* 2006; **17**: 459–463.

Tocolysis

Characteristics

- Use of pharmacological agents to relax the uterine myometrium and to abolish uterine contractions to benefit the mother or the fetus.
- Used in preterm labour, external cephalic version, fetal surgery, uterine hyperstimulation, cord prolapse, prior to and during CS, shoulder dystocia, retained placenta due to retraction ring, acute puerperal uterine inversion.

Key points

- Halogenated anaesthetic agents have been replaced by β-sympathomimetic agents (ritodrine or terbutaline), magnesium sulphate, nitroglycerin, oxytocin antagonists (atosiban), calcium channel blockers (sublingual nifedipine) and cyclo-oxygenase inhibitors.
- Maternal side effects include tachycardia, hypotension and pulmonary oedema; IV nitroglycerin administration may cause vasodilatation and hypotension.

Reference

Chandraharan E, Arulkumarans S. Acute tocolysis (Review). *Current Opinion in Obstetrics and Gynecology* 2005; **17**: 151–156.

Transposition of great vessels

Characteristics

- Congenitally corrected transposition: discordant atrioventricular and ventriculoarterial connections. Associated with ventricular septal defects, pulmonary outflow obstruction, tricuspid valve (systemic) deformity and rhythm disturbances. The anatomical RV with the tricuspid valve is the systemic ventricle; the anatomical LV becomes the pulmonary ventricle thus producing a physiological blood circulation.
- Surgically palliated transposition (Mustard's or Senning's) where baffles redirect venous blood into the LV and pulmonary veins are directed to the systemic RV.

- Main physiological concern in both situations is the morphologically non-systemic RV to sustain systemic pressures and CO.
- Patients are prone to heart failure, arrhythmias, baffle leak with cyanosis and baffle obstruction with SVC obstruction.

Key points

Antenatal

- Regular review by cardiologist looking for early signs of cardiac failure.

Delivery

- Early epidural analgesia to decrease catecholamine release and decrease cardiac work.
- Avoid aorto-caval compression, hypovolaemia and hypervolaemia.
- Invasive monitoring for haemodynamic instability. Central venous monitoring may be difficult to interpret if cardiac anatomy is grossly abnormal.
- Risk of bacteraemia and endocarditis associated with central venous cannulation must be weighed against the benefits of monitoring filling pressures.
- Bacterial endocarditis prophylaxis recommended.
- Bolus (rapid) administration of oxytocin should be avoided.

References

Drenthen W *et al.* Risk of complications during pregnancy after Senning or Mustard (atrial) repair of complete transposition of the great arteries. *European Heart Journal* 2005; **26**: 2588–2595.

Schabel JE, Jasiewicz RC. Anesthetic management of a pregnant patient with congenitally corrected transposition of the great arteries for labor and vaginal delivery. *Journal of Clinical Anesthesia* 2001; **13**: 517–520.

Truncus arteriosus

Characteristics

- Rare congenital cardiac malformation in which only one artery arises from both ventricles.
- Four types are described. Type IV is agenesis of pulmonary arteries where pulmonary perfusion is provided by the bronchial arteries.
- Associated with VSD, right-sided aortic arch and truncal valve.
- Clinical manifestations depend on pulmonary blood flow.

Key points

Antenatal

- Haemodynamic changes during pregnancy, labour and puerperium cause impairment of balance between pulmonary and systemic blood flows.
- Right to left shunt progressively worsens due to decrease in SVR. Net effect is deterioration of arterial oxygenation.
- Require regular cardiology review.

Delivery

- Avoid reduction in SVR (due to histamine release or vasodilator drugs), rise in PVR (due to hypoxia, hypercarbia, acidosis or high inflation pressures), fall in CO (due to reduced VR).

Reference

Bosatra MG *et al.* Caesarean delivery of a patient with truncus arteriosus. *International Journal of Obstetric Anesthesia* 1997; **6**: 279–284.

Urticaria pigmentosa

Characteristics

- Cutaneous manifestation of mastocytosis, proliferation and accumulation of mast cells in various organs.
- Precipitants include trauma or mechanical irritation to the skin, psychological stress, extremes of temperature, spicy foods, alcohol, histamine-releasing drugs, snake and bee venom.
- Symptoms include weakness, fatigue, urticaria, grand mal seizures, anaphylaxis, cardiovascular collapse, etc.

Key points

Antenatal

- Full assessment of drug-related problems with plan for labour analgesia.
- Premedication with H_1 and H_2 antihistamine agents and benzodiazepine to reduce anxiety.
- Close collaboration with obstetric team for the timely administration of prophylactic medications.

Delivery

- Effective analgesia to decrease anxiety—regional analgesia recommended.
- Core temperature maintenance.
- Repositioning should be kept to a minimum.
- If mast cell degranulation is suspected, corticosteroids, antihistamine drugs and adrenaline should be used.
- Avoid histamine-releasing drugs.
- Resuscitation equipment should be available for the duration of labour, delivery and postpartum period to treat unanticipated hypotension and shock.

Reference

Villeneuve V *et al.* Anesthetic management of a labouring parturient with urticaria pigmentosa. *Canadian Journal of Anaesthesia* 2006; **53**: 380–384.

Valve replacements

Characteristics

- The need for anticoagulation with metallic values presents a dilemma in pregnancy. The use of warfarin is still recommended despite the risk of warfarin embryopathy (especially with doses >5mg daily to maintain INR in the therapeutic range).
- The practice of substituting heparin for warfarin in the first trimester potentially eliminates the risk of fetal embryopathy, but increases the risk of thromboembolism and the long-term problems of UFH use, e.g. thrombocytopenia and osteoporosis.

- The use of LMWH is associated with an increase risk of valve thrombosis and is not currently recommended.

Key points

- The American Heart Association/American College of Cardiology Task Force report in 1998 recommended the use of warfarin until week 35, following which UFH should be substituted in anticipation of labour and delivery.
- Warfarin crosses the placenta causing significant anticoagulation of the fetus.
- Careful dose adjustment of anticoagulation with aggressive monitoring of trough and peak levels of heparin is needed.
- Percutaneous mitral balloon valvuloplasty is currently recommended for mitral stenosis, when pharmacological therapy is ineffective during decompensated valvular disease in pregnancy.

References

ACC/AHA. 2006 guidelines for the management of patients with valvular heart disease: a report of the American College of Cardiology/American Heart Association Task Force on Practice Guidelines. *Circulation* 2006; **114**: e84–e231.

Dua S *et al.* Anesthetic management for emergency Caesarean section in a patient with severe valvular disease and preeclampsia. *International Journal of Obstetric Anesthesia* 2006; **15**: 250–253.

Varicella

Characteristics

- Varicella zoster virus causes a primary contagious and usually benign illness commonly known as varicella or chickenpox.
- Virus can lie dormant in the dorsal root ganglia and may be reactivated to cause localized cutaneous eruptions called 'herpes zoster' ('shingles').

Key points

- Possibility of introducing the virus into the CNS during the placement of the regional block, resulting in meningitis or encephalitis, especially during the primary infection when viraemia is present.
- Secondary bacterial superinfection, acute cerebellar ataxia, encephalitis aseptic meningitis and Guillain–Barré syndrome have been reported.
- GA is the anaesthetic of choice if there are active or infected lesions on the skin at the site for placement of a spinal or epidural block.
- Exposure of medical personnel to an infectious patient should be avoided or minimized.
- Consider use of IV aciclovir for severe infection.

Reference

Brown NW *et al.* Anaesthetic considerations in a parturient with varicella presenting for Caesarean section. *Anaesthesia* 2003; **58**: 1092–1095.

Ventriculoperitoneal shunts

Characteristics

- An artificial shunt to drain CSF into the peritoneum with various configurations.

Key points

Antenatal

- Headaches and other symptoms of shunt failure (vomiting, reduced level of consciousness, seizures) need MRI to evaluate ventricular dilatation.

Delivery

- Mode of delivery is determined by obstetric reasons.
- A shortened second stage of labour may be desirable.
- Risk of intra-abdominal infection and adhesion formation around the distal end of the ventriculoperitoneal shunt catheter after CS.
- Meticulous aseptic technique is essential for regional anaesthesia, and prophylactic antibiotics are generally recommended.

Reference

Littleford JA *et al.* Obstetrical anesthesia for a parturient with a ventriculoperitoneal shunt and third ventriculostomy. *Canadian Journal of Anaesthesia* 1999; **46**: 1057–1063.

Von Hippel–Lindau disease

Characteristics

- Rare autosomal dominant disease, causing diffuse haemangioblastomas of the CNS, mostly cerebellum, retina and viscera.
- Associated with renal cell carcinoma, pancreatic cyst and tumours, and phaeochromocytoma

Key points

- Review of medical notes and MRI scans essential.
- Epidural anaesthesia has been used successfully without neurological sequelae.
- The choice of anaesthesia technique should be made after careful evaluation of the extent of the patient's disease.

Reference

Wang A, Sinatra RS. Epidural anesthesia for cesarean section in a patient with von Hippel–Lindau disease and multiple sclerosis. *Anesthesia and Analgesia* 1999; **88**: 1083–1084.

Von Willebrand's disease (See Chapter 4, p 117–118)

Characteristics

- Inherited deficiency of vWF, a carrier protein for factor VIII required for platelet adhesion to damaged endothelium.
- Three types described based on level and function.

Key points

Antenatal

- Close review and management by haematologist.
- Regular measurement of vWF in pregnancy. The amount of vWF is determined by measuring the vWF:Ag level, whereas the Ricof level is a measure of its functional activity. The 'normal' vWF:Ag level is >50%. A 'normal' Ricof level is quoted as >50% which is reduced in vWD. If the level is <10%, there is a significant risk of bleeding.
- Pregnancy increases the level of vWF into the normal range in most patients.
- In a small number, levels remain low and regional anaesthesia is not advised. There is not an absolute consensus on the Ricof level that is safe for regional anaesthesia.
- Analgesic/anaesthetic options need to be discussed in detail in the antenatal period.

Delivery

- Level of vWF falls rapidly following delivery.
- If an epidural catheter has been inserted during labour it must be removed immediately after delivery.
- There is an increased risk of PPH.
- Desmopressin is used therapeutically to boost the level of vWF production.

References

Kujovich JL. von Willebrand disease and pregnancy (Review). *Journal of Thrombosis and Haemostasis* 2005; **3**: 246–253.

Stedeford JC, Pittman JA. Von Willebrand's disease and neuroaxial anaesthesia. *Anaesthesia* 2000; **55**: 1228–1229.

Wegener's granulomatosis

Characteristics

- Wegner's granulomatosis is an uncommon systemic disease characterized by a necrotizing granulomatous vasculitis of the upper and lower respiratory tracts, with or without glomerulonephritis and disseminated small vessel vasculitis.

Key points

- Pulmonary haemorrhage is life threatening.
- Pre-eclampsia and prematurity associated with corticosteroids or prior renal diseases are the most serious complications.
- Head and neck manifestations of the disease may present a difficult airway problem.

Reference

Auzary C *et al.* Pregnancy in patients with Wegener's granulomatosis: report of five cases in three women (Review). *Annals of the Rheumatic Diseases* 2000; **59**: 800–804.

Wolff–Parkinson–White syndrome

Characteristics

- Pre-excitation syndrome where activation of an accessory atrioventricular conduction pathway leads to early and rapid ventricular contractions.
- Short PR interval, anomalous QRS complexes and a delta wave may be seen.
- Paroxysmal supraventricular tachycardias are common.

Key points

- Haemodynamic, hormonal and emotional changes predispose to arrhythmias.
- The tachycardia in pregnancy along with an underlying WPW syndrome may induce unidirectional block in the re-entrant circuit, resulting in atrioventricular tachycardias.
- Tachyarrhythmias causing haemodynamic changes require immediate treatment.
- Vagal stimulation, sedation, propranolol, digoxin, calcium antagonists and adenosine have been used.
- Adenosine is preferred due to its very short half-life.
- Electrical cardioversion during pregnancy has also been successful.

Reference

Robinson JE *et al.* Familial hypokalemic periodic paralysis and Wolff–Parkinson–White syndrome in pregnancy. *Canadian Journal of Anaesthesia* 2000; **47**: 160–164.

Index

B

C

D

E

Q

R

S

T

U

V

W

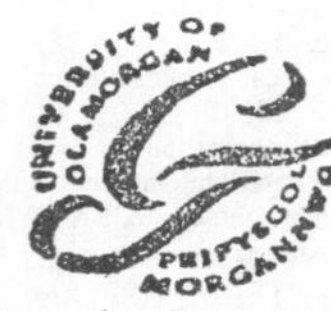